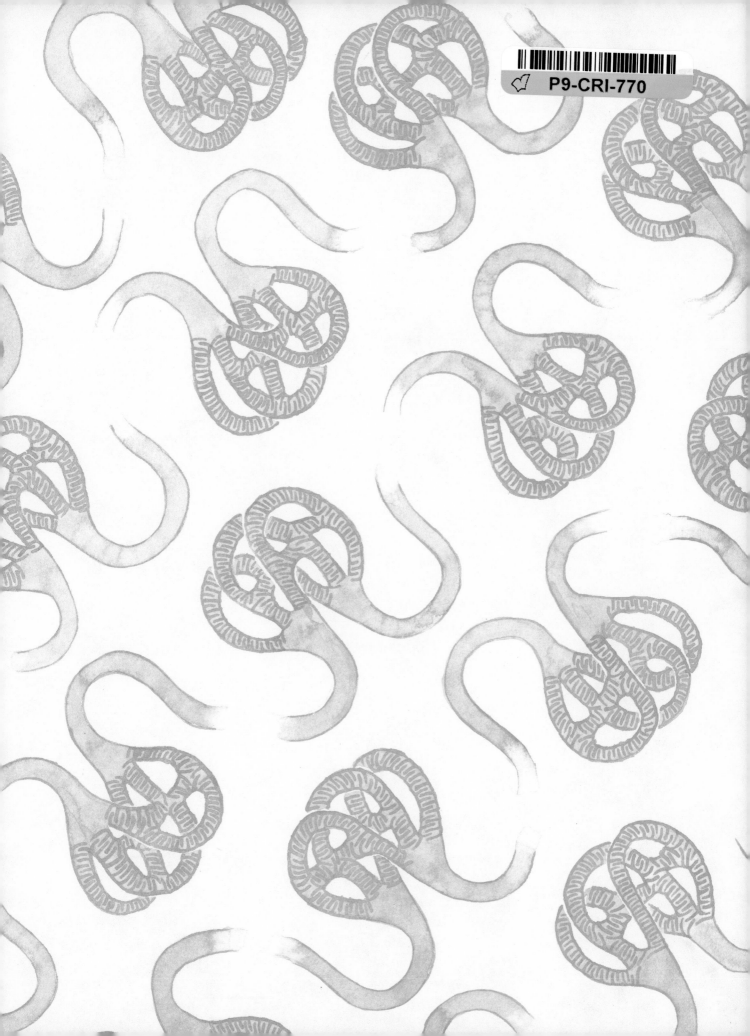

NURSE'S CLINICAL LIBRARY™

# RENAL AND UROLOGIC DISORDERS

*NURSING84* BOOKS™
SPRINGHOUSE CORPORATION
Springhouse, Pennsylvania

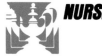
## NURSING84 BOOKS™

The clinical procedures described and
recommended in this publication are based
on research and consultation with medical
and nursing authorities. To the best of our
knowledge, these procedures reflect currently accepted clinical practice; nevertheless, they can't be considered absolute
and universal recommendations. For indi-
vidual application, treatment recommendations must be considered in light of the
patient's clinical condition and, before administration of new or infrequently used
drugs, in light of latest package-insert information. The authors and the publisher
disclaim responsibility for any adverse effects resulting directly or indirectly from the
suggested procedures, from any undetected errors, or from the reader's misunder-
standing of the text.

**Library of Congress Cataloging in
Publication Data**
Main entry under title:
Renal and urologic disorders.
  (Nurse's clinical library)
  "Nursing84 books."
  Bibliography: p.
  Includes index.
1. Urological nursing.   I. Springhouse
Corporation. II. Series. [DNLM:
1. Nephrology—nurses' instruction.
2. Urology—nurses' instruction.
WJ 300 R3913]
RC874.7.R46 1984   616.6   84-14104
ISBN 0-916730-74-3

*Cover:* Color-enhanced X-ray of renal
and urologic system. Photograph by
Howard Sochurek.

*Inside front and back covers:* Renal
glomeruli.

# CONTENTS

# CONTRIBUTORS AND CLINICAL CONSULTANTS

## Contributors

*At the time of publication, the contributors held the following positions:*

**Carole J. Akerly, RN, BSN**
Assistant Head Nurse, Urology Intermediate Care Unit, Duke University Medical Center, Durham, N.C.

**Charold L. Baer, RN, PhD**
Professor, Department of Adult Health and Illness, School of Nursing, Oregon Health Sciences University, Portland

**Terrie H. Blalock, RN, BSN**
Clinical Instructor, Nursing Inservice Education, Duke University Medical Center, Durham, N.C.

**Judy E. Carlson, RN**
Head Nurse, Urology Clinic, Duke University Medical Center, Durham, N.C.

**Jeanette K. Chambers, RN, MS, CS**
Renal Clinical Nurse Specialist, Riverside Methodist Hospital, Columbus, Ohio

**Lynn Bennett Deminski, RN, BSN**
Formerly Staff Urology Nurse, Duke University Medical Center, Durham, N.C.

**Ann Fagerness, RN, BSN, CCRN, CNRN**
Critical Care Educator, Pacific Northwest In-Service Specialists, Seattle, Wash.

**Mary-Frances Jett, RN, BSN, PhD**
Assistant Professor of Physiology in Nursing and Instructor of Physiology in Medicine, Schools of Nursing and Medicine, Vanderbilt University, Nashville, Tenn.

**Larry E. Lancaster, RN, MSN, EdD**
Academic Director and Associate Professor, School of Nursing, Vanderbilt University, Nashville, Tenn.

**Peggy J. Reiley, RN, MS**
Head Nurse, Beth Israel Hospital, Boston

**Sandra Small, RN, MSN, CCRN**
Director of Critical Care, Baptist Medical Center, Little Rock, Ark.

## Clinical Consultants

*At the time of publication, the clinical consultants held the following positions:*

**Charold L. Baer, RN, PhD**
Professor, Department of Adult Health and Illness, School of Nursing, Oregon Health Sciences University, Portland

**Leonard Crowley, MD**
Clinical Assistant Professor, Department of Laboratory Medicine and Pathology and Department of Family Practice, University of Minnesota, Minneapolis; Pathologist, St. Mary's Hospital, Minneapolis

**Harold J. Hoppmann, MD**
Private Practice, Urology, Fairview Southdale Hospital, Edina, Minn.

**Robert L. Klaus, MD, FACS**
Chief, Urology, Albert Einstein Medical Center, Philadelphia

**Kristine M. Kroner, RN, BSN, MHA**
Nurse Manager, Albert Einstein Medical Center, Philadelphia

**Judy E. Riley, RN**
Lithotriptor Coordinator and Urologic Nurse Clinician, Massachusetts General Hospital, Boston

**Grannum R. Sant, MD, FRCS**
Assistant Professor of Urology, School of Medicine, Tufts University, Boston

**Michael I. Sorkin, MD**
Assistant Professor of Medicine, University of Pittsburgh; Director, Peritoneal Dialysis Programs, University of Pittsburgh; Chief, Dialysis Unit, Veterans Administration Medical Center, Pittsburgh

**June L. Stark, RN, BSN, CCRN**
Critical Care Instructor/Renal Nurse Consultant, New England Medical Center, Boston

# FOREWORD

Wherever you encounter renal and urologic disorders, you'll be challenged to recognize and assess them accurately and to provide effective nursing care. It isn't easy. Because the renal system affects the rest of the body in so many ways, it's often difficult to decide if the patient's illness is primarily renal (as in acute or chronic renal failure), primarily urologic (as in urinary tract infections), or primarily in some other system (as in neurogenic bladder). What's more, many patients with chronic renal failure remain asymptomatic until extensive and irreversible damage has occurred.

But recognizing these often elusive disorders is not the only challenge. Managing them correctly requires carefully planned nursing care. For example, the care plan must take into account the patient's psychological response to his disorder. The kidney transplant patient must cope with the presence of a "foreign" organ; the dialysis patient may become psychologically dependent on the machine and the care giver, impeding rehabilitation efforts; and the patient with incontinence or retention may experience embarrassment and social isolation, requiring psychological support to restore an impaired self-concept.

To help the patient recover and regain independence, nursing care must include patient teaching to ensure compliance with essential procedures. Besides providing specific patient care, nurses must coordinate the efforts of other members of the health-care team to minimize the widespread debilitating effects of these disorders.

To meet these varied responsibilities as primary care giver, educator, and coordinator of renal and urologic care, nurses need reliable, up-to-date information. This volume, RENAL AND UROLOGIC DISORDERS, supplies both theoretical and practical information that will help nurses at all professional levels. The introductory chapters review renal and urologic anatomy and physiology and the mechanisms of renal failure. They also contain complete information on assessment, with guidelines for developing nursing diagnoses; and a review of diagnostic tests, including urine and blood studies, radiography, ultrasonography, endoscopy, and tissue biopsy.

The remaining chapters are divided into two sections: renal disorders and urinary tract disorders. Each chapter, in turn, consists of three major parts. *Pathophysiology* covers the origins of each disorder and its distinguishing signs and symptoms, abnormal physiology, and impact on the body. *Medical management* summarizes appropriate diagnostic tests and findings, current treatment, and prognosis. *Nursing management,* organized according to the nursing process, offers detailed guidelines for accurate assessment and includes characteristic findings and their implications. It details the nursing diagnoses that can be deduced from those findings, outlines the goals of nursing care and interventions for attaining those goals, and includes guidelines for evaluating the effectiveness of those interventions.

This volume contains more than 150 anatomic drawings, graphs, charts, and diagrams, many in full color. Special graphic devices call attention to patient-teaching aids and emergency management of life-threatening complications, such as septic shock. In addition, three practical appendices provide a wealth of information about drug therapy. The first lists drugs most often used to treat renal and urologic disorders. The second lists nephrotoxic drugs—how they work, what effects they produce, and how to prevent or treat toxic reactions. The third specifies dosage adjustments in renal failure for three glomerular filtration rates, reflecting mild, moderate, and severe renal failure.

This volume of practical and theoretical information will help nurses meet the challenge of caring for patients with renal and urologic disorders confidently and effectively.

CHAROLD L. BAER, RN, PhD
Professor, Department of Adult Health and Illness
School of Nursing
Oregon Health Sciences University
Portland

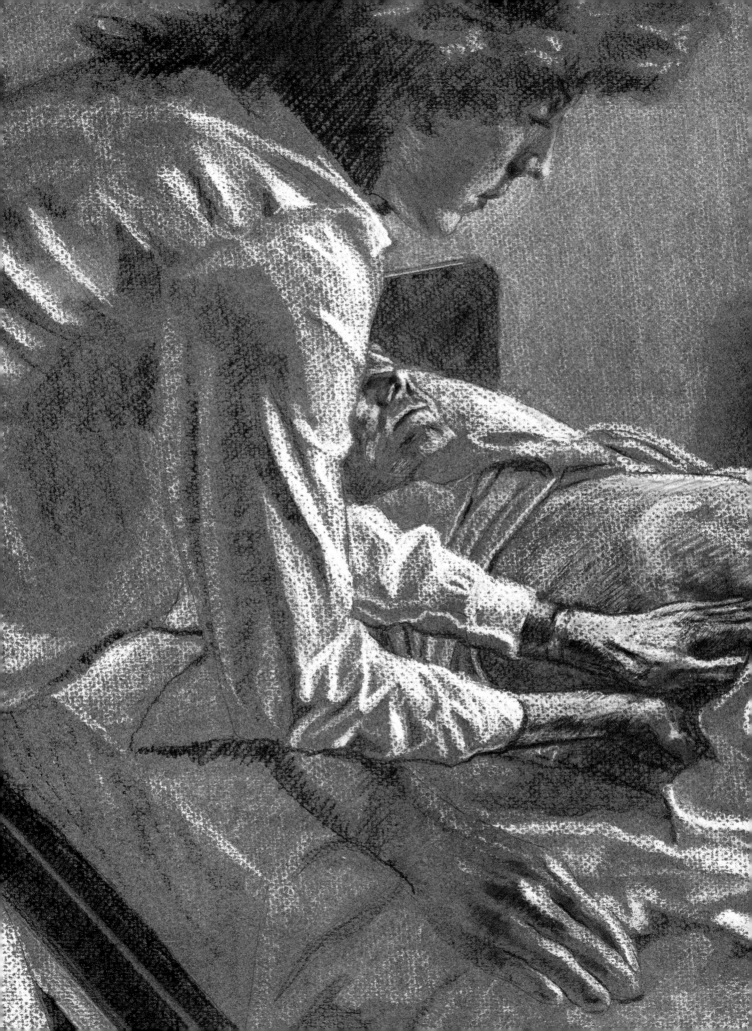

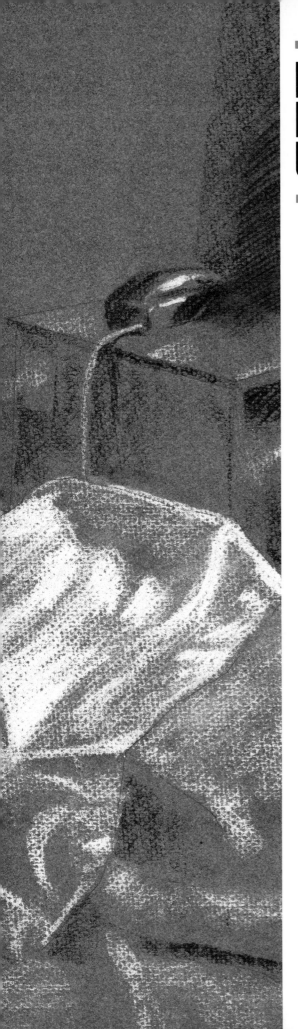

# FUNDAMENTAL RENAL AND UROLOGIC FACTS

# 1 REVIEWING FUNDAMENTAL PRINCIPLES

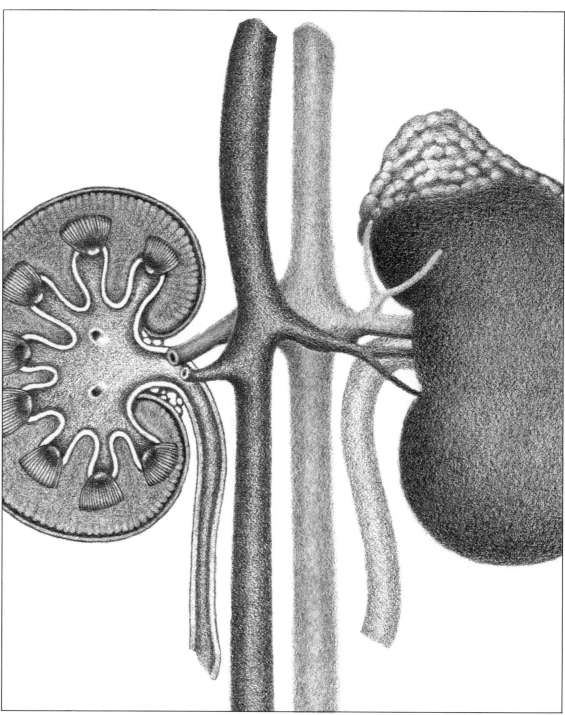

Normal kidneys

Renal and urologic disorders may strike anyone, at any age, at any time. They afflict more than 8 million Americans, and about 78,000 die from them each year. About 200,000 patients are hospitalized annually to remove renal calculi. Nearly 70,000 require treatment with some form of dialysis; the number of patients who require dialysis is growing by about 5,600 a year. An increasing number of patients receive treatment with renal transplantation, which has become more effective with the development of better agents to combat tissue rejection.

Despite more effective dialysis and transplantation therapy, more accurate diagnostic methods, and new drugs, the mortality for renal and urologic disorders has remained about the same for the last 50 years. Concrete gains made in treating specific disorders and prolonging life have been counterbalanced by an apparently greater incidence resulting from more accurate diagnostic techniques and the vulnerability of an increasingly elderly population to renal disease. The implications for nursing are obvious: you can expect the challenges of advancing technology and increasing numbers of patients who need specialized care. To meet these challenges, you'll need a comprehensive understanding of renal and urologic impairments and their widespread systemic effects. In this chapter, we'll review basic structure and physiology, followed by an overview of the many different causes of renal and urologic disorders. In subsequent chapters, we'll discuss the pathophysiology and medical and nursing management strategies of specific disorders.

## THE KIDNEYS AND URINARY TRACT
The renal-urologic system includes the kidneys, ureters, urinary bladder, and urethra. The kidneys, the major organs of this system, receive about 20% of the body's blood volume and process about 180 liters of blood per day. From this blood flow, the kidneys produce and excrete 1,200 to 1,500 ml of urine per day. The kidneys detoxify the blood and eliminate wastes; regulate volume, acid-base balance, and electrolyte concentration of body fluids; regulate calcium balance through vitamin D metabolism; regulate blood pressure; and stimulate new red blood cell (RBC) production (erythropoiesis).

The normal adult kidney is bean-shaped, about 4⅓" (11 cm) long, 1" (2.5 cm) thick, 2" (5 cm) wide, and weighs 4 to 6 oz (113 to 170 g). Together, the kidneys account for about 0.4% of total body weight.

The kidneys are located retroperitoneally in the lumbar area. The right kidney lies somewhat lower than the left because of displacement by the liver; the left kidney is slightly longer than the right and lies closer to the midline. The kidneys assume different locations to accommodate changes in body position, and they move downward and upward during inspiration and expiration with the motion of the diaphragm. Connective tissues (renal fasciae) anchor the kidneys to surrounding structures and help maintain their normal position (see *The renal-urologic system,* page 10).

Enclosed by a fibrous capsule, the kidneys' functional elements (parenchyma) consist of an outer *cortex* and an inner *medulla* (see *Inside the normal kidney,* page 12). The medulla is divided into about 18 to 20 triangular wedges, the *renal pyramids,* which open into the *renal calyces.* The kidneys' basic functional units, the *nephrons,* form the urine (see *The nephron: Basic functional unit,* page 13). Each kidney contains about 1.5 million nephrons.

Urine collects in the renal calyces and pelvis and flows through the ureters to the urinary bladder, where it is stored until expelled by micturition through the urethra. The bladder can store 300 to 500 ml of urine.

## Renal blood supply and innervation
The kidneys receive their blood supply from the renal arteries, which branch to the left and right from the abdominal aorta. Before reaching the kidneys, the renal arteries divide further into anterior and posterior branches. Within the kidneys, the arteries divide into five segmental arteries that enter the renal parenchyma between the renal pyramids to become *interlobar arteries.* Arching around the bases of the pyramids, they branch further into *interlobular arteries* that serve the cortex tissue and kidney capsule. Other interlobular branches serve the glomerular capsules of the nephrons as *afferent arterioles.* At this point they form clumps of capillaries, the *glomeruli,* which are surrounded by *Bowman's capsule.* From the glomeruli, *efferent arterioles,* of smaller diameter than the afferents, emerge from the capsule to form another network of capillaries, the *vasa recta,* around the convoluted tubules and *Henle's loop.* Finally, these capillaries merge into *venules,* which carry the filtered blood back to a system of veins

# The renal-urologic system

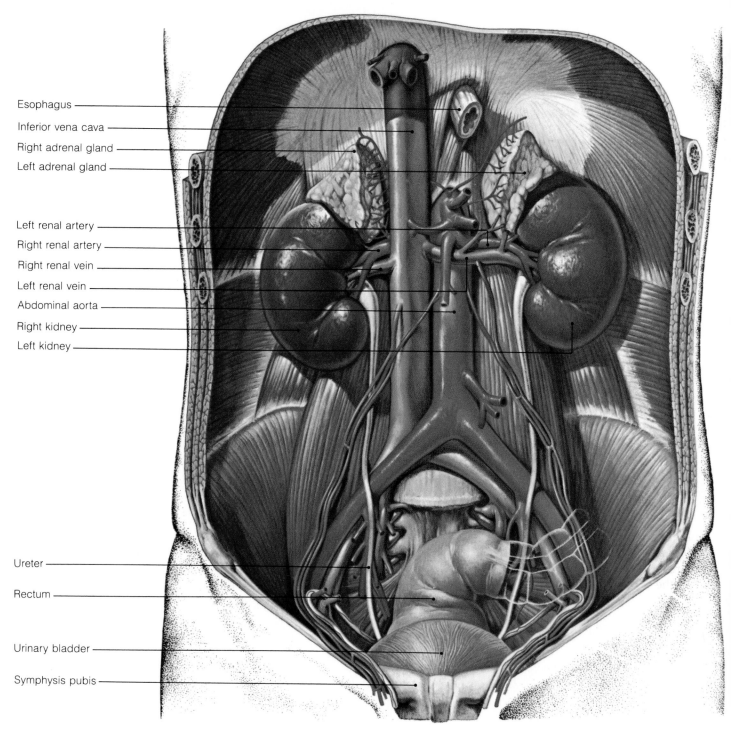

Esophagus
Inferior vena cava
Right adrenal gland
Left adrenal gland

Left renal artery
Right renal artery
Right renal vein
Left renal vein
Abdominal aorta
Right kidney
Left kidney

Ureter

Rectum

Urinary bladder

Symphysis pubis

As this frontal view suggests, the kidneys constitute the major portion of the renal-urologic system. These bean-shaped organs lie near and on either side of the spine at the small of the back, with the left kidney positioned slightly higher than the right. (Note that the *adrenal glands* perch atop the kidneys. These glands affect the renal system by influencing blood pressure and the retention of sodium and water by the kidneys.)

The kidneys receive waste-filled blood from the *renal artery*, which branches off the *aorta*. After passing through a complicated network of smaller blood vessels

and nephrons (see page 13), the filtered blood returns to the circulation via the *renal vein*, which empties into the *inferior vena cava*.

Waste products extracted from the blood by the nephrons are excreted by the kidneys, along with other fluids that constitute the formed urine; this urine passes through the *ureters* by peristalsis to the *urinary bladder*.

When the bladder has filled, nerves in the bladder wall relax the *sphincter* (the micturition reflex), and, consonant with a voluntary stimulus, the urine passes into the urethra and is expelled from the body.

that follow a pattern similar to that of the arteries; this venous network leads to the *renal veins,* which carry the blood to the *inferior vena cava.*

Lymph drainage from the kidneys and upper ureters flows into the aortic and para-aortic nodes and finally into the thoracic duct.

The kidneys are innervated by sympathetic branches from the celiac plexus, the upper lumbar splanchnic and thoracic nerves, and the intermesenteric and superior hypogastric plexuses. These join to form a surrounding renal plexus.

### The lower urinary tract

The lower urinary tract consists of the ureters, the urinary bladder, and the urethra.

The *ureters* are a pair of retroperitoneally located, mucosa-lined, fibromuscular tubes that transport urine from the renal pelvis to the urinary bladder. They are 12″ to 13″ (30 to 33 cm) long and vary in diameter from 2 to 8 mm, with the narrowest portions occurring at the ureteropelvic junction, the site where they enter the bony pelvis, and the uretero-vesical junction. The ureters have no sphincters, but their oblique entrance into the bladder creates a mucosal fold that may act as a sphincter. The ureters transport urine by peristalsis, which may reduce the risk of ascending infections.

The *urinary bladder* is a spherical, hollow muscular sac with a normal adult capacity of 300 to 500 ml. It is located in the pelvis, anterior and inferior to the peritoneal cavity and posterior to the pubic bones. When distended, it projects above the symphysis pubis.

The gross structure of the urinary bladder includes the fundus; apex; body; ureteral orifices; and neck, or urethral orifice. The ureteral orifices are located in the body, whereas the urethral orifice constitutes the most inferior portion of the bladder. These three orifices together constitute a triangular area called the trigone.

The *urethra* is the hollow tube that conveys urine from the bladder to the urinary meatus for excretion. The male urethra is approximately 7⅞″ (20 cm) long, and much of it is external to the torso. The female urethra is 1⅛″ to 2″ (3 to 5 cm) long and about 6 mm wide. It lies within the torso and is relatively close to the anal and vaginal orifices.

The blood supply to the ureters usually stems from the renal artery. However, in their course from the kidneys to the urinary bladder, the ureters may also receive blood from the iliac arteries and from the aorta itself. The ureteral veins follow the arteries and drain into the renal vein and the inferior vena cava and its tributaries.

The urinary bladder's arterial blood supply arises from a fanlike division of vessels arising from the common iliac arteries. Venous drainage derives from short vesical veins that unite to form the pudendal plexus, which ultimately empties into the iliac veins.

Lymph drainage from the middle and lower ureters flows into the common and external iliac nodes and the hypogastric nodes. Lymph drainage from the bladder and urethra flows into the hypogastric, external iliac, and deep sublingual nodes.

The ureters are profusely innervated, and there seem to be similar numbers of sympathetic and parasympathetic fibers. Parasympathetic fibers in the bladder are actively involved in micturition, coordinating bladder contraction, and relaxation of the sphincters.

## FILTRATION, REABSORPTION, AND SECRETION

The renal system's main function is to maintain the body's internal homeostasis. It does this through glomerular filtration and tubular reabsorption and secretion.

### Glomerular filtration

Filtration begins as the blood enters the glomerulus, under fairly high pressure, via the afferent arteriole. This glomerular capillary pressure is opposed by colloidal osmotic pressure and capsular pressure. The difference between these various pressures is called the *net filtration pressure.* The net filtration pressure forces fluid and some solutes of small molecular size through pores in the capillary walls into the lumen of the surrounding Bowman's capsule. The glomerular filtrate is similar to plasma but lacks proteins, which are too large to pass through the capillary pores and so are retained in the blood.

The glomerular filtration rate (GFR), which is normally about 125 ml/minute, depends on three factors: permeability of the glomerular capillary walls, blood pressure, and effective filtration pressure. Alterations in any of these factors will significantly alter the GFR. For example, with a urinary tract obstruction, increased pressure in Bowman's capsule may interfere with glomerular filtration. Or, if cardiac output or blood pressure should fall, renal blood flow and the GFR will fall, too.
*(continued on page 14)*

*(continued on page 14)*

# Inside the normal kidney

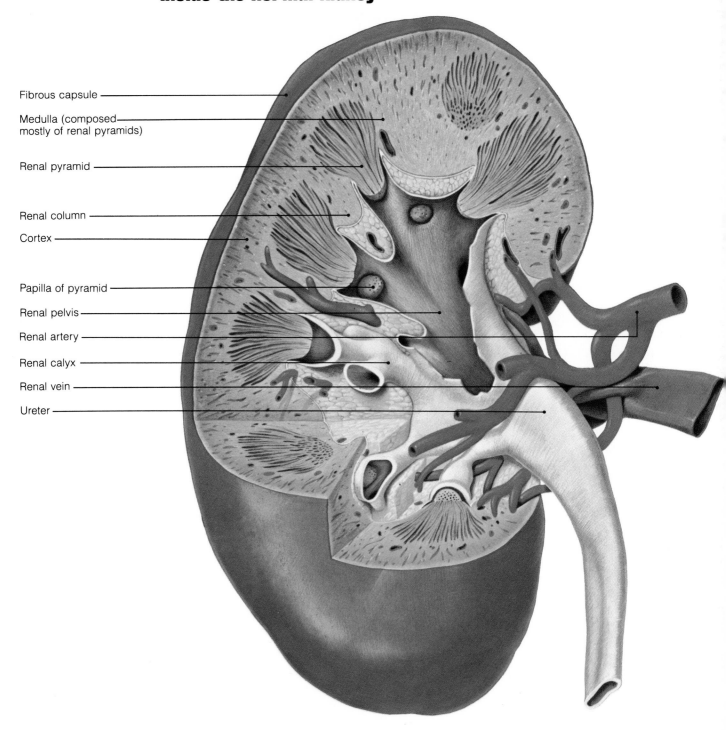

Fibrous capsule

Medulla (composed mostly of renal pyramids)

Renal pyramid

Renal column

Cortex

Papilla of pyramid

Renal pelvis

Renal artery

Renal calyx

Renal vein

Ureter

These drawings reveal the gross structure of the kidney, to the level of its basic units, the nephrons.

Each kidney (above) contains about 1.5 million nephrons, organized into 18 to 20 collection units, the *renal pyramids*, which channel their output into the renal pelvis for excretion. Protected by a *fibrous capsule* and by layers of perinephric fat, the renal parenchyma consists of an outer *cortex* and an inner *medulla*. The medulla contains the renal pyramids, composed mostly of tubular structures. The tapered portion of each pyramid empties into a cuplike *calyx*. The calyces chan-

nel formed urine from the pyramids into the renal pelvis.

Blood is supplied to the kidney by the *renal artery*, which subdivides into several branches. Some of these are responsible for distributing blood within the kidney, while others nourish the kidney cells themselves.

Of the blood brought to the kidney for filtration, about 99% returns to general body circulation through the *renal vein*. The remaining 1% undergoes further processing, resulting in urine-containing waste products that flow to the calyx and renal pelvis. From the pelvis, the urine enters the *ureter*.

## Pyramids of the nephrons

This section of kidney tissue (at top) shows how the glomeruli and proximal and distal tubules of the nephrons are located in the cortex, while the long Henle's loops, together with their accompanying blood vessels and collecting tubules, are formed into renal pyramids in the medulla. Here, countercurrent multiplication maintains the relative osmolality of the urine and interstitial fluid. The tapered end of each pyramid forms a *papilla*, where the collecting tubules empty the urine into the renal pelvis.

## The nephron: Basic functional unit

The nephrons are the kidneys' structural units. They consist of a glomerulus (inside Bowman's capsule), a tubular apparatus, and a collecting duct.

The nephrons perform two main activities: mechanical filtration of fluids, wastes, electrolytes, acids, and bases into the tubular system; and selective reabsorption/secretion of ions.

Blood is brought to and carried away from the glomerular capillaries by two small blood vessels, the *afferent* and *efferent arterioles*. The glomerular capillaries act as bulk filters and pass protein-free and red-blood-cells-free filtrate to the proximal convoluted tubules.

The proximal convoluted tubules have freely permeable cell membranes. This allows reabsorption of nearly all the filtrate's glucose, amino acids, metabolites, and electrolytes into nearby capillaries and the circulation. As these substances return to the circulation, they passively carry large amounts of water.

By the time the filtrate enters the descending limb of Henle's loop, located in the medulla, its water content has been reduced by 70%. At this point, the filtrate contains a high concentration of salts, chiefly sodium. As the filtrate moves deeper into the medulla and into Henle's loop, osmosis draws even more water into the extracellular spaces, further concentrating the filtrate.

Once the filtrate enters the ascending limb, its concentration is readjusted by transport of ions into the tubule. This transport continues until the filtrate enters the distal convoluted tubule.

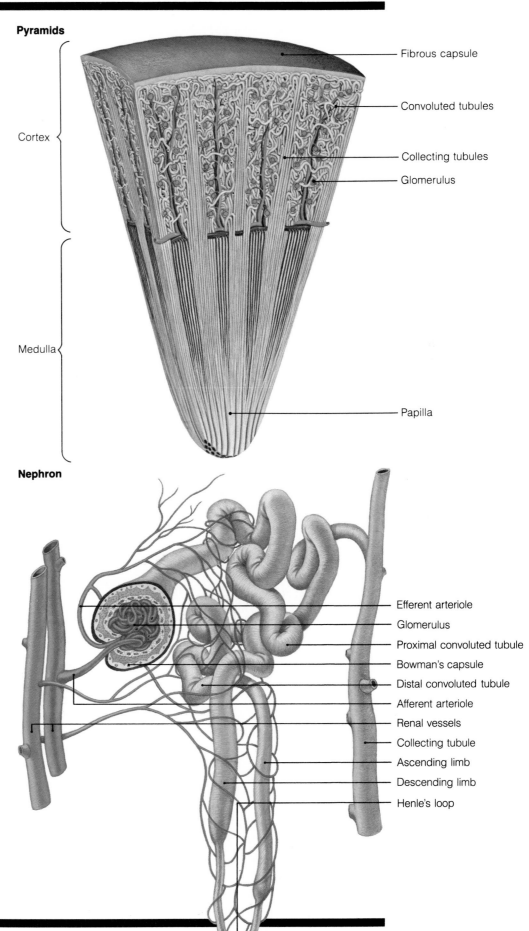

**Pyramids**

Fibrous capsule

Convoluted tubules

Collecting tubules

Glomerulus

Cortex

Medulla

Papilla

**Nephron**

Efferent arteriole

Glomerulus

Proximal convoluted tubule

Bowman's capsule

Distal convoluted tubule

Afferent arteriole

Renal vessels

Collecting tubule

Ascending limb

Descending limb

Henle's loop

## Clearance relates to the GFR

Clearance is the volume of plasma that can be cleared of a dissolved substance by the kidneys per unit of time. The clearance of any dissolved substance from the plasma depends on how the renal tubular cells react to that substance in the glomerular filtrate. Tubular cells can react to dissolved substances in four different ways to affect clearance:

• If the substance is filtered by the glomerulus but not reabsorbed or secreted by the tubules, clearance *equals* the GFR.

• If the substance is filtered by the glomerulus and reabsorbed by the tubules, clearance is *less than* the GFR.

• If the substance is filtered by the glomerulus and secreted by the tubules, clearance is *greater* than the GFR.

• And, finally, if the substance is filtered by the glomerulus and reabsorbed and secreted by the tubules, clearance may be *less than, equal to,* or *greater than* the GFR, depending on the rates of secretion, excretion, and reabsorption of the substance.

Based on these principles, the *creatinine clearance test* is the best method for accurately assessing glomerular filtration. Creatinine, a stable metabolite of protein occurring in blood, is filtered by the glomerulus but is not significantly reabsorbed or secreted in the tubular system. In the test, serum and urine creatinine levels are compared to measure the amount "cleared," or removed, by the kidneys. (See Chapter 3, IMPLEMENTING THE DIAGNOSTIC WORKUP.) Results of this test accurately reflect renal function since creatinine is formed and excreted in constant amounts by the body.

## Tubular reabsorption

Except for proteins of large molecular weight and RBCs, all substances in the extracellular fluid are freely filtered through the glomerulus. These substances (including even useful ones, such as small plasma proteins, amino acids, glucose, hormones, and vitamins) would be lost if not for selective reabsorption by the tubular system. Renal tubules normally reabsorb about 99% of the glomerular filtrate. At the normal GFR of 125 ml/minute, the glomeruli produce about 180 liters of filtrate per day. But because most of this volume is retained during tubular reabsorption, only about 1 to 1.5 liters of filtrate is excreted as urine. The rest is returned to the bloodstream.

Tubular reabsorption is achieved by active and/or passive transport mechanisms. Active transport requires energy to move substances against a concentration or electrochemical gradient. Sodium, potassium, glucose, calcium, phosphates, and amino acids are actively reabsorbed. Passive transport requires no energy since it takes advantage of established concentration gradients. Urea, water, chloride, some bicarbonates, and some phosphates are passively reabsorbed.

Most reabsorption occurs in the proximal tubule, which conserves needed substances but does not reabsorb metabolic waste products. The remaining filtrate passes to Henle's loop, the distal tubule, and the collecting duct, where variable amounts—depending on bodily needs—of the remaining water and electrolytes are reabsorbed.

## Aldosterone, ADH, and water reabsorption

Antidiuretic hormone (ADH) governs water reabsorption from the distal tubule and collecting duct. This hormone increases the permeability of tubule and duct walls to water, promoting its reabsorption as part of the final step in urine concentration. In ADH deficiency, the walls of the distal tubule and collecting duct become less permeable to water, which is excreted, producing a dilute urine.

Aldosterone, an adrenocortical hormone, also significantly influences tubular reabsorption, primarily by regulating sodium retention and helping to control potassium secretion by tubular epithelial cells. To a lesser extent, aldosterone increases tubular secretion of hydrogen ions in exchange for reabsorbed sodium. Thus, increased aldosterone levels result in sodium retention, which leads to expansion of extracellular fluid, increased blood pressure, and, possibly, hypokalemia. Metabolic alkalosis may result from hydrogen ion secretion, but it tends to be mild.

## Tubular secretion

In tubular secretion, substances move by active transport or passive diffusion out of the peritubular blood, through the tubular epithelium, into the lumen. Substances secreted by the tubules include potassium, hydrogen, ammonia, uric acid, exogenous substances (such as drugs), substances that are excreted unchanged (such as para-aminohippuric acid) or are slowly or incompletely metabolized (such as thiamine), and other wastes.

Drugs that are normally secreted by the tubules sometimes compete for transportation into the lumen. This effect is sometimes used to enhance drug therapy. For example, pro-

# The renin-angiotensin feedback system

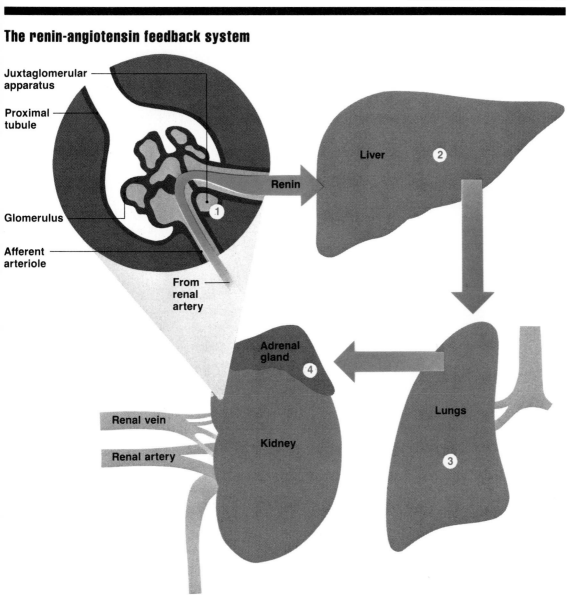

The renin-angiotensin system is an important homeostatic device for regulating the body's sodium and water levels and blood pressure. In this sequence, juxtaglomerular cells (1) near each of the kidney's glomeruli secrete the enzyme *renin* into the blood. The rate of renin secretion depends on the rate of perfusion in the renal afferent arterioles and on the amount of sodium in the serum. A low sodium load and low perfusion pressure (as in hypovolemia) increase renin secretion; a high sodium load and high pressure decrease it.

Renin circulates throughout the body, and, in the liver (2), it converts angiotensinogen to angiotensin I. In the lungs, angiotensin I is converted by hydrolysis (3) to angiotensin II, a potent vasoconstrictor that acts on the adrenal cortex to stimulate production of the hormone aldosterone (4). Aldosterone acts on the juxtaglomerular cells in the nephron to increase sodium and water retention and to stimulate or depress further renin secretion, completing the feedback cycle that automatically readjusts homeostasis.

benecid can block renal excretion of penicillin, causing it to accumulate and, thereby, enhancing its effects.

## Maximal tubular transport capacity

The amount of reabsorption or secretion of a substance depends on the *maximal transport capacity* (Tm) of the tubule for that substance. The Tm is the point or threshold at which the tubular membrane carrier that transports the substance becomes saturated with it and cannot accept more. Renal tubules have different transport thresholds for different substances. Once the Tm is reached, the substances normally reabsorbed are excreted (and substances normally secreted remain in the plasma). The end result for the patient is that homeostasis is interrupted until the filtered load level of the substance falls below the Tm for that substance. For example, the

GFR of glucose varies proportionately with the concentration of glucose in plasma. If the plasma glucose level increases above a critical level, as in diabetes mellitus, it exceeds the tubular Tm for glucose and is then excreted.

## RENAL REGULATORY MECHANISMS

The kidneys' primary functions are filtration of wastes and conservation of essential solutes. In implementing these functions, they also exert an important influence on regulation of electrolytes and water, blood pressure, acid-base balance, calcium and phosphate balance, and erythropoiesis. Each of these aspects will be reviewed.

### Electrolyte regulation

Normally, in most tubule segments, positive ions—such as sodium, potassium, calcium, and magnesium—are actively transported

# The countercurrent multiplying system

How does the kidney concentrate urine? Physiologists have proposed a theory of *countercurrent multiplication* to explain this process.

Part of this theory involves a countercurrent multiplying system operating within—and around—each juxtamedullary nephron. Though much remains to be understood about this system, enough is known to provide a general explanation of concentration mechanisms.

As its name suggests, the system assumes the presence of two side-by-side tubes, each with a current flowing in opposite directions. It further assumes that the two tubes are joined at one end in a U-shape. Because tubular material is transported osmotically from one tube to another across the membrane separating them, *the concentration of material in the U-joint is greater than that entering or leaving the tubes.*

This model describes the nephron. When the nephron's countercurrent multiplying system operates normally, sodium is actively transported out of the solution in the proximal convoluted tubule, with water flowing passively.

So the solution that enters the nephron's descending limb is *isotonic*—that is, it can bathe cells without extracting water. At this point, however, sodium from the extracellular fluid enters passively, so that when the solution within the limb reaches Henle's loop, it's highly concentrated and *hypertonic*—that is, able to extract water from cells.

When the solution enters the ascending limb, it flows along membranes impermeable to water. However, the membranes do allow the active transport of chlorine and the passive flow of sodium. So when the solution enters the distal convoluted tubule, it is *hypotonic*, which allows additional sodium and chlorine to be pumped out actively, with water flowing passively.

Next, the solution enters the collecting tubule. Here the action of antidiuretic hormone (ADH) makes the membrane permeable to water and urea. This leaves a hypertonic solution that enters the renal pelvis as urine.

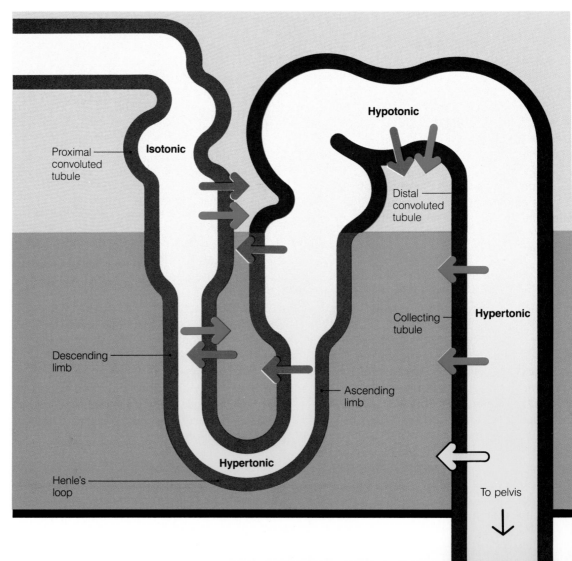

Proximal convoluted tubule — Isotonic — Hypotonic — Distal convoluted tubule — Descending limb — Ascending limb — Collecting tubule — Hypertonic — Henle's loop — Hypertonic — To pelvis

through the tubular epithelium, and negative ions—such as chloride, bicarbonate, and phosphate—are passively transported due to electrical differences that develop across the epithelial membrane when the positive ions are transported. Less than 1% of filtered sodium appears in the urine; most of it is reabsorbed in the proximal tubule. (Remember that sodium reabsorption is an active process, regulated by aldosterone.) Chloride is passively reabsorbed in most parts of the tubular system and tends to follow sodium.

Most filtered potassium is reabsorbed in the proximal tubule. The potassium that's present in the urine usually results from distal tubular secretion, which, in turn, depends on the amount of potassium ingested; the concentrations of hydrogen ions secreted by the tubules; the level of intracellular potassium; the amount of sodium in the distal tubule; serum aldosterone levels; and on the GFR.

## Water regulation

The concentration or dilution of urine excreted by the kidneys depends on regulation within the tubules through the action of ADH on the collecting tubules and on countercurrent multiplication and exchange mechanisms set up between the ascending and descending limbs of Henle's loop and the vasa recta, the network of tubular arterioles and venules.

**ADH and water regulation.** ADH release increases when high blood osmolality stimulates osmoreceptors in the hypothalamus. ADH increases renal reabsorption of water; conversely, low blood osmolality inhibits ADH release and diminishes reabsorption. Thus, the kidneys excrete excessive amounts of water when the blood is too dilute and lesser amounts of water when the blood is too concentrated.

**Countercurrent multiplication and exchange.** This mechanism allows the kidneys to concentrate urine. It's a complicated interaction between the long Henle's loops and their accompanying blood vessels in the medullary interstitium, the vasa recta. This mechanism consists of two processes: multiplication in Henle's loop (see *The countercurrent multiplying system*) and countercurrent exchange between the ascending and descending portions of the vasa recta.

In *multiplication*, urine is concentrated (made hyperosmolar) by the combined action of four different factors:

• active transport of chloride ions (plus passive absorption of sodium ions) into the med-

ullary interstitial fluid by the thick portion of the ascending Henle's loop
• active transport of ions from the collecting duct into the interstitium (caused by the action of ADH on the inner medullary portion of the collecting duct)
• passive diffusion of large amounts of urea from the collecting duct into the interstitium
• transport of additional sodium and chloride into the interstitium from the thin segment of Henle's loop (this transport may be passive).
These four factors interact to produce hyperosmolality in the medullary interstitium.

Ordinarily, the flow of blood through the interstitium tends to remove excess solutes, keeping osmolality down. But medullary blood flow through the vasa recta is too slow to exert this effect very strongly. In addition, the vasa recta act as countercurrent exchangers to maintain interstitial osmotic gradients.

In *countercurrent exchange,* solutes pass easily between the closely adjacent ascending and descending portions of the vasa recta; this ready exchange between the two opposing blood currents allows high concentrations of solutes to exist in the tip of the vasa recta. As blood flows back from the medulla to the cortex, most of the extra sodium, chloride, and urea diffuses out of the blood back into the interstitial fluid, while water diffuses back into the blood. Thus, blood leaving the medulla is only slightly more concentrated than it was before it entered. The countercurrent multiplication and exchange mechanisms allow intricate and precise control of solute and water exchange and transport, which maintains the normal functions of urine concentration and dilution.

## Blood pressure and volume regulation

The kidneys help regulate blood pressure by means of the *renin-angiotensin system* (see *The renin-angiotensin feedback system,* page 15). This enzyme-hormone feedback system involves the liver, the lungs, the adrenal glands, and the nephrons. It responds initially to decreased extracellular fluid volume, which is detected by juxtaglomerular cells in the afferent arteriole supplying the glomerulus, or to changes in sodium levels, which are detected by cells in the adjacent *macula densa.* These stimuli trigger the release of renin, a proteolytic enzyme, from the juxtaglomerular cells. In the liver, renin acts as a catalyst and splits an inactive decapeptide, angiotensin I, from a plasma protein, angiotensinogen. In the lungs, angiotensin I is further split by a converting enzyme to form an active octapeptide, angiotensin II, which is a potent vasoconstrictor. In the circulation, angiotensin II constricts arterioles and, to a lesser extent, veins. Arteriolar constriction increases peripheral resistance, which increases arterial pressure; mild vasoconstriction increases mean circulatory filling pressure up to 20%, which promotes increased venous return to the heart and helps it to pump against the increased pressure load.

Angiotensin II also stimulates the adrenal cortex to release aldosterone. Completing the feedback cycle, aldosterone acts on the distal tubules to increase sodium and water retention to restore effective blood volume, thereby decreasing the initial stimulus for renin release.

### Acid-base regulation
The body's acid-base balance must be regulated as carefully as its fluid and electrolyte balances to allow bodily enzymes to function properly. These enzyme functions occur only in a narrow range of pH: 7.35 to 7.45. This means that any marked change—pH falling lower than 7.3 (acidosis) or rising above 7.5 (alkalosis)—may be life-threatening. Three regulatory components maintain this delicate balance: body fluid buffers, the respiratory system, and the renal system.

**Buffers.** These pairs of weak acids and related weak bases can donate or accept hydrogen ions in solution. In seconds, they combine with strong acids or bases, which would sharply decrease or increase pH, to create weaker acids or bases that affect pH less severely. Body fluid buffers include bicarbonate, phosphate, and protein.

**The respiratory system.** Acting within 1 to 3 minutes, this system interacts with medullary respiratory centers to control the level of plasma carbon dioxide ($PCO_2$). Since the level of $CO_2$ in plasma determines the amount of carbonic acid and hydrogen ions produced, any rise in the $PCO_2$ level lowers pH, and any drop in the $PCO_2$ level raises pH. The lungs and medullary centers control the pH level by altering respiratory rate and depth to eliminate more or less $CO_2$ at the same rate that cells produce it.

**The renal system.** This system maintains normal pH by retaining or excreting hydrogen ions and by regenerating lost buffers. In hours or days, the kidneys excrete acids the lungs can't excrete and excrete hydrogen ions or

reabsorb bicarbonate to correct acidosis; they reverse these processes to correct alkalosis.

Generally, the lungs and the kidneys interact as complementary mechanisms. For example, in respiratory acidosis, the kidneys conserve bicarbonate and excrete more hydrogen ions; they reverse this process in respiratory alkalosis. In metabolic acidosis, the lungs vent more $CO_2$ to help lower body fluid pH; in metabolic alkalosis, they conserve $CO_2$.

### Calcium and phosphate regulation
The kidneys help regulate calcium and phosphate balance by filtering and reabsorbing the 50% of serum calcium not bound to proteins, by activating vitamin $D_3$ and utilizing phosphate from the buffer system. (See *Calcium phosphate imbalance in renal failure,* page 20.)

**Reabsorption of free calcium.** The nephrons actively reabsorb 99% of free calcium; normally, the 1% that is excreted equals the amount ingested daily. However, this normal balance of calcium reabsorption and excretion is vulnerable to rapid change in response to an increased filtered calcium load and to the action of parathyroid hormone (PTH) on the renal tubules. In turn, PTH production responds directly to the extracellular calcium concentration: decreased serum calcium levels stimulate PTH secretion; increased levels suppress it. Elevated serum PTH levels increase renal tubular reabsorption of calcium and inhibit calcium excretion; simultaneously maintaining a reciprocal relationship between calcium and phosphate, PTH inhibits tubular reabsorption of phosphate, thus promoting phosphate excretion.

**Activation of vitamin $D_3$.** This vitamin, the major stimulant to calcium absorption in the small intestine, is essential for normal calcium metabolism. To be useful, vitamin $D_3$ must be converted to its active form in the liver and the kidneys. PTH allows the kidneys to convert the liver-activated form of vitamin $D_3$ to an even more active form, 1,25-dihydroxycholecalciferol, which promotes intestinal calcium absorption.

### Erythropoiesis regulation
The kidneys also participate in the production of RBCs. In response to decreased oxygen tension in the renal blood supply, the kidneys secrete a hormone, *erythropoietin,* that stimulates the bone marrow to produce RBCs. Although erythropoietin is not the only marrow stimulant, it has a significant impact on overall RBC production.

## URINE TRANSPORT AND EXCRETION

Urine, the end product of renal filtration, reabsorption, and secretion, is collected in the renal pelvis, then propelled by peristalsis through the ureters to the urinary bladder. When the bladder fills, stretch receptors in the bladder walls respond to the filling pressure and initiate the *micturition reflex,* which stimulates bladder wall contraction. Contractions last about a minute; if the urine pressure created by this reflex isn't enough to force the bladder neck (posterior urethra) to open, the reflex subsides. As the bladder fills, these reflexes occur more frequently and more powerfully, until the internal sphincter is forced open. This triggers another reflex, which relaxes the external sphincter; if this reflex is more powerful than voluntary control signals from the brain, urination occurs. If not, voluntary control keeps the external sphincter closed until the patient's desire to void allows signals from the brain to activate a micturition reflex. This reflex relaxes the external sphincter and perineal muscles and expels the urine from the bladder through the urethra and urinary meatus.

## RENAL PATHOPHYSIOLOGY

The kidneys are vulnerable to many disorders, ranging from infection and inflammation, which may cause transient dysfunction, to congenital and immune diseases, which may result in total renal failure. Because the kidneys play such a critical role in maintaining homeostasis, their dysfunction or failure adversely affects all other body systems.

Renal pathology leads to varying levels of dysfunction, which are broadly classified as *acute* or *chronic* renal failure. In acute renal failure (ARF), normal kidney function deteriorates rapidly, then gradually recovers. Also, the parenchymal basement membranes usually aren't permanently damaged, so damaged cells can regenerate. In chronic renal failure, parenchymal cellular function is slowly but irreversibly lost. A patient may lose all function of one kidney and two thirds of the other before he begins to show signs and symptoms of chronic renal failure.

## CAUSES OF ACUTE RENAL FAILURE

ARF is the sudden inability of the kidneys to maintain homeostasis (water, electrolyte, and acid-base balances) and to remove metabolic waste materials. Etiologies of ARF can be classified as primary or secondary.

**Primary causes.** These *intrarenal* causes directly involve the renal parenchyma.

*Acute tubular necrosis* is the most common primary cause. In this condition, the proximal tubule, distal tubule, or, frequently, all parts of the tubular system develop reversible lesions and become temporarily dysfunctional.

Acute tubular necrosis commonly results from ischemia (due to hypovolemia, cardiogenic shock, or endotoxic shock); nephrotoxicity (due to the use of aminoglycoside antibiotics, heavy metals, organic solvents, glycols, anesthetics, or radiographic contrast media); intravascular hemolysis following transfusion reactions or toxic hemolysis; and rhabdomyolysis following muscle trauma, muscle disease, seizures, strenuous exercise, or prolonged coma.

Other causes of parenchymal damage include glomerulonephritis, vasculitis, interstitial nephritis, and renal vascular disease.

*Glomerulonephritis* may result from immune complex disorders, collagen tissue destruction, viral lesions, and bacterial infections. Examples of such causes include acute poststreptococcal glomerulonephritis, systemic lupus erythematosus, Goodpasture's syndrome, and bacterial endocarditis.

*Vasculitis* involves inflammation of renal blood vessel walls, which leads to scarring, atrophy, inelasticity, and microaneurysms. Examples include periarteritis and hypersensitivity angiitis.

*Interstitial nephritis* involves fibrosis of the tissue surrounding the nephron as a result of infection, allergic response, abnormal electrolyte levels, or neoplasms. Examples of interstitial nephritis are acute pyelonephritis, allergic nephritis, hypercalcemia, uric acid nephropathy, and renal myeloma.

*Renal vascular disease* results from conditions that narrow or occlude the renal arteries or veins. Examples are renal artery occlusion and renal vein thrombosis.

**Secondary causes.** These indirectly involve the kidney through *prerenal* or *postrenal* (uropathic) causes.

*Prerenal causes* are directly related to hypoperfusion and are typically associated with hypovolemia or cardiovascular failure. In these instances, the decreased blood supply reduces the GFR, which depresses overall renal function. Hypovolemia may result from vascular losses (hemorrhage), gastrointestinal losses (vomiting or diarrhea), renal losses (excessive use of diuretics or osmotic diuresis), and integumentary losses (burns or severe diaphoresis). Cardiovascular failure

## Calcium phosphate imbalance in renal failure

Calcium phosphate is the major mineral of bones and teeth. The bone concentration of calcium also serves as a storage compartment for calcium and is a source of replenishment of serum calcium when a balance between this ion and serum phosphate cannot be maintained by either increased gut absorption or decreased kidney excretion. Serum calcium and phosphate concentrations are regulated by parathyroid hormone (PTH) and activated vitamin D.

The product of $Ca^{++}$ and $PO_4^=$ in the serum is constant. If levels of one ion change, the other rises or falls inversely. This balance must be maintained so that the product of $Ca^{++}$ and $PO_4^=$ doesn't exceed the solubility product for calcium phosphate. When this happens, the mineral precipitates in many body tissues, including the brain, lungs, joints, blood vessels, and skin. This diagram shows what happens when the balance is upset by renal failure.

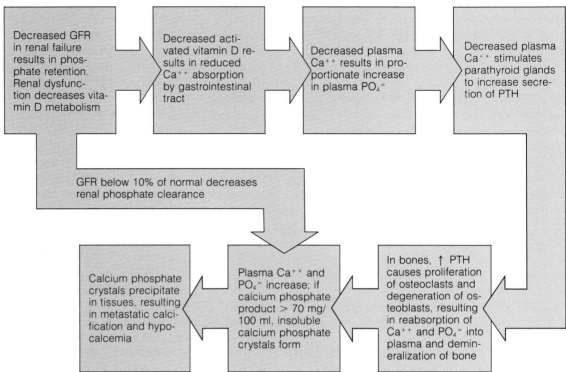

may result from myocardial infarction, cardiac tamponade, vascular pooling (as in sepsis), and vascular occlusions due to thromboses or emboli.

*Postrenal causes* are directly related to obstructions of urinary outflow (uropathies). These uropathies produce renal dysfunction when the obstruction allows urine to accumulate and back up the lower urinary tract to the kidney, eventually causing dilatation and pressure atrophy of tissues above the obstruction. Bilateral urine obstruction can cause ARF. Examples of postrenal uropathies include ureteral problems, such as fibrosis, calculi, crystals, clots, strictures, and accidental ligation; bladder neoplasms; urethral strictures; and compression due to prostatic hypertrophy. Also, parenchymal infections such as pyelonephritis can result from postrenal obstruction and subsequent urine stasis.

Normally, secondary pathologies are reversible because no intrinsic renal damage has occurred. Correcting these extrarenal pathologies may resolve the problem completely.

### PATTERN OF PROGRESSION
ARF is usually a self-limiting, reversible condition that lasts about 10 to 25 days. During the clinical course, the ARF patient progresses through four phases: onset, oliguria, diuresis, and convalescence.

### First phase: Onset
The onset phase extends from the precipitating event to the development of oliguria or, rarely, anuria. This phase typically lasts from a few hours to 2 days, but it can be prolonged an extra 3 to 5 days in some cases of nephrotoxic insult.

### Second phase: Oliguria
During the oliguric phase, the patient's urinary output is less than 400 ml/day. Oliguria usually lasts from 8 to 14 days but can be longer. The longer oliguria persists, the poorer the prognosis.

Research suggests that five pathophysiologic mechanisms interact to produce and maintain oliguria in ARF: increased renal vasoconstriction, cellular edema causing decreased blood flow, decreased glomerular capillary permeability, intratubular obstruction, and the back leak of glomerular filtrate. These mechanisms probably operate in concert but may function separately; they seem to vary according to the cause and severity of ARF.

Some ARF patients maintain normal urinary output or even develop polyuria, but because of nephron dysfunction, their urine lacks appropriate wastes and solutes. Thus, renal failure ensues despite an adequate urine volume. This disorder is often called *nonoliguric* renal failure.

## Third phase: Diuresis

The diuretic phase of ARF occurs in two stages: early and late (functional recovery). The early stage begins when urine volume increases from 400 ml/day and ends when the patient's blood values stop rising. The late diuretic, or functional recovery, stage begins when blood values begin to decline and ends when they stabilize. The entire diuretic phase lasts about 10 days.

## Fourth phase: Convalescence

The convalescent phase begins when blood values stabilize and ends with maximal recovery of renal function. This phase usually lasts from 2 to 6 months or more. The degree of maximal recovery varies from a return to completely normal function to mild, moderate, or severe levels of residual impairment.

## CHRONIC RENAL FAILURE: DIVERSE ORIGINS

The sources of CRF can be roughly grouped into eight disease categories: glomerular, infectious or interstitial, vascular, tubular, obstructive, collagen-related, hereditary metabolic, and congenital. Of these, glomerular diseases are the leading cause of chronic renal failure, followed by infectious or interstitial diseases and vascular diseases.

• *Glomerular diseases* usually result from immune complex diseases, inflammatory processes, or the interactive effects of other systemic diseases. These conditions create lesions in the glomerular capillary basement membrane, followed by accumulation of necrotic cellular debris, with eventual scarring and atrophy. The lesions increase glomerular permeability, allowing normally nonfiltered substances, such as plasma proteins and RBCs, to pass into the filtrate. This impaired filtration reduces serum osmolality, predisposing the patient to edema. The severity of the edema depends on the relationship of the colloid osmotic pressure and the hydrostatic pressure in the vessels. Chronic glomerulonephritis and nephrotic syndrome are the most common glomerular diseases.

• *Infectious or interstitial diseases* result in inflammation of interstitial tissue, leading to accumulation of cellular infiltrate composed primarily of lymphocytes and plasma cells, followed by varying degrees of fibrosis and scarring of the renal parenchyma. Interstitial inflammation can also result from adverse drug reactions, tuberculosis, or other infectious and systemic disorders. Examples of interstitial diseases include pyelonephritis and analgesic nephropathy.

• *Vascular diseases* primarily involve sclerosis and narrowing of the afferent and efferent arterioles and the glomerular capillaries. As pathology progresses, renal blood flow diminishes, leading to a decreased GFR, deficient cellular oxygen and nutrition, and overall renal dysfunction. Vascular diseases include arteriosclerosis (often due to hypertension) and Kimmelstiel-Wilson syndrome.

• *Tubular diseases* result from hereditary cellular membrane defects and chronic electrolyte imbalances that result in deterioration of tubular epithelial cells. The basement membrane is also injured. As a result, the tubular system becomes filled with necrotic cell debris (and sometimes crystalline precipitates) and loses its capacity for normal excretion and secretion. Tubular diseases include proximal and distal tubular acidosis, calcium nephropathy, and hypokalemic nephropathy.

• *Obstructive diseases* are likely to cause CRF if they are allowed to impede urinary outflow for extended periods. As the blocked urine accumulates, it backs up the ureters and finally ascends to the kidney, where it dilates the collecting system and compresses functioning kidney structures. This leads to decreased renal blood flow and GFR, renal ischemia, and dysfunctional nephrons. At the same time, urine stasis predisposes the patient to infection. Such an infection, superimposed on an already impaired renal system, enhances and hastens the progression of renal failure. Obstructive conditions include ureteral and urethral strictures, cysts, neoplasms, calculi, foreign bodies, congenital anomalies, and prostatic hypertrophy.

• *Collagen-related diseases* seem to have a special affinity for highly vascularized tissue and readily attack the renal system. These diseases result in hypertrophy and hyperplasia of collagen fibers, vascular lesions, inflammation, and tissue necrosis. Collagen diseases that cause chronic renal failure include scleroderma, systemic lupus erythematosus, polyarteritis nodosa, and necrotizing angiitis.

• *Hereditary metabolic diseases* result from inborn errors of metabolism that significantly affect the renal system. Most of these diseases inhibit or destroy renal function by producing fibrous glycoprotein deposits, calculi, crystals, or precipitates in the glomerulus or other nephron structures. Such diseases include primary and secondary amyloidosis, sarcoidosis, and hyperoxaluria.

• *Congenital diseases* include anatomic defects and hereditary renal diseases that are present from birth. Congenital anomalies, such as aplastic or hypoplastic kidneys, result from abnormal development of the renal vasculature, tubules, collecting system, or drainage apparatus.

Most commonly, hereditary diseases are cystic or glomerular. In polycystic kidney disease and medullary cystic kidney disease, large cysts develop in the kidney, enlarging it and compressing functional tissue. In hereditary glomerular diseases, such as hereditary glomerulonephritis, pathology is similar to that of other glomerular diseases.

## PATTERN OF PROGRESSION
Unlike ARF, the chronic form, whatever its causes, tends to develop in three major stages: decreased renal reserve, renal insufficiency, and irreversible renal failure.

**Decreased renal reserve.** In this stage, the kidneys respond to injury with mild to moderately decreased function. This does not adversely affect homeostasis since some compensatory alterations occur. Renal dysfunction can be detected at this stage only by careful assessment.

**Renal insufficiency.** In this stage, azotemia (retention of nitrogenous compounds), hypertension, anemia, and other symptoms occur but are still mild, even though about 75% of functional renal tissue has been destroyed and the GFR has decreased to 40 to 70 ml/minute. Associated abnormalities may include hyperuricemia, hypertriglyceridemia, and impaired urine concentration. These abnormalities typically produce few overt physiologic effects, but renal reserve is so low that any stress—infection, dehydration, or other trauma—will further impair renal function. If the source of physiologic stress can be corrected quickly, renal function may be restored to more stable levels. But if the stress continues so that the nephron mass deteriorates and the GFR falls below 5 ml/minute, the patient will experience overt renal failure.

**End-stage renal disease.** At this final stage, the GFR has fallen below 5 ml/minute, and 90% of renal tissue has been destroyed. The patient in this condition experiences severe impairment of all body systems.

## SYSTEMIC RESPONSES TO RENAL FAILURE
The systemic physiologic responses to acute and chronic renal failure are similar regardless of etiology, but their effects vary according to the severity and duration of renal dysfunction. (See also Chapter 4, COMBATING ACUTE RENAL FAILURE, and Chapter 5, COMPENSATING FOR CHRONIC RENAL FAILURE.)

### Fluid and electrolyte responses
Renal dysfunction quickly leads to electrolyte imbalances because excess ions can't be excreted and deficient ions can be neither conserved nor generated. Hyponatremia results from excessive sodium and water retention, and edema results from excessive sodium and water intake. Similarly, when the kidneys can't concentrate urine or excrete fluids, accumulating fluid leads to hypervolemia.

The most perilous serum electrolyte imbalances are hyperkalemia, hypocalcemia, and hypermagnesemia. Metabolic acidosis is also a major problem.

### Metabolic responses
Renal failure affects metabolic mechanisms in various ways, including glucose intolerance, hyperlipidemia, hyperlipoproteinemia, and elevated blood urea nitrogen (BUN) and creatinine levels.

**Glucose intolerance.** The primary endocrine response to renal failure is glucose intolerance. This effect results from peripheral insensitivity to insulin, due to uremia, and prolonged insulin half-life resulting from its impaired metabolism. Renal glucose intolerance is clinically insignificant unless the patient has preexisting glucose intolerance; must take drugs, such as corticosteroids, that affect glucose levels; or is receiving extra glucose, as in hyperalimentation therapy.

**Hyperlipidemia and hyperlipoproteinemia.** Serum cholesterol levels remain normal in renal failure, except in nephrotic syndrome. Serum triglyceride levels rise in uremia because of increased production and decreased excretion. Increased triglyceride levels are related to peripheral insulin resistance and elevated serum insulin levels, which promote increased glyceride synthesis in the liver. Increased triglyceride levels also result from reduced activity of lipoprotein lipase due to insulin resistance.

**Elevated metabolites.** Diminished renal function causes protein metabolism products to accumulate, as reflected in rising BUN levels. Elevated urea, nitrogen, and other protein metabolite levels are mainly responsible for the uremic syndrome and its various manifestations.

## Cardiovascular responses

The effects of renal failure on the cardiovascular system include hypertension; congestive heart failure (CHF); dysrhythmias; uremic pericarditis; and systemic edema.

**Hypertension.** One of the most common complications of uremia, hypertension results from several different pathophysiologic mechanisms. Excessive levels of fluid and sodium are major contributors to hypertension, but inappropriate activation of the renin-angiotensin system may also be involved. Normally activated by reduced blood supply to the nephrons, this system may also be triggered by reduced vascular flow resulting from edema, accumulation of cellular debris, sclerosis, or scarring. Thus, even when the nephron blood supply is adequate, the underlying pathology may stimulate the renin-angiotensin system. This inappropriate response promotes vasoconstriction, aldosterone secretion, and sodium and water retention; all contributing to hypertension.

**Congestive heart failure.** Although CHF may be acute, it's generally a chronic disorder associated with salt and water retention by the kidneys. CHF ensues when the stress of fluid retention and the pathology accompanying hypertension burden the cardiovascular system beyond its ability to compensate.

**Dysrhythmias.** Electrolyte imbalances—especially hyperkalemia, hypocalcemia, and hypernatremia—induced by renal failure may result in cardiac dysrhythmias. Of these imbalances, hyperkalemia has the most rapid, profound, and perilous effects.

**Uremic pericarditis.** This form of pericarditis is more common in chronic than in acute renal failure. It occurs when uremic toxins in the plasma irritate the pericardial membrane, increasing its permeability and resulting in an influx of fluid into the pericardial sac. Eventually, this fluid compresses the ventricles and impairs cardiac function. Untreated, the condition may lead to cardiac tamponade. Uremic pericarditis may recur after treatment and is common in hemodialysis patients.

**Systemic edema.** This condition often develops in renal failure as a result of decreased serum osmolality and the increased hydrostatic pressure caused by fluid overload. Coexisting CHF (particularly right ventricular) increases the risk of systemic edema.

## Hematopoietic responses

Renal failure affects the hematopoietic system, resulting in anemia, coagulation defects, and increased susceptibility to infection.

**Anemia.** Decreased renal mass and uremic toxins reduce production of erythropoietin; accumulating uremic toxins adversely affect RBC survival time, platelet integrity, and folic acid activity. In addition, uremic toxins create hypertonic serum, which causes crenation (shrinkage) of RBCs.

RBCs are also lost through the gastrointestinal tract, mucous membranes, and dialysis.

These losses seem insignificant if one considers each one individually, but their cumulative effect over time can be considerable. Thus, the anemia associated with renal failure can be quite severe and does not respond well to nutritional or drug therapy.

**Coagulation defects.** Uremic toxins may cause platelet dysfunction by altering platelet surfaces and interfering with aggregation. Hypocalcemia in renal failure may also contribute to this dysfunction since calcium normally acts as a coagulation catalyst. Remember, however, that many renal failure patients are "normally" acidotic and thus have a proportionately increased amount of ionized calcium available. In such patients, the ionized calcium level is unlikely to drop to levels that could impair coagulation.

**Increased susceptibility to infection.** Infection complicates 30% to 70% of all cases of ARF and significantly increases morbidity and mortality in both acute and chronic renal failure. In fact, septicemia is the number one cause of death in ARF patients. Research suggests that uremic serum impairs the phagocytic and chemotactic activities of leukocytes, which, in turn, inhibits acute inflammatory responses and decreases delayed hypersensitivity reactions.

## Respiratory responses

Potential manifestations of renal failure in the respiratory system include pulmonary edema, pneumonia or pneumonitis, and Kussmaul's respirations. Pulmonary edema and Kussmaul's respirations are more common in acute than in chronic renal failure patients, which probably reflects the CRF patient's adaptation to chronic systemic changes.

**Pulmonary edema.** In renal failure, this condition results from fluid overload due to renal dysfunction; left ventricular dysfunction due to continuous excessive demand on the cardiovascular system; and increased pulmonary capillary permeability related to uremic toxins in the serum.

*(continued on page 26)*

# How renal compensation regulates blood pH

Normally, blood pH is maintained between 7.35 and 7.45. A variation of only 0.4 of a pH unit in either direction (acidosis or alkalosis) can be fatal. The body regulates the pH of its fluids through three mechanisms. *Blood buffers* neutralize excess acids or alkalies that form as a result of metabolic processes; the *lungs* act within minutes to regulate the volatile carbonic acid in the blood through exhalation or retention of carbon dioxide; and the *kidneys* respond, as explained here.

The kidneys play a major role in maintaining blood pH by conserving or excreting various acids and bases to maintain effective buffer ratios. When arterial blood pH decreases, the kidneys excrete more hydrogen ions and reabsorb more bicarbonate into the blood to overcome the rising acidity. Conversely, when arterial blood pH increases, the kidneys overcome alkalinity by excreting more bicarbonate.

At far right, nonrenal buffering mechanisms are shown in the diagram. These include, from top, buffering of anions and $CO_2$ in arterial blood, carried out mainly by red blood cells and by plasma proteins; interstitial fluid buffering of acids (A) from tissue and bone; and respiratory control of arterial blood pH.

### Three mechanisms
In renal compensation, three compensatory mechanisms operate simultaneously along the nephron. From the top, they are *bicarbonate reabsorption, titratable acid excretion,* and *ammonia excretion.* The basic reactions taking place in the blood (left column), in the renal tubular cell (center column), and in the tubular lumen (right column) are shown arranged similarly for the three mechanisms. Blood and urine both flow from the top of the diagram to the bottom. Note that in each compensatory mechanism, the enzyme *carbonic anhydrase* (CA), found inside the renal tubular cell and in the tubular epithelial cell, catalyzes the formation and breakdown of carbonic acid, which results in the secretion of hydrogen ions into the urine and the reabsorption of bicarbonate ions into the blood.

### Bicarbonate reabsorption
Here, the tubular epithelial cells combine carbon dioxide and water under the influence of CA to form carbonic acid, which dissociates into bicarbonate ion and hydrogen ion. The hydrogen ion is secreted into the lumen of the tubule, and the sodium ion that dissociates from the sodium bicarbonate in the tubule passively diffuses into the tubular epithelial cell and is actively reabsorbed into the blood to maintain electroneutrality. The hydrogen ion then combines with the bicarbonate ion to form carbonic acid. This dissociates to form water, which is excreted, and carbon dioxide, which enters the tubular epithelial cells to be reused to form carbonic acid. The sodium ion that was reabsorbed from the tubule is secreted into the extracellular fluid (blood), where it combines with the bicarbonate ion that the epithelial cell has reabsorbed to form sodium bicarbonate. In the end, one hydrogen ion has been lost, and the bicarbonate has been conserved. Bicarbonate reabsorption is a key mechanism, along with respiratory control of arterial blood $CO_2$ (far right), in maintaining the proper buffer ratios in body fluids.

### Titratable acid excretion
Here, the tubular cells secrete hydrogen ions into the urine in exchange mainly for sodium ions from the glomerular filtrate. Because of glomerular filtration, the urine contains buffers, such as phosphate, some of which are destined for excretion. The secreted hydrogen ions titrate these buffers in the acid direction. For example, they convert monohydrogen phosphate ($HPO_4^=$) to the more acid dihydrogen phosphate ($H_2PO_4^-$). In this reaction, a hydrogen ion replaces a sodium ion that accompanies the monohydrogen phosphate in the dihydrogen phosphate salt. The sodium ion passively diffuses through the luminal membrane into the tubular cell and is pumped by the peritubular membrane into the peritubular fluid. The bicarbonate ion generated in the cell passively accompanies the sodium ion into the peritubular fluid and eventually into the blood.

For each secreted hydrogen ion that combines with phosphate (or other buffers) to form titratable acid, an equivalent quantity of bicarbonate is generated by the tubular cell and added to the blood. Thus, by excreting hydrogen ions as titratable acid, the kidney conserves the bases in body fluids and restores plasma bicarbonate.

### Ammonia excretion
Here, ammonia ($NH_3$), synthesized mainly from glutamine in the tubular cells by transamination and deamination, diffuses readily into the tubular urine. If the urine is acid, ammonia combines with a hydrogen ion to form an ammonium ion ($NH_4^+$), as shown here. Ammonium, unlike ammonia, penetrates cell membranes poorly because of its electrical charge, so it's trapped in the urine and excreted.

As long as free hydrogen ions are present in the tubular urine, ammonia will be converted to ammonium, promoting diffusion of $NH_3$ into the urine rather than toward the blood. Conversely, in alkaline urine, the lack of hydrogen ions to bind ammonia shifts the diffusion of ammonia toward the blood. For each hydrogen ion excreted with ammonia, an equivalent quantity of sodium bicarbonate is added to the blood.

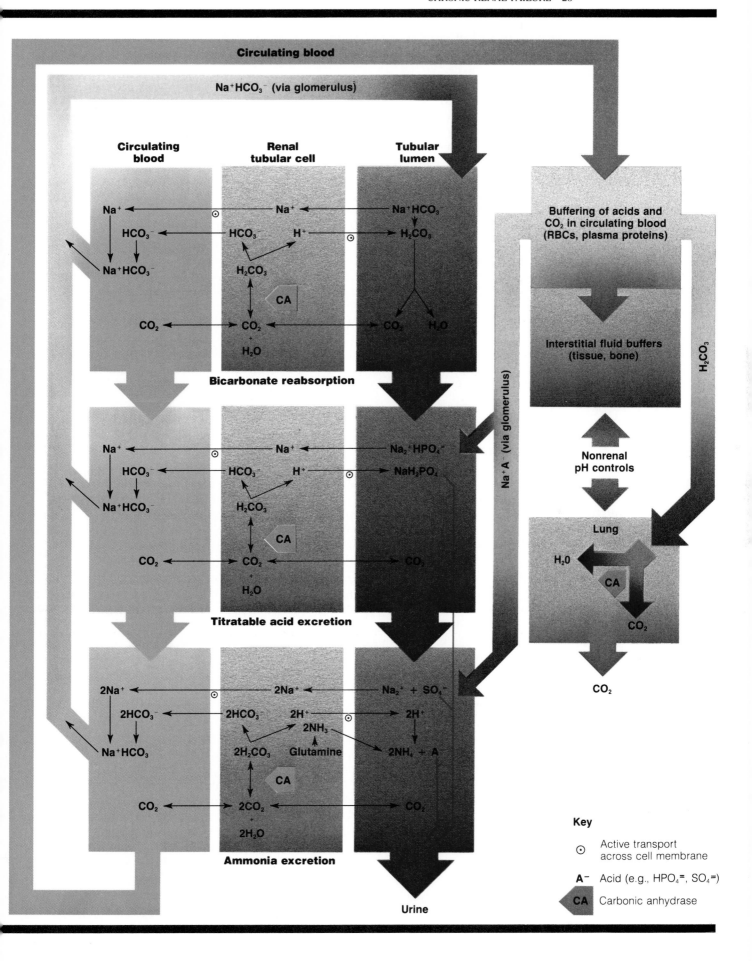

**Pneumonia or pneumonitis.** Renal failure increases susceptibility to pneumonia or pneumonitis. Contributing factors may include the presence of thick, tenacious oral secretions due to decreased fluid intake; the tendency of such secretions to trap bacteria within the respiratory system; impairment of pulmonary macrophage activity by uremic toxins; fluid overload, which may lead to dyspnea and ineffective breathing; a depressed cough reflex associated with uremia; and a weakened, lethargic state due to uremia.

**Kussmaul's respirations.** To compensate for metabolic acidosis, the rate and depth of respirations (Kussmaul's respirations) are increased, which helps to vent more $CO_2$ and lower plasma pH. Kussmaul's respirations commonly occur in ARF or in acute exacerbations of CRF. Note that these respirations are a compensatory mechanism; they're frequently misinterpreted as "respiratory distress" and dealt with inappropriately.

## Gastrointestinal responses

Renal failure causes multiple distressing gastrointestinal symptoms, including anorexia, nausea, emesis, uremic fetor, stomatitis, gastritis, bleeding, diarrhea, and constipation. These symptoms interfere with adequate nutrition and exacerbate the uremia.

**Anorexia, nausea, and emesis.** Uremic toxins and ammonia, released by decomposing urea, irritate the GI mucosa, producing anorexia, nausea, and emesis. Dehydration intensifies the patient's discomfort, especially in the early morning.

**Uremic fetor and stomatitis.** Affected by the same irritants as the GI mucosa, the oral mucosa develops small, painful ulcerations. Decomposing urea taints the patient's breath with the odor of urine (uremic fetor) and interferes with his sense of taste. He may complain that foods taste metallic or are otherwise disagreeable. Inflammation from stomatitis may also cause him to taste blood. These changes depress the patient's appetite and nutritional intake, which can result in, and accelerate, protein catabolism.

**Gastritis and GI bleeding.** Chronic irritation of the GI mucosa by the uremic toxins and ammonia can result in small ulcerations similar to those produced by stress. Typically, the resultant bleeding and increased capillary fragility produced by the toxins lead to slow GI oozing of blood. However, if the patient is severely uremic and critically ill from multisystem dysfunction, the oozing may escalate to a full-blown GI hemorrhage or uremic colitis. Fortunately, these instances of severe bleeding are uncommon.

Usually, GI bleeding is mild and can be monitored adequately with daily stool guaiac testing. Remember, however, that blood is protein, and as it is reabsorbed from the GI tract, it will be metabolized to produce urea and other metabolites that accentuate the uremia. To minimize this hazard, cleansing enemas (typically soapsuds) have *sometimes* been administered to control protein metabolism from this source. However, this type of therapy is of questionable benefit and is now used infrequently.

Keep in mind also that GI bleeding will accentuate hyperkalemia as a result of the destruction of RBCs.

**Bowel dysfunction.** Bowel function is rarely normal in patients with renal failure. Actually, most CRF patients need a lot of help in establishing an effective bowel regimen to combat constipation. The presence of uremic toxins and abnormal electrolyte levels (especially of potassium) produces significant changes in bowel function. Hyperkalemia is frequently associated with hypermotility and diarrhea; hypokalemia and other electrolyte abnormalities may produce hypomotility and constipation. Restricted fluid intake, reduced dietary bulk, diminished physical activity, and drug therapy may all contribute to constipation.

## Neuromuscular responses

The effects of renal failure on the neuromuscular system include drowsiness, confusion, irritability, tremors, twitching, convulsions, coma, and peripheral neuropathy. These abnormalities are commonly intermittent and of varying severity. However, as renal failure advances, neurologic abnormalities become more severe and distinct.

As uremic toxins accumulate and eventually cross the blood-brain barrier, they produce uremic encephalopathy. This, together with the depressive effects of metabolic acidosis, produces drowsiness, confusion, and irritability. If the encephalopathy is not treated, coma follows. Electrolyte imbalances may combine with uremic encephalopathy to produce tremors, twitching, and convulsions.

**Peripheral neuropathy.** Varying degrees of peripheral neuropathy result from the depressive effects of uremic toxins on both sensory and motor nerve conduction. Three stages of peripheral neuropathy are recognized.
• Restless leg syndrome, the first stage, in-

volves general paresthesia as well as burning or tingling sensations that occur mainly in the lower extremities. This stage may occur in acute or chronic renal failure, but the next two stages occur only in CRF.
• Motor involvement, the second stage, is manifested by footdrop and concomitant impairment of mobility.
• Motor nerve disruption, the third stage, may rarely progress to paraplegia.

## Psychosocial responses
Psychosocial abnormalities associated with renal failure include altered mentation, such as confusion, loss of recent memory, decreased ability to concentrate, and altered perception. Some patients' coping ability may be so impaired by the physiologic stress of renal failure that they develop frank psychoses. The underlying physiologic mechanisms include uremic encephalopathy, electrolyte imbalances, central nervous system depression related to metabolic acidosis, and cerebral edema resulting from high levels of uremic toxins and fluid retention.

Decreased libido, impotence, and infertility associated with CRF often cause major psychosocial maladaptations stemming from threatened body image and increasingly negative feelings of self-worth.

## Integumentary responses
Renal failure also has significant effects on the skin, hair, and nails. These effects include pallor and yellowness, dryness, pruritus, hair loss, brittle nails, purpura and ecchymoses, secondary skin infections, and uremic frost. Except for uremic frost, which occurs only in critically or terminally ill patients, all of these effects may appear in acute or chronic renal failure patients.

## Skeletal responses
The skeletal system is severely assaulted during renal failure, resulting in such disorders as hypocalcemia, osteodystrophy, and soft tissue calcification. These disorders cause bone and joint pain, spontaneous fractures (especially of the ribs), impaired bone growth in children, and calcification of soft tissues.

**Hypocalcemia.** This disorder results from hyperphosphatemia created by decreased renal excretion of phosphates and decreased gastric reabsorption of calcium due to decreased renal conversion of vitamin D to its active metabolite. Hypocalcemia overstimulates PTH, which leads to osteodystrophy.

**Osteodystrophy.** This disorder, which is more common in growing children than in adults, is marked by increased PTH secretion, which stimulates osteoclastic bone reabsorption activity. This produces a loss of calcium and phosphorus into the bloodstream, elevating the serum levels of these electrolytes.

**Soft tissue calcification.** As a result of increased osteoclastic activity and mobilization of phosphorus and calcium from the bone, soft tissues (such as small and medium-sized blood vessels), periarticular tissues, lungs, myocardium, eyes, and skin may develop metastatic calcifications.

## Reproductive responses
Because of its short duration, ARF doesn't usually cause reproductive abnormalities. However, chronic renal failure often causes infertility, decreased libido, and impotence. In both sexes, accumulated uremic toxins cause infertility by depressing ovulation and sperm production and by producing menstrual irregularities. Reduced libido probably results from combined physiologic and psychological effects of uremia. Although male impotence shares these origins, it may be aggravated by drug therapy, especially with some antihypertensive agents. Adequate dialysis or transplantation partially reverses reproductive dysfunction.

## Nursing implications
Every case of renal or urologic disease is a little different from the next. Not only do these disorders have multiple causes, but they also may be acute or chronic, obvious or insidious, reversible or irreversible. They may also occur as complications of many other disorders. Nursing care can make an important difference to each patient.

Advances in medical technology mean that an increasing number of patients will need specialized renal care, and your role as teacher and counselor will become more important than ever before. Patients and their families, who may have to deal with the devastating effects of advanced renal failure, will need accurate information about short- and long-term management, the importance of proper home care, and the availability of support groups to help them cope with changes in life-style. Only if you understand renal and urologic anatomy, physiology, and pathophysiology will you be able to convey this complicated information in a way that's most helpful to patients and their families.

**Points to remember**

• The kidneys detoxify the blood and eliminate wastes; regulate fluid volume, acid-base balance, and electrolyte concentrations in body fluids; regulate calcium and phosphorus (bone) metabolism; control blood pressure; and stimulate erythropoiesis.
• The kidneys process about 1,700 liters of blood a day and excrete about 1,200 to 1,500 ml of urine a day.
• The basic functional unit of the kidney is the nephron, consisting of a glomerulus, Bowman's capsule, tubular structures, and a collecting duct. Each kidney contains about 1.5 million nephrons.
• The glomerular filtration rate depends on the permeability of the glomerular capillary walls, blood pressure, and filtration pressure.
• Clearance represents the volume of plasma that can be cleared of a substance per unit of time.
• The amount of tubular reabsorption or secretion of a substance depends on the maximal transport capacity of the renal tubule for that substance.
• Antidiuretic hormone (ADH) controls water reabsorption from the distal tubule and collecting duct. Increased ADH activity decreases urine volume and increases solute concentration. Aldosterone regulates sodium retention and helps control potassium secretion in the renal tubules.
• Acute renal failure may arise from intrarenal, prerenal, or postrenal (uropathic) causes. Chronic renal failure has various causes: glomerular, tubular, vascular, infectious or interstitial, obstructive, collagen-related, hereditary metabolic, and congenital diseases.
• Systemic responses to renal failure involve every major body system.

# 2 ASSESSING RENAL AND UROLOGIC FUNCTION

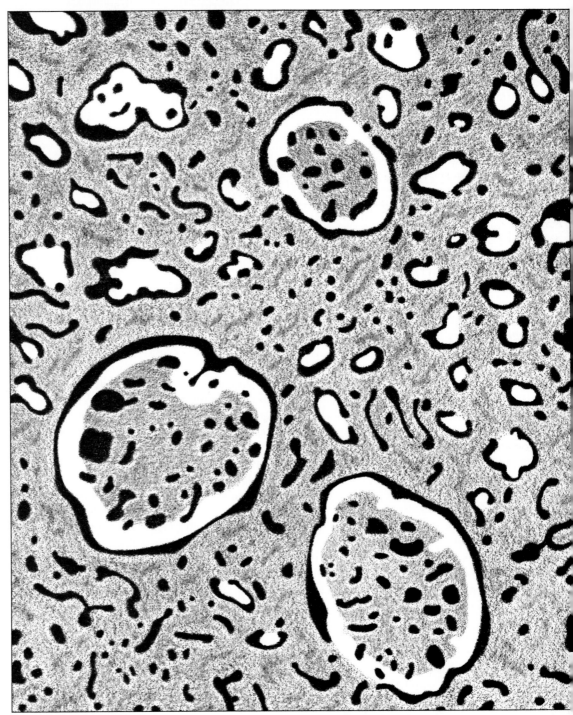

Interstitial edema in renal cortex

Because the kidneys are so profoundly involved in maintaining homeostasis, you may uncover clues to renal dysfunction in *any* body system when you assess your patient's renal system. So assessment for renal or urologic disorders requires that you consider a wide range of signs and symptoms. Recognizing such disorders is especially difficult because it's not easy to know *when* to assess the renal system. Consider, for example, chronic renal disease, in which the patient may look and feel well—even though his kidneys have lost 75% of their normal function. His body finds ways to compensate as the disease slowly progresses, and he may have a brief and unremarkable medical history, with few signs and symptoms.

To assess renal status reliably, you'll have to take an especially detailed history and observe the patient for characteristic but sometimes subtle signs. You'll have to take stock of physical factors, such as obesity, that influence the condition of his kidneys. You may have to weigh him each morning for gain or loss of fluid. And you'll have to be prepared to perform a variety of fairly simple diagnostic tests. This chapter will provide you with all the information you need to perform a thorough renal assessment, from preparing the patient and taking the medical history, to determining the patient's chief complaint and performing the physical examination, and, finally, to interpreting your findings—the nursing diagnosis.

### Gather the equipment
For renal system assessment you'll need a thermometer, stethoscope, ophthalmoscope, scale, sphygmomanometer, lubricating jelly and gloves, reflex hammer, cotton, and a safety pin. An electrocardiograph is also needed to assess heart function and electrolyte status.

Make sure the examination room is private, quiet, well lit, and at a comfortable temperature. If the assessment must be done in the patient's hospital room, draw the drapes or close the door to eliminate extraneous noise.

### Prepare the patient
Before you begin the assessment, explain to the patient what you will do and why you will do it. Try to determine the patient's physical and mental condition. If he's in pain or fatigued from lack of sleep, postpone the assessment, if possible. If he's anxious, try to make him feel comfortable by approaching him with a calm, confident, and concerned manner. Encourage him to ask questions and to voice his concerns.

You may allow a family member or close friend to accompany the patient if he desires or if he is too confused or anxious to give you adequate information. Find out who the most appropriate person is—sometimes a patient's son or daughter may know more about his illness than his wife. If another person is present, always check with the patient before beginning the interview. There may be portions of the interview he doesn't want the other person to hear, either because he's too embarrassed or because he doesn't want to alarm the other person. After you've prepared the patient adequately, begin a detailed assessment.

### THE NURSING HISTORY
Careful observation and skillful interview techniques will help you gather reliable information about the patient and his health status. You may want to complete your nursing history over several sessions to avoid overtaxing an acutely ill patient.

Ask open-ended questions when you want the patient to give you more than one-word answers. For example, if you say, "Tell me about your night," the patient will probably give you a fuller response than if you ask, "How did you sleep last night?"

Also be sure to listen closely to the patient's answers: be alert for verbal and nonverbal cues that can guide your questioning to elicit specific information. Pay attention to facial expressions, hand placement, posture, tone of voice, and other mannerisms.

### Form an initial impression
As you interview the patient, assess his overall appearance. Does the patient look healthy or sick? What's his general state of hygiene? Is his skin color normal? Yellowish or gray skin may indicate retention of uremic wastes. Pallor often means anemia.

Does he look cyanotic? Is his skin sweaty or dry? Look at his eyes. Are they discolored? Does he seem edematous or dehydrated?

Assess body size and development. Is he overweight or underweight? Are his extremities normal in size and shape? Observe his posture and movements. Does he have trouble lying flat? Does he keep changing position? Note any physical handicaps.

Ask the patient how old he is. Does he look

his age? Adults with renal disease may look older than their age. Children with renal disease may look younger than their age because the disease inhibits their growth by changing growth hormone levels and calcium absorption rates.

Note the patient's racial and cultural background. Race is related to the incidence of some renal disease; for example, nephrosclerosis and renal failure can result from malignant hypertension, a condition common among blacks. Cultural factors can also influence a patient's response to illness. For example, a man whose culture does not allow men to display pain may deny its presence.

As you talk to the patient, evaluate his emotional and mental states. Does he seem anxious or upset? Does he seem able to concentrate? How long is his attention span? Does he seem alert and oriented to time and place? Does he respond appropriately to your questions? The uremic patient is likely to show difficulty in concentration and other symptoms of mental impairment.

Does the patient have any speech impediments? Does he speak too rapidly or too slowly?

### Define the chief complaint

Ask the patient to describe his chief complaint—that is, his reason for seeking health care—and record his description in his own words. Consider the chief complaint as a subjective explanation, not a diagnostic statement. For example, a patient with a history of abdominal aneurysm may be experiencing anuria or flank pain and mistakenly may state that his problem is the aneurysm when, in fact, he may have renal calculi. By accepting his diagnosis, you could set the tone and focus of the interview in the wrong direction.

Encourage him to describe his complaint in detail. Ask about its onset, quality, location, duration, and any aggravating or alleviating factors. Have his symptoms changed over time? Find out about prescribed drugs, previous treatments or hospitalizations, medical visits, or surgical procedures relating to the chief complaint, and list them in chronologic order.

### Ask about voiding, incontinence

After the patient defines his chief complaint, find out if he's experiencing other signs and symptoms of renal and urologic dysfunction. Ask especially about his voiding habits. How frequently and in what amounts does he urinate? Be sure to ask about fluid intake before judging his output abnormal. Has he experienced any change in intake or output? If so, when did he notice the change? Ask if he has pain or burning during urination or difficulty starting a stream. Does his bladder feel full after he urinates? Does he urinate during the night? How often? Nocturia is significant unless his fluid intake before bedtime is large. Ask if he experiences incontinence or dribbling of urine. If so, does it occur when he's straining, as during exercise, coughing, or defecating? Ask about the color of his urine. A dark amber color indicates highly concentrated urine, usually associated with decreased volume. Clear, watery urine is associated with increased volume. Brown or bright red urine may contain blood. Other color changes may result from taking certain drugs. (See *Interpreting color variations in urine,* page 32.) Ask whether he's noticed any foul or unusual odor emanating from his urine.

Has the patient experienced genital itching or injury? Does he feel flank pain or suprapubic pain? If so, does repositioning relieve it? Position changes don't relieve pain from renal colic, but lying down does reduce inflammatory pain.

Encourage him to be as specific as possible about all symptoms, and ask about factors that alleviate or aggravate them.

### Review medical history

Obtaining a medical history of the patient's family sometimes provides important clues to the present illness. Find out if anyone in the patient's family has or ever had chronic renal failure, diabetes, hypertension, polycystic kidney disease, Goodpasture's syndrome, Alport's syndrome (hereditary nephritis), renal tubular acidosis, or cystinosis. Also ask about a family history of noninherited renal disorders, such as urinary tract infections, congenital anomalies, and urinary calculi, which tend to recur in some families.

Ask the patient about his previous illnesses, operations, or injuries, especially those that could result in urologic or renal disorders, such as urinary tract infections, streptococcal infections, diabetes, tuberculosis, hypertension, and systemic lupus erythematosus. Ask if he's ever had a sexually transmitted disease and whether it was treated. Ask if he's had gout, kidney or bladder stones, or a recent blood transfusion. Ask women about renal problems during pregnancy.

# Systemic effects in renal disease

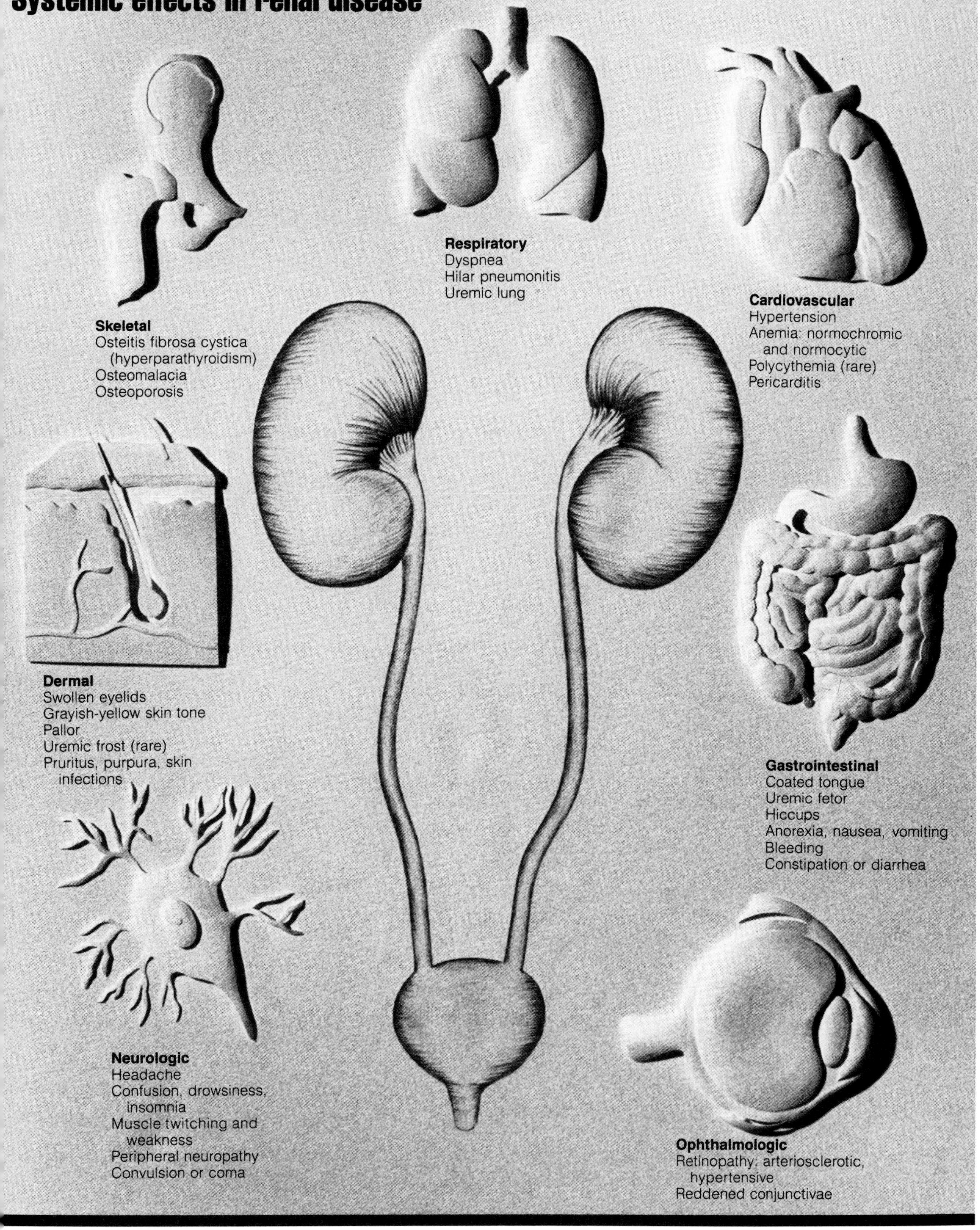

**Respiratory**
Dyspnea
Hilar pneumonitis
Uremic lung

**Cardiovascular**
Hypertension
Anemia: normochromic
   and normocytic
Polycythemia (rare)
Pericarditis

**Skeletal**
Osteitis fibrosa cystica
   (hyperparathyroidism)
Osteomalacia
Osteoporosis

**Dermal**
Swollen eyelids
Grayish-yellow skin tone
Pallor
Uremic frost (rare)
Pruritus, purpura, skin
   infections

**Gastrointestinal**
Coated tongue
Uremic fetor
Hiccups
Anorexia, nausea, vomiting
Bleeding
Constipation or diarrhea

**Neurologic**
Headache
Confusion, drowsiness,
   insomnia
Muscle twitching and
   weakness
Peripheral neuropathy
Convulsion or coma

**Ophthalmologic**
Retinopathy: arteriosclerotic,
   hypertensive
Reddened conjunctivae

## Interpreting color variations in urine

| Color | Causes |
| --- | --- |
| Straw-colored (dilute urine) | Anxiety, diabetes insipidus, diabetes mellitus, overhydration |
| Dark yellow or amber (concentrated urine) | Febrile state, dehydration |
| Cloudy | Pus, blood, epithelial cells, fat, phosphate, chyle, spermatozoa, prostatic fluid, bacteria, colloidal particles, urates, all-vegetable diet |
| Red or red-brown | Porphyrin, hemoglobin, myoglobin, erythrocytes, pyrvinium pamoate (Povan) |
| Orange-red or orange-brown | Drugs such as phenazopyridine (Pyridium) |
| Yellow-brown or green-brown | Bilirubin, phenol |
| Dark brown or black | Methylene blue, blood, porphyrin, phenol, dehydration |

Find out what drugs, prescription or non-prescription, the patient is taking. For example, chronic self-medication with over-the-counter combination analgesics may lead to kidney failure; so may nonsteroidal anti-inflammatory agents, such as indomethacin.

Find out why he's taking each medication, how often, and how much; and if he experiences any side effects from it. Some immune-complex reactions can cause tubular damage. Find out if the patient has allergies, for example, to iodine. This would preclude urologic diagnostic tests using iodine-based contrast dye, such as excretory urography.

### Define habits and life-style

Get general information about the patient's life-style, such as smoking and drinking habits. Cigarette smoking is associated with many diseases, including bladder cancer in women. Excessive alcohol intake can cause liver damage, which can lead to hepatorenal syndrome.

Ask the patient about his sleeping habits—when he retires, when he wakes up, if he wakes frequently during the night, and if he thinks he gets enough sleep. Ask if he is frequently tired during the day.

Find out what the patient normally eats in a day. Does he think he eats enough, too little, or too much? Does he eat between meals? How much coffee does he drink? Remember that caffeine may irritate the bladder. Try to form an impression of his intake of sodium, potassium, and fluids. Ask also about food preferences and food allergies that should be reported to the hospital dietitian.

Consider that social factors can also influence a patient's mental and physical status. Find out about his economic status and employment history. What type of work does he do? Does he find it satisfying? Does he feel secure in his job? If the patient is retired, ask what type of work he did. Are finances a problem? Does the patient have medical insurance? Ask about his home environment. What does he do in a typical day, and what kinds of leisure activities does he enjoy? What is his health philosophy, and how important is good health to him?

### Conduct a review of systems

Continue the patient interview with questions reviewing the major body systems. Follow a head-to-toe pattern, progressing from general to specific information.

Begin by assessing the patient's energy level since both uremia and anemia can cause fatigue. Can he perform activities of daily living, or does fatigue interfere with his ability to function? Does he ever become short of breath or experience palpitations? If so, what usually brings this on? What does he do when fatigued?

Ask the patient about his skin. Is it excessively dry or oily? Patients with chronic renal failure often have dry, itchy skin, possibly caused by elevated phosphorus levels or uremic toxins. If his skin feels itchy, ask how long ago the itchiness began and what he usually does about it. Make sure it's not caused by a change in laundry detergent or soap.

Find out if the patient experiences any cardiovascular problems, such as pericarditis or hypertension. Does he ever have chest pains or pain during inspiration? Remember that uremic pericarditis can develop from chronic renal failure. If so, does this happen with activity or at rest?

Gastrointestinal disturbances, such as anorexia, nausea, and vomiting, can occur in the patient with uremia. Ask the patient with such symptoms if they recur at a particular time of day or if they are brought on by a particular food. Ask the patient if he experiences recurrent bouts of hiccups. Does he have any trouble tasting food, and do food smells appeal to him? Patients with renal failure often have a metallic taste in their mouths that causes nausea and interferes with their ability to eat.

Ask the patient if he's had recent constipation, diarrhea, or abdominal cramping. Find out if he uses a stool softener or laxative; patients taking aluminum hydroxide (Amphojel) often experience constipation.

Ask the patient if he ever feels bone pain or if he's experienced recent joint pain. Disturbances in calcium-phosphorus balance can cause bone and joint disease in patients with chronic renal failure.

Since renal and urologic disorders can interfere with sexual function, ask the patient if he's experienced recent changes in his sexual activity or drive. Ask the female patient if she menstruates normally and if she's noticed any abnormal genital discharge.

Next, assess the patient's mental status. This is important because uremia often produces nervous system changes. Ask if he's felt confused or irritable or if he's noticed mood swings, recent memory loss, or difficulty concentrating. Has he experienced frequent headaches or episodes of dizziness?

Carefully assess the patient's sensory system because patients with renal failure often develop neuropathy. Ask the patient if he's noticed blurred vision or spots before his eyes? Has he had difficulty hearing? Find out especially if he's felt numbness, tingling, or burning in his extremities.

## THE PHYSICAL EXAMINATION

Having assembled your subjective data from the nursing history, you can go on to the physical examination. You'll perform the renal examination as you would any physical assessment, using inspection, auscultation, palpation, and percussion.

Begin by weighing the patient and comparing the results to a baseline weight, if one is available. Weigh the patient daily at the same time, and make sure he is wearing the same type of clothing. If maintaining these constants isn't possible, document whatever's different about each weigh-in. Measuring weight gains and losses is important, and often difficult, in renal and urologic assessment. Patients with renal failure may show a 10-lb (4.53-kg) gain from fluid retention or a 10-lb loss from anorexia and vomiting. Significant weight gain or loss within 24 to 48 hours indicates a change in fluid weight, not body mass.

### Check vital signs

When you've made the patient relaxed and comfortable, take his vital signs. Generally, a fever suggests a viral, bacterial, or parasitic infection, but in the patient with renal or urologic disorders it may mean pyelonephritis or bladder infection. When you monitor the patient with a fever, try checking his temperature at night, even if you have to wake him briefly, because that's when temperature spikes normally occur.

Next, take the patient's blood pressure in both arms since there may be a difference. However, if the patient is on hemodialysis, remember to avoid taking the blood pressure in the arm with a fistula or shunt.

Determine if there's any difference in blood pressure readings when the patient is lying down and when he's sitting up. If blood pressure drops when the patient sits up (postural hypotension), he could have volume depletion.

If the patient has hypertension, be alert for other signs of renal disease. Hypertension can result from increased vascular volume caused by sodium and water retention or from disruption in the renin-angiotensin-aldosterone system. Renin, an enzyme produced by ischemic kidneys, directly raises blood pressure. Be aware, also, of extreme hypotension, which can lead to renal shutdown.

Check the patient's apical and peripheral pulses, and note any difference. A patient with renal disease may have abnormal altered heart rates and rhythms if he's developed congestive heart failure or hyperkalemia.

### Examine the integument

Feel the patient's skin to assess temperature. Is it noticeably hot or cold? Are his extremities cooler than the rest of his body? This could indicate peripheral vascular disease.

As you did in your initial patient assessment, note his skin color. A patient with renal

## Recognizing signs of calcification

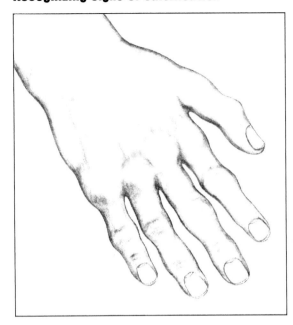

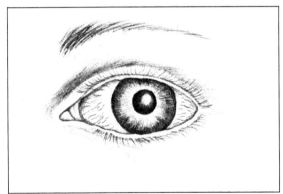

Low calcium levels in patients with renal failure stimulate the parathyroid to release calcium from bones. So when you assess patients with renal failure, you may see calcium deposits in soft tissue throughout the body.

Look for bony calcium deposits around the joints of hands. Look also in the eyes, where calcium deposits cause conjunctivitis and keratopathies.

Calcium deposits, shown by radiography, can also accumulate in joints, in the renal tubules (nephrocalcinosis), in the lungs, in the heart, in large vessels such as the aorta, and in small coronary arteries.

failure often has characteristic yellow-tan, sallow skin resulting from the retention of urochrome, a urine pigment normally excreted by the kidneys. The patient with renal failure also commonly looks pale from anemia.

Note the texture of the skin and determine if it is smooth, rough, scaly, or dry. A patient with renal failure often has rough, scaly, dry skin, probably caused by atrophied sweat and oil glands. You may also notice signs of chronic skin irritation from repeated scratching, a sign of pruritus.

Look for uremic frost, a film of white or yellow urate crystals on the skin. Uremic frost occurs only in severe renal failure and is now rare because of recent advances in renal diagnosis and treatment.

**Check the patient's skin.** Look for bruising, purpura, petechiae, or ecchymoses, which can result from clotting abnormalities in patients with acute and chronic renal failure. Check also for ulcers, sores, or other signs of secondary infection, especially if the patient has diabetes, since diabetics are prone to develop peripheral vascular disease. Check the patient's toes since ulcers often develop there.

**Palpate skin and soft tissue.** Check for subcutaneous calcium deposits. These can also form in the eyes, joints, and cardiac muscle, and radiologic studies may be needed to detect them. These deposits are calcium phosphate crystals, which form in patients with renal failure when serum phosphorus levels rise. The elevated phosphorus levels reciprocally lower serum calcium levels, which, in turn, stimulates the parathyroid gland to release calcium from the bones. Such stimulation of the parathyroid gland, in its severe form, can cause calcium phosphate crystals to form in soft tissues throughout the body. (See *Recognizing signs of calcification.*)

**Examine fingernails and toenails.** A patient with renal failure may have thin, brittle, pitted nails with characteristic red bands. Check his nail beds for color by pressing two or more fingernails and releasing them. Color should return to normal immediately. Pallor or cyanosis in the nail beds may indicate anemia, peripheral vascular disease, or respiratory dysfunction.

**Evaluate skin turgor.** If the patient's skin doesn't fall immediately back into place when you lift it, and he is not old and hasn't recently lost weight, he is probably dehydrated. Dehydration often occurs in the diuretic phase of various renal dysfunctions. To check skin turgor in an elderly patient, try lifting skin in the shoulder area. Skin in this area retains elasticity the longest.

### Assess fluid status

Measure and compare intake and output daily, and report changes in output. Because of insensible loss from skin and lungs, output should equal only about two thirds of intake over 24 hours. The normal hourly output is 30 to 100 ml; normal 24-hour output, 720 ml to 2,400 ml. When measuring output, be sure to consider fluid loss from diarrhea, vomiting, fever, or wound drainage.

Use daily intake-output records and weights

## Reviewing EKG changes in hyperkalemia

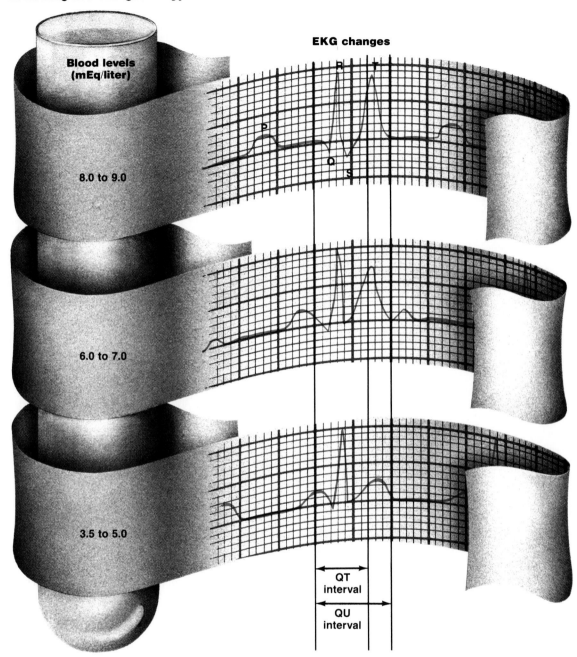

**Blood levels (mEq/liter)**

8.0 to 9.0

6.0 to 7.0

3.5 to 5.0

**EKG changes**

QT interval

QU interval

You can expect to see some characteristic changes in a patient's EKG as his serum potassium level rises. Initially, the T wave increases in magnitude; with increasing serum potassium levels, the ST segment becomes depressed, the U wave disappears, and the QRS duration and PR interval increase. As hyperkalemia worsens, often the P wave will disappear; ventricular fibrillation or asystole is likely to occur.

to validate each other. One ml of water weighs 1 g, so if a patient's intake exceeds his output by 1,000 ml in 24 hours, his weight should increase by about 1 kg. If his output exceeds his intake, the negative fluid balance should produce weight loss.

### Assess for edema
Edema is common in renal patients who gain fluid weight from sodium and water retention.

**Check dependent areas first.** Look for edema in the ankles and feet; if the patient is bedridden, in the sacral area. Inspect his neck veins for distention. To do this, have him lie flat.

When his neck veins are distended, raise the top of the bed 45°. Normally, venous distention should disappear. Dependent or total body edema accompanied by distended neck veins indicates fluid overload.

**Check for pitting.** A shiny, taut appearance to a patient's extremity confirms the presence of edema. Evaluate the degree of edema by pressing the swollen area with your finger for 5 seconds. Then remove your finger quickly. If a small depression remains (pitting), the area is edematous and can be described on a 4-point scale (or whatever measuring standard your hospital uses). A barely perceptible

## Assessing breath sounds

Normal breath sounds are divided into three categories, according to type and location: *bronchial, bronchovesicular,* and *vesicular.* You should normally hear bronchial sounds, which are harsh, loud, and high-pitched, over the trachea. Bronchovesicular sounds are soft and breezy, about two notes lower than bronchial sounds. You'll normally hear these anteriorly, near the main-stem bronchi in the first and second intercostal spaces, and posteriorly, between the scapulae. You should hear vesicular sounds, which are soft and low-pitched, over normal lung parenchyma but not over the presternum or the scapulae.

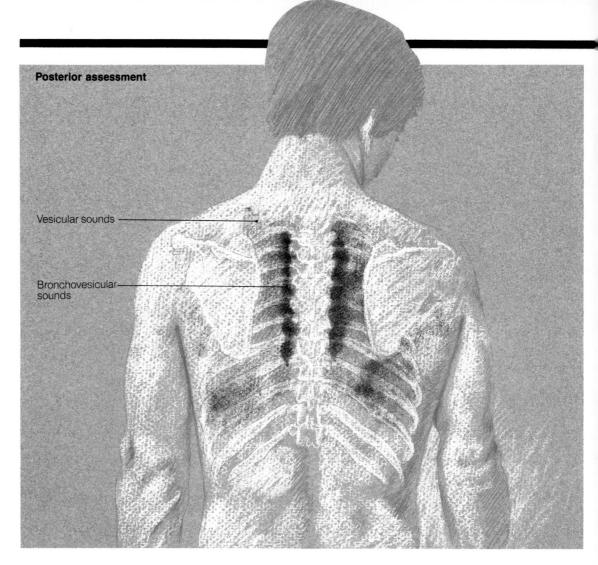

**Posterior assessment**

Vesicular sounds

Bronchovesicular sounds

---

pit is a 1+. A deep pit that takes over 30 seconds to rebound is a 4+.

Check the eyes for puffiness, another sign of fluid overload.

**Inspect the head**
Include in your inspection examination of the hair, face, eyes, nose, oral mucosa, and gums.

**Examine the hair.** Is it shiny or dull, oily or dry? The patient with renal failure commonly has dry, brittle hair, resulting from deterioration of sebaceous glands that normally lubricate the hair. Check the scalp for dandruff, scaliness, or sores.

**Observe the face.** Check for shape, markings, and expression. The patient receiving steroid therapy may have a characteristic moon face and acne, a common steroid side effect. The patient with systemic lupus erythematosus may show the characteristic butterfly rash. The patient with scleroderma may have the rigid, expressionless face characteristic of this disease.

**Examine the eyes.** Inspect the conjunctiva for paleness, which can result from anemia,

and for redness, which can result from calcium deposits. Check the sclera for redness, which can result from calcium-phosphorus imbalance.

Next, examine the eye internally with an ophthalmoscope. Inspect the retina for abnormalities, such as arteriolar changes that indicate malignant hypertension: retinal arteriolar walls may become thickened, with small areas of infarction or hemorrhage. Check also for papilledema; cotton-wool patches from edema; and dilated, tortuous veins.

**Examine the nose.** Check for epistaxis and mucous membrane color.

**Inspect the oral mucosa and the gums.** If the patient has anemia, both are usually pale. Examining the mucosa can also help you evaluate hydration. Dry mucosa indicates mild dehydration; very dry mucosa (associated with cracked lips and sunken eyes) indicates severe dehydration.

Check for gum swelling, redness, or bleeding, and check for tongue or lip sores. Assess for ammoniac or urinelike breath odor (uremic fetor), which often accompanies uremia.

**Anterior assessment**

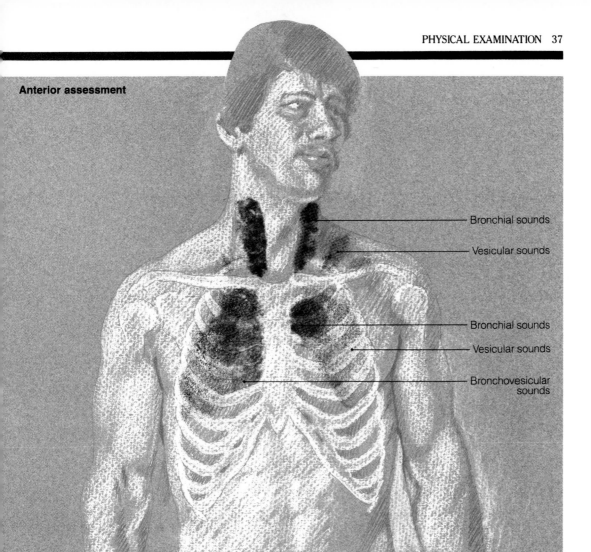

Bronchial sounds

Vesicular sounds

Bronchial sounds

Vesicular sounds

Bronchovesicular sounds

## Assess cardiovascular function

Assess the patient's cardiac rate and rhythm by auscultating the heart, palpating the pulse, and running a standard 12-lead EKG. Changes in cardiac rate and rhythm, especially in the patient without underlying cardiac disease, often indicate severe fluid or electrolyte imbalance. A gallop rhythm, for example, suggests fluid overload.

**Watch for hyperkalemia.** The most profound conduction disorders result from an elevated serum potassium level, or hyperkalemia (see *Reviewing EKG changes in hyperkalemia,* page 35). This is a common complication of acute renal failure; normally, potassium is rapidly excreted, but impaired renal function causes a buildup of potassium in the extracellular fluid. Hyperkalemia is confirmed by serum potassium levels greater than 5.5 mEq/liter and urine potassium levels less than 10 mEq/24-hr urine.

In hyperkalemia, the patient's EKG undergoes characteristic changes:
A tall, peaked T wave indicates early hyperkalemia.

• A prolonged PR interval above 0.20 second indicates increased cardiac involvement.
• Lack of a P wave and a widened QRS complex indicate severe hyperkalemia.

In the final stages of cardiac involvement, undetected hyperkalemia can trigger ventricular fibrillation or asystole, which requires life-saving measures.

**Auscultate the heart for murmurs.** Remember that murmurs can occur in many areas of the heart during systole or diastole. A systolic murmur may indicate anemia from renal failure. Murmurs stemming from aortic and mitral insufficiency sometimes accompany hypertension, anemia, or fluid overload.

**Listen for pericardial friction rubs.** These harsh, rasping sounds, usually heard over the precordium, result from friction between inflamed pericardial and visceral layers of the heart. A friction rub may indicate uremia, which causes inflammation and fibrous changes in the pericardium. Remember that pericardial friction rubs can be audible during both diastole and systole but are usually louder during systole.

## Palpating the kidneys

To palpate the kidney bi-manually, place one hand under the patient's rib cage and iliac crest. Place your other hand on her abdomen in the same place, with fingertips pointing toward her umbilicus. Then press your hands together each time your patient inhales. Increase pressure with each inhalation until you reach maximum palpation depth. Ask the patient to inhale as deeply as possible; you should note the kidney's contour and size. Check also for lumps, masses, or tenderness.

If you have trouble palpating this way, try "capturing" the kidney: position your hands as you normally would, then ask the patient to breathe deeply. At the peak of inspiration, quickly but gently press your hands together, exerting slightly more pressure anteriorly than posteriorly. Ask the patient to exhale as slowly as possible. When she's exhaled completely, slowly release your hands. You should feel the kidney slide into place.

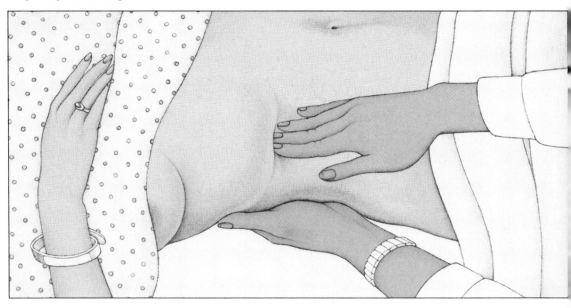

### Evaluate respiration

Listen closely to the patient's breathing pattern. Is it fast or slow, labored or calm? Does it change when he sits up, lies down, or sits forward? Time the interval between inspirations and expirations. Also compare the quality of inspirations to that of expirations; if inspiration is more labored than expiration, suspect uremic pericarditis.

Notice if the patient is coughing and, if so, whether his cough is productive. Patients with renal disease are more susceptible to upper respiratory infections because uremic toxins impair white blood cell function.

Check chest expansion for symmetry during breathing. Unequal expansion usually indicates respiratory abnormality. Determine if the patient uses accessory muscles, such as the sternocleidomastoids, to aid breathing. If he does, his breathing is labored. Determine if he's experiencing retractions, which usually indicate restricted air flow to the lungs.

**Auscultate the lungs.** This is the crucial part of respiratory assessment since patients with renal failure may produce various abnormal breath sounds.

Ask the patient to sit upright and to take deep breaths through his mouth. This will make the breath sounds easier to hear. With your stethoscope, begin auscultating at the apex and—comparing left side to right—move down the chest. Listen for one full inspiration and expiration before moving the stethoscope to the next position. Remember that you are listening for the normal flow of air in and out of the tracheobronchial tree and for abnormal breath sounds signifying fluid or mucus in the chest (see *Assessing breath sounds*, pages 36 and 37).

**Listen carefully for rales or rhonchi.** These suggest fluid overload. Rales are discrete crackling sounds that may be heard on inspiration. Rhonchi and wheezes are low-pitched musical sounds heard on inspiration and expiration. They result from air passage through partially obstructed bronchi, as in pulmonary edema. Listen also for louder-than-normal, high-pitched breath sounds, resembling bronchial sounds, at the periphery of the lungs. They could mean uremic pneumonitis.

After auscultation, tell the patient to cough and breathe deeply. Let him rest for a few minutes. Then listen again to areas where you heard any abnormal breath sounds. Note any changes. Sometimes coughing can clear rales and rhonchi, but it can't clear wheezes and friction rubs.

### Assess the abdomen

With the patient lying supine, examine his abdomen for striae, rashes, discolorations, and surgical scars. Determine whether the general size and shape of the abdomen is normal or abnormal. Note any distention, marked by a protruding umbilicus and tense, glistening abdominal skin. Distention can result from ascites or from accumulated feces in the intestinal tract.

If you find distention, percuss the abdomen to determine if the distention results from accumulation of air, fluid, or solids. A dull tone indicates solids (such as a sigmoid colon filled with stool) or fluid; a tympanic tone indicates air (as in gaseous bowel distention).

**Check for ascites.** When ascites is present, you'll also detect dullness when you percuss the patient's flanks. Another test for ascites is the fluid wave test. Ask the patient or another person to press down slightly on the patient's abdominal midline with the palm of his hand. Then place one of your palms on one of the patient's flanks and sharply tap the opposite flank. If you feel a moving wave in your resting palm, fluid is present.

**Inspect the skin.** If the patient has a peritoneal dialysis catheter, inspect the area around it for redness, swelling, or discharge. If he has an ileal loop diversion or a ureterostomy, remove the collection bag and inspect the site. Note any skin irritation or excoriation.

**Palpate the abdomen.** Check for masses and for tender areas. Palpate the liver for location and tenderness. Normally, the liver is palpable 1″ to 2″ (2.5 to 5 cm) below the right costal margin. If it is palpable below this level, the patient could have hepatomegaly, a result of circulatory overload that sometimes accompanies renal failure. Also note tenderness of the liver, which may indicate inflammation or, possibly, hepatitis.

**Auscultate the abdomen.** Listen for bowel sounds, which normally occur 5 to 35 times a minute. Note their pitch, frequency, duration, and location, and ask the patient if pain or cramping accompanies these sounds. Hypoactive bowel sounds may occur in patients with ascites, peritonitis, or an ileus. Peristalsis also diminishes in patients with uremia. Hyperactive bowel sounds occur if the patient has diarrhea.

### Examine the kidneys
Abdominal asymmetry, fullness, or bulging may indicate an enlarged kidney. Edematous or erythematous skin over the flanks may indicate the patient has an inflammation, such as a perinephric abscess.

**Palpate the kidneys.** Ask the patient to sit up. Then palpate for size and tenderness. Normal kidneys are difficult to palpate, but, if the patient is very thin, you may feel the lower pole of his right kidney and, rarely, the tip of his left one. (See *Palpating the kidneys.*) If a kidney is easily palpable, it's probably enlarged. Suspect polycystic kidneys, hydronephrosis, or a neoplasm.

To perform bimanual deep palpation, have the patient lie in a supine position. To palpate

## Percussing the kidneys

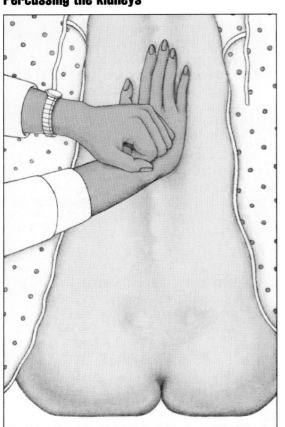
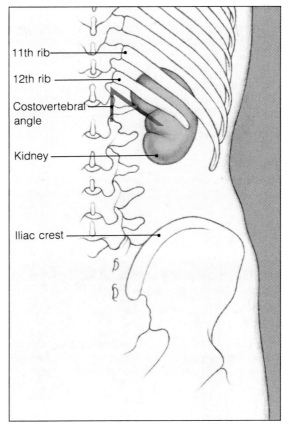

11th rib
12th rib
Costovertebral angle
Kidney
Iliac crest

Before you percuss the kidneys, explain to the patient what you are going to do so you don't startle him.

Then, with the patient lying on his side or in a sitting position (as shown), place the palm of one hand on the patient's back over the area of the costovertebral angle. Strike the back of that hand with the ulnar surface of your other fist.

## Listening for bruits: Pinpointing arterial obstruction

Bruits are vascular sounds that resemble heart murmurs. Bruits over the renal arteries, especially in hypertensive patients, indicate renal artery stenosis. Bruits over the aorta, iliac arteries, or femoral arteries signal arterial insufficiency to the legs. The illustration shows the best place to listen for each sound.

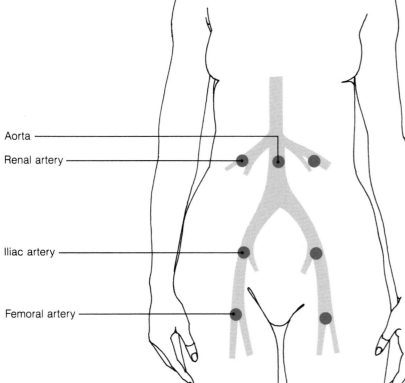

Aorta

Renal artery

Iliac artery

Femoral artery

the right kidney, place your right hand anteriorly between his lower costal margin and iliac crest, with your fingertips pointing toward his umbilicus. Place your left hand in the same location under his right flank. Ask the patient to breathe normally, and press your hands together each time he inhales, increasing the pressure gently with each breath. When you reach maximum palpation depth, ask the patient to breathe deeply. As he does, you should feel the lower pole of the kidney move down between your hands. Note its contour and size. Check for lumps, masses, and tenderness. Repeat the procedure with the left kidney. Normal kidneys feel firm and are roughly the same size. If one kidney seems

significantly smaller than the other, suspect kidney malfunction.

**Percuss to assess pain.** To percuss the kidneys, ask the patient to sit or to lie on his side. Place the palm of your hand on his back over the costovertebral angle, and strike the back of your hand with your fist. (See *Percussing the kidneys,* page 39.) Normally, the patient will feel the thud, but no pain. Pain usually signals infection, such as pyelonephritis. When percussing, remember that the spleen sounds dull; the kidneys, resonant.

**Auscultate for bruits.** Using your stethoscope, auscultate the renal arteries for the blowing or swishing sounds that could indicate partial obstruction of the renal arteries (see *Listening for bruits: Pinpointing arterial obstruction*).

### Assess bladder, genitalia, and prostate

First, ask the patient to empty his bladder. Percuss the area over the bladder, beginning 2″ (5 cm) above the symphysis pubis and moving downward. A tympanic sound indicates a normal bladder; a dull sound may mean the bladder is retaining urine.

Next, palpate the patient's bladder bimanually, beginning at the midline of the abdomen about 1″ to 2″ (2.5 to 5 cm) above the symphysis pubis. A normal, empty bladder is not palpable. If you suspect retained urine, palpate just above the symphysis pubis; if the bladder feels smooth and firm, it contains urine.

Excessive urine retention causes abdominal distention. Inspect the patient's lower abdomen and pelvic area for signs of swelling. A severely distended bladder will feel smooth, rounded, and fluctuant. Estimate the bladder's location and size, and note any lumps, masses, or tenderness. (Remember that bladder palpation and percussion usually stimulate the micturition reflex.)

Inspect the patient's genitalia, noting any redness, tenderness, swelling, or discharge. Check the male patient for enlargement of the scrotum and testes. If he's experiencing signs and symptoms of obstruction, such as dribbling, frequency, urgency, or pain, perform a rectal examination and palpate the prostate for enlargement. In the female patient, when a vaginal exam is needed to rule out extrinsic obstruction, it is performed by a specially trained nurse.

### Assess the musculoskeletal system

Examine the patient's extremities for symmetry and size, and assess overall body growth

# Assessment guide for fluid and electrolyte status

| Body system | Assessment | Cause |
|---|---|---|
| Cardiovascular | Altered pulse rate | Fluid volume deficit |
| | Bounding pulse | Fluid volume excess |
| | Decreased blood pressure | Fluid volume deficit |
| | Narrow pulse pressure | Fluid volume deficit |
| | Cardiac dysrhythmias | Potassium deficit, potassium excess |
| | Jugular vein distention | Fluid volume excess |
| Gastrointestinal | Abdominal cramps | Potassium excess |
| | Nausea, vomiting, diarrhea | Magnesium excess |
| | < 5% weight loss | Mild dehydration |
| | > 5% weight loss | Moderate dehydration |
| | > 15% weight loss | Severe dehydration |
| | < 5% weight gain | Mild overhydration |
| | > 5% weight gain | Moderate overhydration |
| | > 15% weight gain | Severe overhydration |
| | Sticky, dry mucous membranes | Fluid volume deficit, sodium excess |
| | Increased viscosity of saliva | Sodium deficit |
| | Longitudinal furrows on tongue | Sodium deficit |
| Integumentary | Increased temperature | Sodium excess |
| | Decreased temperature | Fluid volume deficit |
| | Decreased skin turgor | Fluid volume deficit |
| | Warm, moist skin | Fluid volume excess |
| | Flushing | Magnesium deficit |
| | Dry, cracked lips | Fluid volume deficit |
| | Edema of dependent body parts, such as sacrum and lower extremities | Fluid volume excess |
| Musculoskeletal | Muscle weakness | Potassium deficit, calcium excess |
| | Hypertonia | Calcium deficit, metabolic alkalosis |
| Neurologic | Depressed CNS activity | Fluid volume deficit |
| | Increased intracranial pressure | Sodium deficit |
| | Positive Babinski's sign | Magnesium deficit |
| | Disorientation or confusion | Acidosis, alkalosis |
| Ophthalmic | Dry conjunctivae | Fluid volume deficit |
| | Decreased tearing | Fluid volume deficit |
| | Periorbital edema | Fluid volume excess |
| | Sunken eyes | Fluid volume deficit |
| Renal | Oliguria | Sodium deficit, sodium excess |
| Respiratory | Moist rales, rhonchi | Fluid volume excess |
| | Increased respiratory rate | Fluid volume excess |
| | Dyspnea | Fluid volume excess |
| | Pulmonary edema | Fluid volume excess |
| | Shallow, slow breathing | Metabolic alkalosis, respiratory acidosis |
| | Deep, rapid breathing | Metabolic acidosis, respiratory alkalosis |

# Testing peripheral sensation

Here are a few simple tests for evaluating sensory function in your patient's feet. This will help you to determine the integrity of his peripheral nervous system.

To evaluate the patient's sensation of light touch, touch the sole of his foot with a cotton wisp, firmly enough to stimulate sensory nerve endings but not so firm as to dimple the skin (right). Does he feel it?

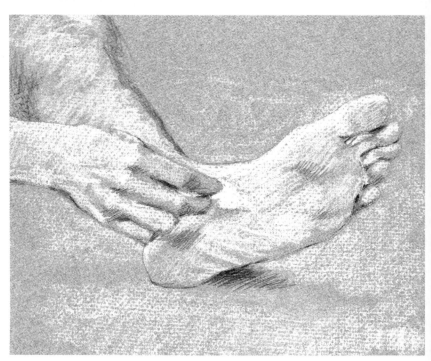

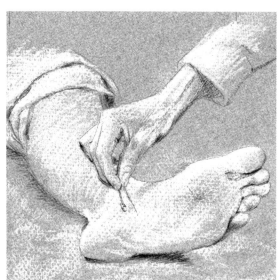

Evaluate for superficial pain by touching the sole of his foot alternately with the sharp and dull ends of a safety pin (above). Does he feel pain?

To test his sensitivity to vibration, apply the base of a vibrating tuning fork to the ankle (right). Does he feel the vibration?

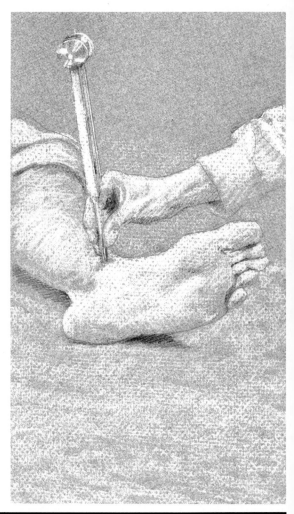

and muscle strength. Watch for atrophied muscles and delayed growth, which are common in patients with renal failure. Assessing growth rate is especially important in children, in whom impaired calcium and phosphorus metabolism harms skeletal development.

As you know, renal failure causes phosphorus retention, bringing on high phosphorus and low calcium levels. This leads to hyperparathyroidism and the leaching of calcium from bones, which can result in osteodystrophy.

Examine the joints for swelling, redness, or tenderness, which may result from calcium deposition in bursas and other periarticular structures. Also check for signs of gout, such as inflammation of joints, which may result from retention of uric acid.

Ask the patient to walk across the room while you watch for leg pain and limited range of motion. Determine whether his gait is steady or unsteady, and ask if walking causes pain. Ask the patient how far he can walk without becoming fatigued.

### Evaluate neurologic status

Neurologic assessment is particularly important because chronic renal failure can lead to accumulation of uremic toxins and electrolyte imbalances, which produce neurologic impairment.

**Determine state of consciousness.** Is the patient alert and oriented? Patients with renal failure commonly have altered states of consciousness, ranging from slight confusion to coma, which result from the accumulation of nitrogenous wastes. Such patients may also exhibit irritability, inability to concentrate, or loss of recent memory.

**Assess speech.** Thick, slurred, or slowed speech is a sign of dysarthria, a possible complication of advanced renal insufficiency. Check for associated signs of neuromuscular irritability, such as fasciculations or persistent hiccups. Ask the patient if he experiences muscle cramps.

**Check for signs of encephalopathy.** Check for trembling and for asterixis (flapping tremor), an early sign of encephalopathy. Do this by asking him to hyperextend his arms and spread his fingers. If asterixis is present, his fingers will start to move irregularly—in a side-to-side, or flapping, motion—after about 30 seconds.

Observe also for motor ataxia, which can occur early in renal failure, and for intense myoclonus (uremic twitching), which develops in late stages of renal disease.

**Check for neuropathy.** Chronic uremia often leads to neuropathy, which typically affects the legs more severely than the arms. Check for loss of feeling in the arms and legs, and ask the patient if he experiences discomfort in his lower legs and feet. (See *Testing peripheral sensation*.) An early sign of neuropathy, called the "restless leg" syndrome, is characterized by lower leg discomfort that worsens at the end of the day and is partially relieved by movement. Often it's accompanied by cramping, itching, a feeling of "pins and needles," or crawling sensations. Ask the patient if he ever feels burning, or paresthesias, of the soles of his feet.

As renal failure progresses, neuropathy may affect motor, as well as sensory, nerves. If you suspect extreme neuropathy, check the patient for foot drop, the most common clinical sign of muscular neuropathy.

## NURSING DIAGNOSIS

After you've collected your assessment findings, remember that many signs and symptoms of renal disorders may also result from disorders of other body systems. Try to identify the factors that, in your judgment, may require further study. If necessary, discuss relevant diagnostic tests with the doctor. Once you're satisfied that your assessment is complete, you can go on to formulate nursing diagnoses.

A nursing diagnosis is based on the subjective and objective data you've gathered throughout your assessment. A typical nursing diagnosis describes a combination of signs and symptoms that indicate an actual or potential health problem requiring nursing intervention.

Keep your nursing diagnoses as simple as possible. Establish baseline assessments using the nursing data base; then write your diagnostic statement, making sure it reflects a problem related to etiology. Your statement should represent a specific problem requiring nursing intervention. If you know the cause of the problem, your nursing diagnosis should clearly describe it.

Carefully applying all assessment steps— the patient history, the physical examination, and integration of objective and subjective findings—can help you recognize subtle physiologic changes that may require early intervention. Skillful assessment is the essential foundation for effective nursing management.

### Points to remember

- A thorough renal assessment includes patient preparation, overall inspection, history taking, physical examination, and formulation of nursing diagnoses.
- The patient interview provides valuable subjective information to help you interpret your examination results. It can help you distinguish renal disorders from those of other body systems. To make the interview successful, put your patient at ease as much as possible. Conduct it in stages, if necessary, to avoid tiring him.
- The physical examination should proceed systematically: weigh the patient; check vital signs; examine the integument and the head; evaluate cardiovascular and respiratory function; assess the abdomen, kidneys, bladder, genitalia and prostate, musculoskeletal system, and neurologic status.
- Thorough knowledge of examination techniques— auscultation, percussion, inspection, and palpation—is necessary for a complete and accurate renal assessment.
- Results of the patient interview and the physical examination allow you to formulate nursing diagnoses—statements of signs and symptoms that indicate actual or potential health problems requiring nursing interventions.

# 3 IMPLEMENTING THE DIAGNOSTIC WORKUP

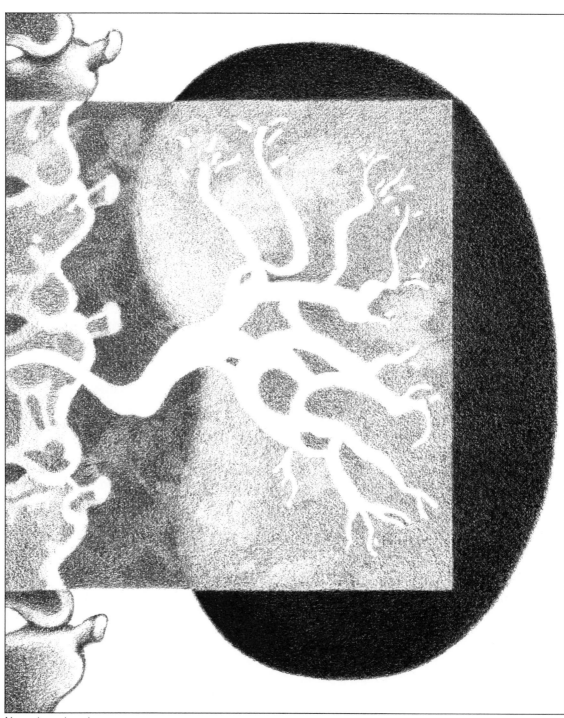

Normal renal angiogram

ortunately, a broad array of diagnostic tests is available to assess the renal system. Today, these tests are safer and more accurate than ever. Technologic advances, such as improved imaging techniques and computer processing, and the combination of tests, such as ultrasonography and excretory urography, help diagnose disorders that previously required the use of invasive methods. Understanding these tests, their indications, the techniques involved, and the significance of abnormal test results is essential for effective nursing management of renal disorders.

### A wide range of tests

Urine and blood studies provide general information concerning the patient's overall state of health. Urine tests also help evaluate the kidneys' diluting and concentrating capacity; blood tests help assess the kidneys' capacity to eliminate waste and maintain homeostasis and also help evaluate glomerular and tubular function. Clearance tests evaluate the kidneys' ability to excrete substances over a period of time. Imaging tests—radiography, radionuclide imaging, and ultrasonography—allow visualization of renal abnormalities. Other specialized tests evaluate renal structure and function: endoscopic tests allow direct visualization of the urethra and bladder and provide a channel for other invasive procedures; biopsy permits histologic examination of kidney tissue; and cystometry allows evaluation of the bladder's neuromuscular mechanisms.

### URINE TESTS

Urine tests begin the diagnostic workup and may reveal abnormal findings before clinical symptoms appear. Abnormal findings suggest the presence of disease and mandate further tests to identify a specific disorder.

### Urine elements

Examination of urine includes an evaluation of volume, color, clarity, and odor; determination of pH, specific gravity, and osmolality; possible measurement of electrolytes; the detection and rough measurement of abnormal constituents, such as proteins and glucose; and the microscopic examination of sediment for red and white blood cells, crystals, casts, and bacteria.

**Volume.** Closely regulated by the kidneys, urine volume reflects overall fluid homeostasis. Actual volume depends on fluid intake; concentration of solutes in the filtrate; cardiac output; hormonal influences; and fluid loss through the lungs, the large intestine, and the skin. To remove excess water and waste products, the kidneys normally produce approximately 1,500 ml of urine/day.

*Polyuria,* urine output that exceeds 1,500 ml/day, may be a normal adaptive response to excess fluid intake, or it may indicate that the renal tubules are not retaining electrolytes and water. This often occurs in the early stages of chronic renal failure and in the diuretic phase following acute renal failure.

*Oliguria,* urine volume under 400 ml/day, can follow certain conditions, such as dehydration due to prolonged vomiting or diarrhea, when the normal kidney responds by reabsorbing water and producing a concentrated urine. Diminished urine flow may also be associated with transfusion reactions, acute glomerulonephritis or pyelonephritis, and terminal chronic nephritis.

*Anuria,* urine volume below 75 ml/day, is always an abnormal finding. Even in chronic renal failure, the kidneys almost always produce more than 75 ml of urine per day. Anuria is associated with the absence of kidneys and obstruction of the urinary tract; it can follow acute tubular necrosis resulting from exposure to toxic agents.

**Color and clarity.** Clear, light yellow urine, with no evidence of sediment, indicates normal urine. Cloudy (turbid) urine may indicate bacterial growth in a urinary tract infection, thereby requiring culture-and-sensitivity tests. Changes in color can result from diet; drugs; and many metabolic, inflammatory, or infectious diseases. For example, yellow-orange or yellow-green urine can result from certain drugs; red-pink or purple urine, from some laxatives; and blue-green urine, from dyes used in certain diagnostic tests. Checking the patient's medications may prevent misdiagnosis. Red urine, which may mimic hematuria, indicates contamination if the specimen is taken during menstruation.

**Odor.** A mild, aromatic odor normally indicates freshly voided urine. A more pungent odor characterizes a concentrated urine; foul-smelling urine may indicate a urinary tract infection or may occur with ingestion of certain foods or drugs.

**pH.** Urine pH reflects the kidneys' ability to maintain a normal hydrogen ion concentration of the body's plasma and extracellular fluid—a normal acid-base balance. Urine pH is normally slightly acidic at 6.0 but may range from 5.0 to 7.0. An alkaline pH is characteris-

# Analyzing urine findings in renal failure

| Urine element | Normal findings | Abnormal findings in renal failure |
|---|---|---|
| Volume | 1,200 to 1,500 ml/day | Polyuria (> 1,500 ml/day) may indicate onset<br>Oliguria (< 400 ml/day) indicates inability to maintain renal function; can follow acute tubular necrosis<br>Anuria (< 75 ml/day) associated with absence of kidneys and obstruction of the urinary tract |
| Color | Clear yellow or amber | Varies with degree of concentration and specific gravity |
| Clarity | Clear or slightly cloudy | Varies with renal infection |
| Odor | Mild, aromatic | Unusual odor with infectious process |
| pH | 5.0 to 7.0 | Increases because of decreased glomerular filtration, causing decreased excretion of phosphate, sulfate, and other acids; or impaired distal tubular function, leading to decreased secretion of hydrogen ion ($H^+$) |
| Specific gravity | 1.003 to 1.030 | Decreases in early stages; later fixed at 1.010 |
| Osmolality | 300 to 900 mOsm/kg of water | Decreases |
| Protein | 0 to < 150 mg/day | > 4 g/day indicates nephrotic syndrome<br>0.5 to 4.0 g/day indicates renal disease<br>< 0.5 to 1.0 g/day indicates chronic glomerulonephritis |
| Glucose | None | Glycosuria varies |
| Electrolytes<br>  Sodium | 50 to 200 mEq/24 hours | Varies, but may increase if tubules fail to reabsorb normally |
|   Potassium | 25 to 125 mEq/24 hours | Decreases |
|   Chloride | 100 to 250 mEq/24 hours | Decreases |
|   Calcium | 2.5 to 15 mEq/24 hours | Decreases with lack of activated vitamin D; increases in renal tubular acidosis |
|   Phosphorus | 1 g/24 hours | Varies |
|   Magnesium | < 150 mg/24 hours | Decreases because of destruction of glomerular function |
| Creatinine | Males: 100 to 150 ml/min<br>Females: 85 to 125 ml/min | Decreases |
| Urea | Approximately 60% of creatinine clearance | Decreases with renal damage |
| Red blood cells | None | If present, may indicate urinary tract infection, renal disease, bladder tumor, ureteral calculi, renal infection |
| White blood cells | None | If present, may indicate renal infection, urinary tract infection, calculi |
| Crystals | None | If present, may lead to calculi and may impede ureteral blood flow |
| Casts | None | If present, may indicate renal infection, inflammation, tubular damage, renal failure |
| Bacteria | < 100,000 organisms/ml | If present, may indicate infection in kidneys or lower urinary tract |

tic of a diet high in vegetables, citrus fruits, and dairy products but low in meat; it may also result from Fanconi's syndrome, urinary tract infection, and metabolic or respiratory alkalosis. An acid pH is typical of a high-protein diet and is associated with renal tuberculosis, pyrexia, phenylketonuria and alkaptonuria, and all forms of acidosis.

Urine pH is quickly determined by using acid-base reagent strips. Testing of urine pH requires a freshly voided specimen, since urea, the chief nitrogenous constituent of urine, breaks down into ammonia after a period of time, producing alkaline urine and a false result.

**Specific gravity (SG).** A urinometer calibrated with water to a specific gravity of 1.001 is used as a standard to determine urine's SG—that is, its weight compared to an equal volume of water. This test estimates the density of urine or the number of solute particles in solution, thereby providing information about the concentrating and diluting ability of the renal tubules. Normal urine has an SG of 1.003 to 1.030. An excess of ingested fluid stimulates the kidneys to excrete more water, indicating a dilute or less concentrated urine. Conversely, in dehydration, the kidneys conserve water and excrete less urine, indicating a concentrated urine.

Depressed SG (1.001 to 1.003) is characteristic of diabetes insipidus, glomerulonephritis, pyelonephritis, acute renal failure, alkalosis, hypercalcemia, and hypokalemia. Elevated SG is characteristic of hepatic disorders, congestive heart failure, dehydration, and nephrosis. Fixed SG, in which values remain relatively constant from specimen to specimen, indicates severe renal damage. In renal failure, the kidneys first lose their ability to concentrate urine and then to dilute it. The SG eventually becomes fixed at 1.010, the same SG as protein-free plasma or glomerular filtrate before tubular activity.

**Osmolality.** This test is more sensitive and precise than SG for determining the kidneys' diluting and concentrating ability. Osmolality expresses the total number of particles in a solution. Plasma osmolality regulates water reabsorption in the tubules by regulating release of antidiuretic hormone (ADH). The distal segment of the renal tubules varies its permeability to water in response to ADH, which, with renal blood flow, determines urine concentration or dilution. Urine osmolality depends on the patient's state of hydration and plasma osmolality. Urine osmolality ranges from 50 to 1,400 mOsm/liter; a normal average is 300 to 900 mOsm/liter. In chronic renal disease, urine osmolality—like the specific gravity—resembles that of protein-free plasma or dilute urine.

**Electrolytes.** Because the kidneys maintain electrolyte balance by selective reabsorption and secretion, certain electrolytes are normally present in urine. These electrolytes include sodium, potassium, chloride, calcium, phosphates, and magnesium. All require a 24-hour urine specimen. However, urine levels of electrolytes are less significant than serum levels and are not routinely measured. Urine electrolyte levels vary, depending on the underlying clinical condition. For example, in renal failure, the kidneys may lose their ability to regulate these electrolytes, thus altering electrolyte excretion.

**Abnormal constituents.** The kidneys filter selected substances through their semipermeable membranes and prevent certain substances from passing through the glomeruli. The following substances are not normally present in urine; their presence usually indicates disease.

*Proteins* are normally too large to pass through glomerular capillaries. Healthy urine contains only traces of proteins (100 to 150 mg/day excreted in urine), which are undetectable by routine screening procedures. Transient proteinuria can result from changes in body position (orthostatic proteinuria) or can be associated with stress, exposure to cold, or fever. Heavy proteinuria, detectable by screening tests, nearly always indicates renal disease. Thus, suspected renal disease requires analysis of a 24-hour urine specimen for protein. Pathologic proteinuria can result from increased glomerular permeability, which can have various causes, including glomerulonephritis, congestive heart failure, renal tubular damage with defective reabsorption of protein, or cystitis.

In most forms of renal disease marked by proteinuria, the most prevalent urine protein is albumin because it's the smallest, the most easily filterable, and the most prevalent of all proteins. As kidney damage progresses, however, proteins of higher molecular weight—including the larger globulins—escape into the urine. The abnormal presence of certain proteins in urine has special diagnostic significance; for example, Bence Jones protein in urine strongly suggests multiple myeloma.

*Glucose* is normally absent since it's filtered at the glomerulus and totally reabsorbed in the proximal tubule. Transient, nonpathologic glycosuria may result from stress or pregnancy and may follow ingestion of a high-carbohydrate meal. In hyperglycemia, glucose may spill into the urine, depending on the renal threshold for glucose (the blood glucose concentration at which the kidneys excrete glucose). This occurs at approximately 170 mg/100 ml. The presence of glucose in the urine, although abnormal, does not necessarily indicate renal failure; however, in the absence of hyperglycemia, it may indicate renal tubular malfunction.

**Microscopic elements.** The presence of cells, crystals, and casts in centrifuged urine sediment can indicate or confirm renal disease. Centrifuged urine may also reveal the presence of bacteria.

*Red blood cells (RBCs)* are normally too large to pass through glomerular capillaries into the tubular system. Hematuria, either microscopic or visible to the naked eye, indicates bleeding within the genitourinary tract and may result from infection, obstruction, inflammation, trauma, tumors, glomerulonephritis, renal hypertension, lupus nephritis, renal tuberculosis, renal vein thrombosis, hydronephrosis, pyelonephritis, scurvy, malaria, parasitic bladder infection, subacute bacterial endocarditis, polyarteritis nodosa, and hemorrhagic disorders.

*White blood cells (WBCs),* if numerous, imply urinary tract inflammation, especially cystitis or pyelonephritis, and require bacteriologic cultures. Since WBCs in the sediment lyse rapidly, reliable evaluation requires careful collection and handling techniques.

*Crystals* in the urine generally represent end products of tissue metabolism. Crystal formation is pH-dependent. Phosphates crystallize in alkaline urine; urates crystallize in acid urine. Crystals are significant when an unusually large number of one type are present and when the crystals are abnormal. Crystals also provide clues to calculus formation.

*Casts* (plugs of gelled proteinaceous material—high-molecular-weight mucoprotein) form in the renal tubules and collecting ducts by agglutination of protein cells or cellular debris and are flushed loose by urine flow. Casts are found in normal urine. Hyaline casts, for example, composed almost entirely of protein, are common and, if found alone, are considered insignificant. All other types of casts are usually associated with renal disease: WBC casts, with inflammation or pyelonephritis; RBC casts, with glomerular disease or acute tubular necrosis; granular and waxy casts, with progressive degenerative changes in the kidney; and broad casts, with advanced renal failure.

*Bacteria* in excess of 100,000 colonies/ml of a single microbe species indicate probable urinary tract infection or pyelonephritis. Counts of 10,000/ml to 100,000/ml are inconclusive and require a repeat culture. Low counts (fewer than 10,000/ml) suggest that the organisms are contaminants. Urine specimens should be cultured within 15 minutes of collection, or they can be immediately refrigerated—up to 48 hours at 39.2° F. (4° C.)—without significant bacterial growth.

## BLOOD TESTS

When considered with findings from urine tests, blood tests help diagnose renal disease and may be a primary source of information in renal failure. Blood tests may include a complete blood count; analyses of blood gases and electrolytes; and measurements of plasma osmolality, serum proteins, plasma glucose, and serum levels of blood urea nitrogen (BUN), creatinine, and uric acid.

### Complete blood count

This series of tests, usually routine in any workup for renal disease, provides important information related to kidney function; it is especially important in patients with chronic renal failure. For example, hematocrit and hemoglobin levels indicate fluid status. Rising serum hemoglobin levels and hematocrit concentrations indicate hypovolemia or dehydration. Conversely, falling hemoglobin and hematocrit levels may mean fluid overload. Frequent monitoring of hemoglobin and hematocrit levels can also determine the need for a blood transfusion to treat chronic anemia due to diminished renal secretion of erythropoietin. Secretion of erythropoietin stimulates production, maturation, and release of red cells from the bone marrow and other blood-forming tissues.

An elevated WBC count may indicate infection associated with increased catabolism and subsequent increase in protein breakdown, which lead to worsening renal failure. The platelet count, prothrombin time, and partial thromboplastin time are also significant in diagnosing renal dysfunction. For example, abnormal platelet function appears to be the major cause of hemorrhage in patients with uremia.

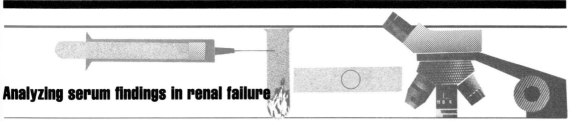

# Analyzing serum findings in renal failure

| Serum element | Normal findings | Abnormal findings in renal failure |
|---|---|---|
| Hematocrit | Male: 40% to 50%<br>Female: 37% to 47% | Decreases; may increase in dehydration |
| Hemoglobin | Male: 14 to 18 g/dl<br>Female: 12 to 16 g/dl | Decreases; may increase in dehydration |
| Total white blood cells | 5,000 to 10,000/µl | Increases in infection, such as pyelonephritis |
| Coagulation factors<br>Platelet count<br>Prothrombin time<br>Partial thromboplastin<br>time | <br>250,000 to 500,000/mm³<br>11 to 18 seconds<br>60 to 85 seconds<br>(activated: 35 to 45 seconds) | <br>Decreases in presence of uremic toxins<br>Decreases in presence of uremic toxins<br>Decreases in presence of uremic toxins |
| Blood gas analysis<br>pH<br>$PCO_2$<br><br>$HCO_3^-$ | <br>7.35 to 7.45<br>35 to 45 mm Hg<br><br>22 to 29 mEq/liter | <br>Decreases because of metabolic acidosis<br>Decreases because of pulmonary hyperventilation, a compensatory response<br>Decreases because of base deficit, resulting from hydrogen ion ($H^+$) retention and bicarbonate ion loss |
| Electrolytes<br>Sodium<br><br>Potassium<br><br>Chloride<br><br>Calcium<br><br>Phosphorus<br><br>Magnesium<br>Alkaline phosphatase | <br>136 to 145 mEq/liter<br><br>3.5 to 5.5 mEq/liter<br><br>98 to 110 mEq/liter<br><br>8.5 to 10.5 mg/dl<br><br>2 to 4.5 mg/100 ml<br><br>1.5 to 1.95 mEq/liter<br>75 to 250 µ/ml | <br>May increase or decrease, depending on the kidney's ability to reabsorb and secrete<br>Usually increases; may decrease because of polyuria in early stages of disease<br>Usually increases; also increases in metabolic acidosis<br>Decreases because of insufficient activated vitamin D<br>Increases because of decreased tubular secretion<br>Increases because of bone destruction<br>Increases because of bone destruction |
| Osmolality | 280 to 295 mOsm/kg of water | Varies |
| Total protein | 6.0 to 7.8 g/100 ml | Decreases in nephrotic syndrome because of increased glomerular permeability |
| Albumin | 3.5 to 5.5 g/100 ml | Decreases in nephrotic syndrome because of increased glomerular permeability |
| Blood urea nitrogen | 9 to 20 mg/100 dl | Increases because of inadequate excretion |
| Creatinine | 0.7 to 1.5 mg/dl | Increases |
| Uric acid | 3.0 to 8.0 mg/dl | Increases |

## Blood gases and electrolytes

Analysis of arterial blood gases (ABGs) evaluates the adequacy of gas exchange in the lungs, the integrity of the ventilatory control system and renal system, and the blood pH and acid-base balance. Measurements of serum concentrations of electrolytes assess the body's acid-base and fluid balance.

Metabolic processes continually form acids, which must be eliminated to maintain acid-base balance. To maintain this balance, the lungs control excretion of $CO_2$, and the kidneys control excretion of hydrogen ions and also reabsorb bicarbonate to keep pH within an acceptable range. Blood gas studies measure the lungs' capacity to regulate $CO_2$ concentration in the blood and determine the kidneys' capacity to retain or excrete metabolic acids and bases. Electrolyte assays determine if abnormalities result from an increase in acid or a loss of base. Because these functions are so closely interwoven, accurate assessment of homeostasis requires simultaneous interpretation of blood gas and electrolyte studies.

**Blood gas analysis.** Routine blood gas analysis measures pH, $PaCO_2$, $PaO_2$, and $HCO_3^-$ (bicarbonate ion) to assess the body's acid-base balance. Together with body fluid and respiratory buffers, the kidneys control acid-base balance, maintaining pH of blood and intracellular fluid within a narrow neutral range.

Renal dysfunction inhibits excretion of the hydrogen ion, which accumulates in the body and causes falling blood pH. The bicarbonate ion, plasma proteins, and a fraction of bone salts act to buffer this excess of hydrogen ions. The respiratory buffering mechanism also acts to decrease the $CO_2$ level, which further reduces the bicarbonate ion content (formed of $CO_2$ and water).

As progressively severe renal failure increases acid retention, this respiratory compensation becomes increasingly essential to maintain blood pH within a range that is compatible with life. Usually in far-advanced renal failure and uremia the patient may show severe hyperventilation and Kussmaul's respiration. In renal failure and metabolic acidosis, ABG analysis shows low pH, low $PaCO_2$, and low $HCO_3^-$. As plasma bicarbonate concentration falls, chloride, another anion, is conserved to maintain electroneutrality, which may lead to hyperchloremia.

**Electrolytes.** In renal failure, serum levels of electrolytes may rise and fall significantly since the kidneys are the primary regulators of fluid and electrolyte balance. The following electrolytes are measured most commonly.

*Sodium,* the major extracellular cation, helps the kidneys regulate body water. Therefore, serum levels of sodium are evaluated in relation to the amount of body water. Decreased sodium levels promote water excretion, and increased levels promote retention. For example, a sodium deficit (hyponatremia) refers to a decreased level of sodium in relation to the body's water level.

In renal failure, the kidneys lose the ability to adjust the amount of sodium reabsorbed to meet the body's needs. In the early stages of renal failure associated with polyuria, serum sodium levels may be low; in later stages with oliguria, serum sodium levels may rise. However, in advanced renal failure, hyponatremia may be dilutional, not reflecting

sodium deficit but its dilution in excessive retained water due to the diseased kidney's inability to excrete it. Hyponatremia in these patients is also related to dietary sodium restriction and possibly to severe diarrhea and vomiting. Because urine sodium determinations are frequently more sensitive to early changes in sodium balance, they should always be evaluated simultaneously with serum sodium findings.

*Potassium,* the major intracellular cation, is vital to homeostasis. Potassium levels are affected by variations in the secretion of adrenal steroid hormones and by fluctuations in pH and in serum glucose and serum sodium levels. A reciprocal relationship appears to exist between potassium and sodium; a substantial intake of one element causes a corresponding decrease in the other. In late stages of renal failure, serum potassium levels increase because the kidneys lose their ability to regulate potassium excretion and secretion. Serum potassium levels must be monitored closely to maintain them within 3.5 to 5 mEq/liter. Potassium levels that occur outside this narrow range may cause fatal cardiac dysrhythmias.

*Chloride,* the major extracellular anion, interacts with sodium to help maintain the osmotic pressure of blood. Chloride levels relate inversely to bicarbonate levels and thus reflect acid-base balance. In renal disease, elevated chloride levels are related to metabolic acidosis. During metabolic acidosis, when bicarbonate is depleted, the kidneys conserve chloride to replace base, which results in elevated chloride levels.

Elevated serum chloride levels (hyperchloremia) may also result from severe dehydration, complete renal shutdown, head injury, or primary aldosteronism. Low chloride levels (hypochloremia) are usually associated with low sodium and potassium levels.

*Serum calcium and phosphorus* also interact inversely. Increasing calcium levels, due to increased levels of parathyroid hormone (PTH) release, decrease serum phosphorus levels and vice versa. To maintain this balance, the renal tubules, under the influence of PTH, selectively reabsorb or filter and excrete phosphorus. The balance of calcium and phosphorus is also influenced by the level of calcium mobilization from other causes. (See Chapter 1 for normal interactions between calcium, phosphorus, vitamin D, and PTH.)

Renal disease interferes with activation of vitamin D and thus inhibits calcium absorption from the intestine. Use of vitamin D requires its conversion to an active metabolite in the kidney. Also, renal failure diminishes the excretion of phosphorus, causing hyperphosphatemia. Together, vitamin D inactivation and hyperphosphatemia decrease serum calcium levels, which, in turn, stimulate PTH activity. Thus, renal failure causes depressed serum calcium, elevated phosphorus, and elevated PTH levels.

### Plasma osmolality

The amount of ADH released by the pituitary gland is regulated by plasma osmolality. Insufficient water intake increases plasma osmolality, thereby triggering pituitary release of ADH. The kidneys respond by reabsorbing water from the distal tubules and producing a more concentrated urine. Conversely, excessive water intake decreases plasma osmolality, thereby inhibiting release of ADH and causing urine to become dilute. Thus, simultaneous determination of serum and urine osmolality can help assess the distal tubular response to circulating ADH. Increased serum osmolality and decreased urine osmolality, measured simultaneously, indicate decreased responsiveness of the distal tubules to circulating ADH.

### Serum proteins

Serum proteins aid tissue anabolism and blood coagulation, act as buffers in acid-base balance, and provide antibodies for immunity. One protein—albumin—constitutes more than 50% of the proteins in serum; a group of proteins (globulins) account for the remainder. Albumin maintains oncotic pressure of plasma, which, in turn, maintains normal distribution of water in the body compartments. A sharp decline in albumin levels leads to edema. In renal dysfunction, failure to excrete nitrogenous products of protein breakdown causes them to accumulate.

### Plasma glucose

Normally, all of the glucose filtered at the glomerulus is reabsorbed through active transport at the proximal tubule. Glucose appears in the urine only when the plasma glucose level exceeds the tubular maximal capacity, as in diabetes mellitus. Chronic renal insufficiency is often accompanied by a varying degree of abnormal glucose intolerance, depending on the degree of renal failure. In chronic renal failure, glucose intolerance results from delayed production and slow degradation (increased half-life) of insulin and

from insensitivity of peripheral tissues to insulin. Serum insulin levels may rise, but peripheral tissue resistance renders insulin ineffective. Also, in certain tubular disorders, renal glycosuria may develop even when the plasma glucose level is normal.

In renal disease, the plasma glucose level may be slightly elevated. However, in renal failure, results from the oral glucose tolerance test are frequently abnormal. This test measures carbohydrate metabolism by monitoring plasma glucose levels after ingestion of a challenge dose of glucose.

### Blood urea nitrogen

This test measures the nitrogen fraction of urea, the chief end product of protein metabolism. Formed in the liver from ammonia and excreted by the kidneys, urea constitutes 40% to 50% of the blood's nonprotein nitrogen. Urea is freely filtered at the glomerulus and reabsorbed to a limited degree in the tubules. Not easily reabsorbed, urea contributes to the osmotic force that promotes water reabsorption from the collecting duct in the presence of ADH. Insufficient excretion of urea results in an elevated BUN level—an elevation in nitrogenous waste products in the blood as reflected by lab tests—called azotemia. Uremia, a term sometimes confused with azotemia, refers to signs and symptoms of all the effects of renal failure. The BUN level reflects protein intake and renal excretory capacity, but it indicates uremia less reliably than the serum creatinine level.

Elevated BUN levels commonly reflect renal dysfunction but may occur in several other conditions even in persons with normally functioning kidneys. Thus, BUN levels must be interpreted in light of other renal function tests. For example, consider that decreased blood flow diminishes urea excretion even in normally functioning kidneys, since elimination of urea depends on blood flow through the renal tubules. Thus, in decreased renal blood flow from dehydration, a fluid challenge reduces the BUN level. Similarly, several other conditions, such as high protein intake, a catabolic state—as in severe trauma or infection—or absorption of blood from the gastrointestinal tract, can elevate BUN levels without renal impairment.

### Serum creatinine

A quantitative analysis of serum creatinine levels, this test measures renal damage more reliably than BUN levels because renal im-

## Interpreting test results

Correlate abnormal test results with your clinical assessment. Keep these points in mind:
• Relate abnormal test results to the patient's condition. A blood urea nitrogen (BUN) level of 50 is abnormally high, according to standard values, but may be acceptable in a patient with renal disease.
• Look for signs and symptoms based on test results. A BUN level of 50 indicates azotemia and should alert you to look for uremia, which usually accompanies azotemia. However, uremic symptoms (such as nausea, vomiting, headache, vertigo, and dimness of vision) may occur at varying times, depending on the patient.

Remember, too, that signs and symptoms may not always correlate with test results because improper collection and labeling of specimens and certain drugs and dietary products can prevent accurate test results.

pairment is virtually the only cause of elevated creatinine levels. Nevertheless, the BUN and serum creatinine tests are usually performed together to provide a broad view of kidney function. Creatinine, a nonprotein end product of creatine metabolism, is freely filtered at the glomerulus and excreted in the urine. Creatinine appears in serum in amounts proportional to the body's muscle mass. Elevated serum creatinine levels indicate severe, persistent renal impairment.

### Serum uric acid

Another nitrogenous waste product found in the blood, uric acid clears the body by glomerular filtration and tubular secretion. In renal failure, decreased renal clearance and tubular secretion of uric acid elevate uric acid levels. However, because normal uric acid levels exist in a wide range and do not rise consistently in renal failure, they're not commonly used to measure renal function. Depressed uric acid levels may indicate defective tubular absorption.

## CLEARANCE TESTS

Abnormal findings from urine and blood tests suggest renal disease or dysfunction. Special tests for filtration, reabsorption, and secretion permit precise evaluation of renal function. Clearance, the volume of plasma that can be cleared of a substance per unit of time, is the test principle used to evaluate these urine-forming mechanisms. Clearance is also a measure of renal plasma flow, which, if diminished by renal disease, impairs renal function.

### Inulin clearance

Inulin, which is administered I.V., is freely filtered at the glomerulus and not reabsorbed or secreted by the renal tubules, so the rate of inulin clearance is nearly an exact measure of the glomerular filtration rate (GFR). The clearance rate of inulin is calculated from measurements of inulin in the plasma and urine. Despite its sensitivity and low incidence of side effects, the inulin clearance test is used infrequently because it's time-consuming, complex, and uncomfortable for the patient.

Depressed inulin clearance is characteristic in congestive heart failure, decreased renal blood flow, acute tubular necrosis, acute and chronic glomerulonephritis, advanced bilateral chronic pyelonephritis, nephrosclerosis, advanced bilateral renal lesions, bilateral ureteral obstruction, and dehydration.

### Creatinine clearance

The creatinine clearance test, which may be the most commonly used test for assessing the GFR, determines how efficiently the kidneys clear creatinine from the blood. Creatinine, an anhydride of creatine, is formed and excreted in constant amounts by an irreversible reaction and functions solely as the main end product of creatine. Creatinine production is proportional to total muscle mass. Although creatinine is freely filtered at the glomerulus and not reabsorbed, the actual rate of creatinine clearance may be slightly lower since some creatinine is secreted by the tubules. After ages 30 to 40, the creatinine clearance rate decreases at about 1 ml/minute/year.

## Understanding the clearance principle

Clearance refers to renal capacity to remove various substances from the plasma. Clearance depends on how efficiently the renal tubular cells handle the substance that has been filtered by the glomeruli. If the tubules don't reabsorb or secrete the substance (such as inulin or creatinine), clearance equals the glomerular filtration rate (GFR). If the tubules reabsorb and/or secrete the substance (such as sodium and uric acid), clearance is less than, equal to, or greater than the GFR.

To calculate plasma clearance for any substance, use this formula:
*Plasma clearance (ml/minute) = urinary concentration (mg/dl) × urinary volume (ml/minute) ÷ plasma concentration (mg/dl).*

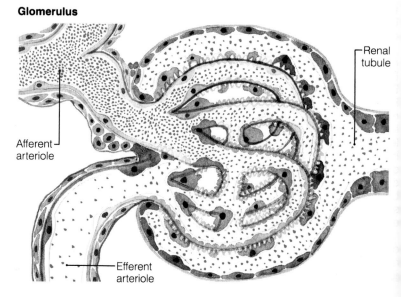

**Glomerulus**

Renal tubule

Afferent arteriole

Efferent arteriole

# BUN and creatinine: Keys to kidney function

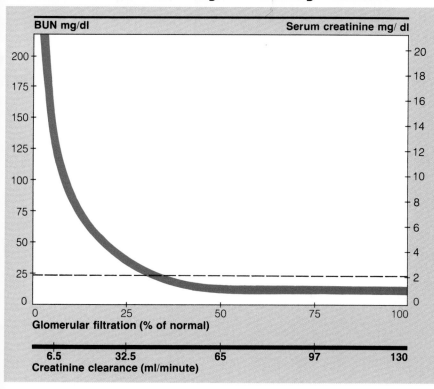

BUN mg/dl

Serum creatinine mg/dl

Glomerular filtration (% of normal)

Creatinine clearance (ml/minute)

The graph shows the correlation among glomerular filtration (in percent of normal as measured by creatinine clearance), BUN, and serum creatinine. The broken horizontal line represents the upper levels of normal BUN and serum creatinine. The curve shows changes in BUN and serum creatinine levels as the GFR decreases. As much as 75% of renal function must be lost before BUN and creatinine levels rise above normal. However, further small losses of renal function cause large increases in BUN and creatinine levels.

Although the kidneys excrete more than 200 nitrogenous waste products daily, urea and creatinine are the two we measure—usually as blood urea nitrogen (BUN) and serum creatinine—for kidney function.

## BUN

Protein—ingested or borrowed from the body—is broken down into amino acids and nitrogenous wastes. Urea nitrogen is the end product of protein metabolism, and urea not circulating in the blood is mostly excreted in the urine.

When urea isn't excreted in proportion to its production, the BUN levels rise. But elevated BUN levels may be misleading. First, the protein metabolism rate isn't constant. It's directly increased (thus raising the BUN levels) by excessive protein intake and by the catabolism of starvation, infection, trauma, surgery, hematoma resorption, bleeding into the gut, corticosteroids or tetracyclines, and even heavy exertion.

Second, urea excretion isn't constant, either. Dehydration or hypovolemia from poor cardiac output or diuretic kidney sodium loss can elevate BUN levels by lowering the glomerular filtration rate (GFR). So can vomiting, diarrhea, systemic or local infections, surgery, trauma, hemorrhage, a sudden drop in a chronic hypertensive patient's blood pressure, or nephrotoxic drugs. Besides, the tiny urea molecule will be reabsorbed into kidney circulation several times before it's excreted.

So BUN levels can express either a rise in the protein metabolism rate or a drop in the GFR. And each of these changes can result from something other than kidney dysfunction. For these reasons, BUN levels must be examined with serum creatinine levels.

### Creatinine

Creatinine, another nitrogenous waste, is the product of muscle metabolism. Unlike BUN, it's unaffected by diet and practically unaffected by fluid intake. The amount produced each day is proportional to the body's muscle mass, which seldom changes rapidly.

The amount of creatinine excreted (normally 0.7 to 1.5 mg/ 100 ml) is roughly proportional to the GFR. A large change in the GFR produces only a small change in serum creatinine levels unless kidney failure has already set in. This "unless" makes creatinine a more reliable assessment tool for kidney function than BUN.

### BUN and creatinine

You need both BUN and creatinine to tell the whole story. The nephrons normally clean the blood of waste products. But at the onset of kidney disease, the nephrons lose this ability, at least in part.

As a result, BUN and creatinine accumulate in the blood. This happens subtly at first, because the nephrons still functioning compensate by performing clearances on larger solute loads. Yet, as more and more nephrons are destroyed, the rise in BUN and creatinine levels becomes more evident.

Their simultaneous rise is the key to a diagnosis. This is true even if the two indicators rise at a rate that maintains their 20:1 ratio. For together, raised BUN and creatinine levels always spell kidney disease.

# Imaging agents

Diagnostic imaging agents in renal disorders include contrast imaging agents and radioactive imaging agents.

## Contrast imaging agents

Contrast imaging agents—radiopaque dyes or drugs—are impenetrable by X-rays and thus allow radiologic visualization of internal structures such as the kidneys. Depending on the structure to be studied, contrast imaging agents may be instilled directly into a site, such as the bladder, or they may be given orally. Some agents have an affinity for a certain organ or tissue and, when given orally, can localize radiopacity, or they can be absorbed and excreted.

## Radioactive imaging agents

Radioactive imaging agents—also called radiopharmaceuticals—are used primarily for diagnosis but may also be used for treatment. These agents contain radionuclides or radioisotopes, which are taken up and metabolized by organs and tissues.

Most radionuclides emit gamma rays. Since gamma rays are highly penetrating, they can—after ingestion—be detected externally with special instruments. Their high penetration and ease of measurement make radionuclides effective as diagnostic tracers. Measuring the emitted radiation can help evaluate a metabolic pathway, indicate the size of an organ, or pinpoint the site of disease.

| Agent | Diagnostic use | Patient preparation |
|---|---|---|
| **Contrast imaging agents** | | |
| **diatrizoate meglumine, methylglucamine, or sodium** *Transurethral:* Cystografin | Retrograde cystourethrography | Laxative the night before test and low-residue diet the day before test are recommended |
| *I.V. push:* Cardiografin, Renografin, Reno-M-60, Renovist* | Venography | Nothing by mouth after midnight; light sedative and local anesthetic required; light general anesthetic may be required |
| | Computerized tomography (CT) scan | Depends on area to be scanned |
| *Continuous I.V. infusion:* Reno-M-30 | Excretory urography | Laxative the night before test and low-residue diet the day before test are recommended |
| *Urethral instillation:* Reno-M-60 | Retrograde pyelography | Low-residue diet the day before test and laxative the night before test are recommended. Nothing by mouth after midnight |
| **iothalamate meglumine or sodium** Angio-Conray, Conray-325 | Excretory urography | Low-residue diet and laxative the day before examination; fluids must be restricted |
| | Venography | Premedication with sedative or tranquilizer, and local anesthetic needed; general anesthetic may be needed. Nothing by mouth from midnight before test. |
| **Radioactive imaging agents** | | |
| **technetium Tc 99m glucoheptonate** | Imaging of kidney function | Variable |

*Several forms of Renografin and Renovist available. Drug selected depends on test. Not all forms of drug appropriate for all tests.

Low creatinine clearance rates may result from reduced renal blood flow (associated with shock or renal artery obstruction), acute tubular necrosis, acute or chronic glomerulonephritis, advanced bilateral chronic pyelonephritis, advanced bilateral renal lesions, or nephrosclerosis. High creatinine clearance rates generally have little diagnostic significance.

### Urea clearance

The urea clearance test also predicts the GFR. This test is an analysis of urine levels of urea, the main nitrogenous component in urine and the end product of protein metabolism. After filtration by the glomeruli, roughly 40% of the urea is reabsorbed by the renal tubules. However, since the reabsorption rate varies with the amount of water reabsorbed, this

Low urea clearance rates may indicate decreased renal blood flow, acute or chronic glomerulonephritis, advanced bilateral chronic pyelonephritis, acute tubular necrosis, or nephrosclerosis. Diminished clearance rates may also result from advanced bilateral renal lesions, bilateral ureteral obstruction, congestive heart failure, or dehydration. High urea clearance rates usually are not diagnostically significant.

### Phenolsulfonphthalein (PSP) excretion

The PSP excretion test evaluates tubular function and is indicated for patients with abnormal urine concentration, one of the earliest signs of renal dysfunction. This test also helps measure renal blood flow because clearance of PSP is proportional to renal blood flow. Decreased excretion usually results from impaired renal perfusion rather than decreased tubular function. When PSP is administered I.V., the kidneys normally clear 95% of the dose in one passage, primarily by proximal tubular excretion.

Depressed PSP excretion may reveal moderate-to-severe renal impairment, renal vascular disease, congestive heart failure, and gout. Elevated PSP excretion is characteristic in hypoalbuminemia, hepatic disease, and multiple myeloma.

## IMAGING TESTS

Imaging techniques used to evaluate renal abnormalities include radiography (with or without contrast medium), radionuclide studies, and ultrasonography. These techniques are used to visualize the number, size, and location of the kidneys, to identify the presence and site of obstruction, to detect and characterize lesions, to visualize renal arteries and veins, and to guide percutaneous diagnostic and therapeutic interventions, such as biopsy and nephrostomy.

### Kidney-ureter-bladder (KUB) radiography

Usually the first step in diagnostic testing of the renal system, the KUB test helps determine kidney position, size, and structure and detects calculi and foreign bodies. A KUB test usually precedes a renal biopsy to determine kidney placement. This test has many limitations and nearly always must be followed by more complex procedures, such as excretory urography or renal computerized tomography (CT) scan.

Abnormal findings may include bilateral or unilateral hypertrophy or abnormally small

---

**Nursing considerations**

After sterile catheterization, the bladder is filled. Reflux or discomfort signals full bladder.

The examination may be performed in the operating room. A special consent form may be required; check your hospital's protocol. Check the patient's history for hypersensitivity to iodine or iodine-containing foods, or to contrast media used in previous diagnostic tests.

The patient must remain completely immobile for the test. A special consent form may be required. Check the patient's history for hypersensitivity to iodine or iodine-containing foods, or to contrast media used in previous diagnostic tests.

Urography is contraindicated in patients with anuria. Make sure the patient has signed a consent form. Check the patient's history for hypersensitivity to iodine or iodine-containing foods, or to contrast media used in previous diagnostic tests.

Post-test oliguria or anuria may develop.

Make sure the patient has signed a consent form. Check the patient's history for hypersensitivity to iodine or iodine-containing foods, or to contrast media used in previous diagnostic tests.
Monitor intake and output following the test. Note: This drug is incompatible with promethazine hydrochloride (Phenergan); precipitate will form.

Check institution protocol for special consent form requirements. Examination may be performed in operating room or special procedures room. Check the patient's history for hypersensitivity to iodine or iodine-containing foods, or to contrast media used in previous diagnostic tests.

The patient must remain completely immobile during the test; a sedative may be necessary for an uncooperative patient.

---

test actually assesses overall renal function; the creatinine clearance test provides a more accurate evaluation of the GFR. The normal range of urea clearance is 64 to 100 ml/minute at a urine flow rate of 2 ml/minute or greater. At flow rates of less than 2 ml/minute, the normal range is 40 to 70 ml/minute. Urea clearance rates below 20 ml/minute are usually associated with symptoms of uremia.

## Visualizing renal abnormalities

Kidney-ureter-bladder (KUB) radiography is usually the first step in diagnostic testing of a patient with urinary symptoms. The KUB helps determine the position, size, and structure of the kidneys and detects gross abnormalities. Calculi are easily identified because of their density. Excretory urography further defines abnormalities. This procedure can demonstrate such disorders as renal cysts, enlarged kidneys due to polycystic disease, horseshoe kidney, and congenital absence of a kidney.

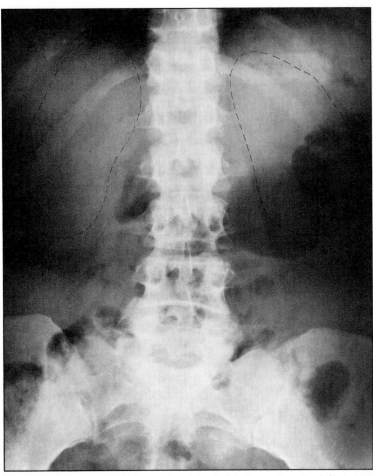

This KUB shows normal kidneys, the right slightly lower than the left.

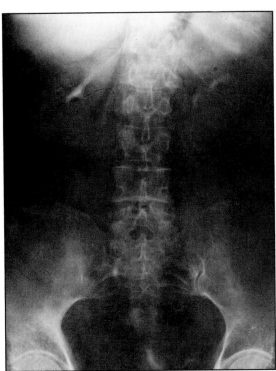

Note the cyst on the right kidney and an abnormally small left kidney in this excretory urogram.

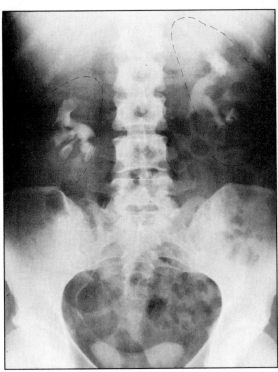

The bilaterally enlarged kidneys shown in this excretory urogram result from polycystic disease.

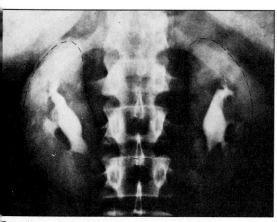

Excretory urography demonstrates congenital anomalies, such as this horseshoe kidney.

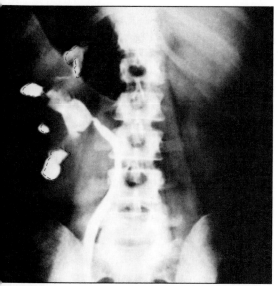

Visualization of the kidneys can reveal abnormalities such as calculi, as shown in this KUB.

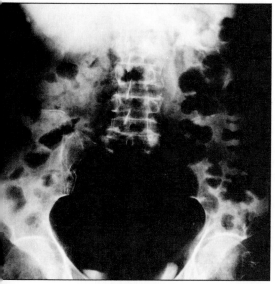

This excretory urogram shows congenital absence of a kidney in a patient with absent abdominal musculature.

kidneys, suggesting end-stage glomerulonephritis or bilateral atrophic pyelonephritis. Decreased size of one kidney suggests possible congenital hypoplasia, atrophic pyelonephritis, or ischemia; renal displacement may be due to a tumor. Obliteration or bulging of a portion of the psoas muscle may result from a tumor, abscess, or hematoma.

KUB radiography may also detect congenital anomalies, such as abnormal location or absence of a kidney. It may show renal axes that parallel the vertebral column, suggesting horseshoe kidney. A lobulated edge or border may suggest polycystic kidney disease or patchy atrophic pyelonephritis. Opaque bodies may reflect calculi or vascular calcification due to aneurysm or atheroma; opacification may also suggest cystic tumors, fecaliths, foreign bodies, or abnormal fluid collection.

### Excretory urography

The cornerstone of a urologic workup, excretory urography allows visualization of the renal parenchyma, calyxes, pelvises, ureters, bladder, and, in some cases, the urethra following intravenous administration of a contrast medium. Known traditionally as intravenous pyelography, this common procedure is more accurately called excretory urography because the test shows the entire urinary tract—not just the renal pelvis, as the prefix *pyelo-* implies.

Timing this examination provides information about various structures. In the first minute after injection (the nephrographic stage), the contrast medium delineates the size and shape of the kidneys. After 3 to 5 minutes (the pyelographic stage), the contrast medium moves into the calyxes and pelvises, allowing visualization of cysts, tumors, and other obstructions.

Excretory urography can demonstrate renal or ureteral calculi; abnormal size, shape, or structure of kidneys, ureters, or bladder; supernumerary or absent kidney(s); polycystic kidney disease associated with renal hypertrophy; redundant pelvis or ureter; space-occupying lesions; pyelonephritis; renal tuberculosis; hydronephrosis; and renovascular hypertension.

### Retrograde pyelography

After injection of a contrast medium through a ureteral catheter during cystoscopy, retrograde pyelography allows radiographic examination of the renal collecting system (calyxes, renal pelvises, and ureters). Although some of the iodine-based contrast medium may be absorbed through the mucous membranes, this test is preferred for patients with hypersensitivity to iodine (in whom I.V. administration of an iodine-based contrast medium, as in excretory urography, is contraindicated). Because this test doesn't depend on renal function, it is also indicated when visualization of the renal collecting system is inadequate because of marked renal insufficiency. Retrograde pyelography may detect obstruction to the flow of urine in the renal collecting system. Such obstruction results from stricture, neoplasm, blood clot, or calculi.

### Renal angiography
After arterial injection of a contrast medium, renal angiography permits radiographic examination of the renal vasculature and parenchyma. As the contrast medium pervades the renal vasculature, rapid-sequence radiographs show the vessels during three phases of filling: arterial, nephrographic, and venous. This invasive procedure risks potential complications that may include embolus or clot formation, vessel injury from arterial puncture or catheter manipulation, allergic reaction to the contrast medium, and injury to the renal tissue from the contrast medium.

Renal tumors usually show hypervascularity; renal cysts typically appear as clearly delineated, radiolucent masses. Renal artery stenosis produces constriction in the blood vessels, usually within the proximal portion of their length, and confirms renovascular hypertension. In renal infarction, blood vessels may appear absent or cut off since normal tissue is replaced by scar tissue; triangular areas of infarcted tissue may appear near the periphery of the affected kidney; and the kidney itself may appear shrunken because of tissue scarring. Renal angiography may also detect renal artery aneurysms and renal arteriovenous fistulas. In severe or chronic pyelonephritis, this test may show destruction, distortion, and fibrosis of renal tissue with areas of reduced and tortuous vascularity. This test may also show increased capsular circulation, suggesting renal abscesses or inflammatory masses.

When angiography is used to evaluate renal trauma, it may detect intrarenal hematoma, parenchymal laceration, shattered kidney, and areas of infarction. It may also help to distinguish pseudotumors from tumors or cysts, to evaluate the volume of residual functioning renal tissue in hydronephrosis, and to evaluate donors and recipients before and after renal transplantation.

Renal venography may be performed to detect renal vein thrombosis and venous extension of renal cell carcinoma. Since renal venography requires injection of a contrast medium against usually heavy renal venous outflow that may distort distribution of the contrast medium, the procedure is sometimes performed with intraarterial infusion of epinephrine to reduce renal blood flow.

### Voiding cystourethrography
In this test, a contrast medium is instilled by gentle syringe pressure or gravity through a catheter introduced through the urethra and into the bladder. Fluoroscopic films or overhead radiographs demonstrate bladder filling, then show excretion of the contrast medium as the patient voids. The test is useful in detecting abnormalities of the urinary tract, such as ureteral strictures and congenital anomalies of the lower urinary tract, and in investigating urinary reflux, chronic urinary tract infections, and incontinence.

This procedure may show urethral stricture or valves, vesical or urethral diverticula, ureteroceles, prostatic enlargement, vesicoureteral reflux, or neurogenic bladder. Their severity and location are then evaluated to determine if surgery is needed.

### Retrograde cystography
Retrograde cystography involves the instillation of a contrast medium into the bladder, followed by radiographic examination. This procedure helps diagnose bladder rupture without urethral involvement since it can determine the location and extent of the rupture. Other indications for retrograde cystography include neurogenic bladder, recurrent urinary tract infections (especially in children), suspected vesicoureteral reflux, vesical fistulas, diverticula, and tumors. Retrograde cystography is also performed when cystoscopic examination is impractical, as in male infants, or when excretory urography has not adequately visualized the bladder. Voiding cystourethrography is often performed concomitantly.

### Retrograde urethrography
Used almost exclusively in males, this radiographic study is performed during instillation or injection of a contrast medium into the urethra. This imaging test permits visualization of its membranous, bulbar, and penile portions.

# Renal angiography: Visualizing renal vasculature and parenchyma

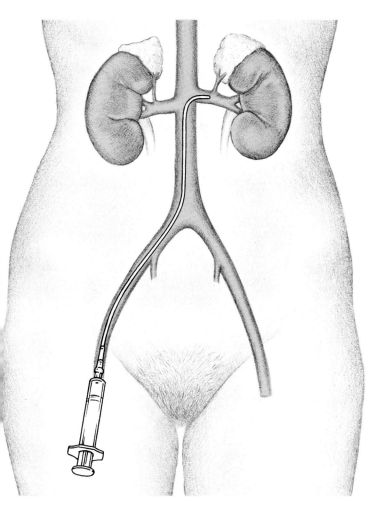

In renal angiography, a catheter is advanced, under fluoroscopic guidance, up the femoroiliac vessels to the aorta, contrast medium is injected, and radiographs show vessels during three phases of filling: arterial, nephrographic, and venous. These renal angiograms show a normal kidney in arterial (bottom, left) and nephrographic (bottom, right) stages of filling, with the catheter visible over the spine. In the arterial phase, the contrast medium clearly delineates the trunk and branches of the arterial tree. The nephrographic phase demonstrates movement of the contrast medium from renal arteries and its diffusion throughout the renal capillary structure, with greatest concentration in the pyramids and cortex. Abnormal conditions might produce local retention of contrast medium (indicating arterial stenosis), bead-and-string filling pattern (arterial dysplasia), displacement or irregular branching of vessels, or unusual diffusion of contrast medium (invasion by tumor or cyst).

**Arterial stage**

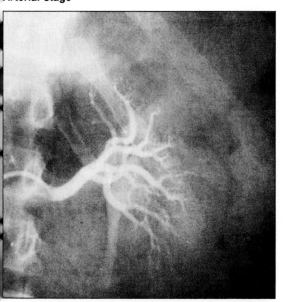

**Nephrographic stage**

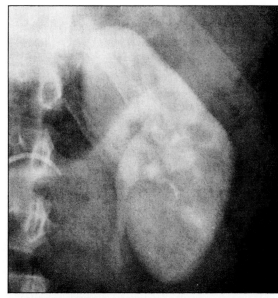

Retrograde urethrography may demonstrate the following abnormalities: urethral diverticula, fistulas, strictures, false passages, calculi, and lacerations; congenital anomalies, such as urethral valves and perineal hypospadias; and, rarely, tumors.

### Renal computerized tomography scan

Renal CT scan provides an image of the kidneys constructed from a series of tomograms, or cross-sectional slices, which are then translated by a computer and displayed on an oscilloscope screen. The density of the image reflects the amount of radiation absorbed by renal tissue and permits identification of masses and other lesions. Renal CT scan is sometimes performed after administration of an I.V. contrast medium that accentuates the density of the renal parenchyma and helps differentiate renal masses. Highly accurate and definitive, this test is usually performed to investigate diseases demonstrated by other diagnostic procedures, such as excretory urography. It may also precede percutaneous biopsy, to ensure accurate needle placement, or may follow kidney transplantation to determine the size and location of the kidney in relation to the bladder.

Renal masses appear as areas of density different from that of normal parenchyma. Renal cysts, for example, appear as smooth, sharply defined masses with thin walls and a lower density than normal parenchyma. Tumors, such as renal cell carcinoma, however, tend to have thick walls and mixed density. With contrast enhancement, solid tumors show a higher density than renal cysts but a lower density than that of normal parenchyma; tumors with hemorrhage, calcification, or necrosis show higher densities; vascular tumors are more clearly defined; and adrenal tumors are confined masses.

Renal CT scan may also identify other abnormalities, including obstructions, calculi, polycystic kidney disease, congenital anomalies, and abnormal accumulations of fluid around the kidneys. After nephrectomy, CT scan can detect abnormal masses such as recurrent tumors.

### Nephrotomography

In nephrotomography, special films are exposed before and after opacification of the renal arterial network with contrast medium. The resulting tomographic slices clearly delineate various linear layers of the kidneys while blurring structures in front of and behind these selected planes. Nephrotomography is performed as a separate procedure or as an adjunct to excretory urography. It is especially useful in identifying lesions, such as cysts and solid tumors, suggested by excretory urography or retrograde pyelography; areas of nonperfusion; and renal lacerations following trauma.

### Radionuclide renal imaging

This test involves I.V. injection of a radionuclide, followed by scintiphotography. Observing the uptake concentration and transit of the radionuclide during radionuclide renal imaging allows assessment of renal blood flow, nephron and collecting system function, and renal structure. Depending on the patient's clinical status, this procedure may include dynamic scans to assess renal perfusion and function or static scans to assess structure. Radionuclide renal imaging may also be substituted for excretory urography in patients with hypersensitivity to contrast agents.

Since approximately 25% of cardiac output goes directly to the kidneys, renal perfusion should be evident immediately following uptake of the radionuclide in the abdominal aorta. The perfusion study can identify impeded renal circulation in patients with renovascular hypertension and abdominal aortic disease, can help differentiate tumors from cysts, and may indicate obstruction of vascular grafts. The function study can detect abnormalities of the collecting system and extravasation of the urine and can localize ureteral obstruction.

Static images can demonstrate lesions, congenital abnormalities, and traumatic injury. They can also detect space-occupying lesions within or surrounding the kidney; identify congenital disorders; and define regions of infarction, rupture, or hemorrhage after trauma. A lower than normal total concentration of the radionuclide suggests a diffuse renal disorder, such as acute tubular necrosis, severe infection, or ischemia. In a patient who has had a kidney transplant, decreased radionuclide uptake generally indicates organ rejection. Failure of visualization may indicate congenital ectopia or aplasia. A definitive diagnosis usually requires the combined analysis of static images with perfusion and function studies.

### Renal ultrasonography

During ultrasonography, high-frequency sound waves are transmitted from a transducer

# Review nursing management in diagnostic testing

When caring for a patient who is scheduled for—or who has undergone—urologic testing, remember these points.

Because many urologic tests are embarrassing to the patient, reassure him and minimize his anxiety by clearly and accurately describing the scheduled procedure. Avoid giving explanations when the patient is in pain or otherwise distracted. Make your explanations clear and concise, and encourage questions. Tell the patient what he is most likely to experience during the test and what he'll be expected to do. Routinely involving the patient in the test procedure promotes compliance, encourages cooperation, and helps ensure accurate test results.

Make sure the fluid intake of a patient with a suspected urinary tract lesion is adequate (except when underlying medical conditions dictate fluid restriction). Adequate hydration is especially important after procedures involving instillation of a contrast medium, because fluids help flush out the contrast medium.

Observe for adverse effects following instillation of the contrast medium. Common effects include abdominal cramps, diarrhea, flushing, iodine hypersensitivity, nausea, vomiting, and pruritus. Be sure to ask the patient about previous X-ray procedures and if he had any reactions to them. Hypersensitivity and other severe reactions are most likely to develop after parenteral administration, which may induce an anaphylactic reaction, with bronchospasm and shock. Keep in mind that sneezing, wheezing, and tissue swelling are often the first signs of a severe anaphylactic reaction. To treat such reactions promptly, be sure that emergency equipment is readily available.

Administer a laxative, as ordered, to a patient scheduled for radiographic tests (such as retrograde pyelography), because overlying gas or feces in the lumen of the gastrointestinal tract may interfere with the quality of X-ray films of the urinary system.

After an invasive test, monitor fluid intake and output. Inability to void may necessitate catheterization. Notify the doctor if hematuria persists after the third voiding; describe its presence and progress accurately.

Watch for signs of urinary sepsis (such as fever, chills, or hypotension) after any test that involves instrumentation of the urinary system (cystourethroscopy, for example).

---

through the kidneys and perirenal structures. The resulting echoes, amplified and converted into electrical impulses, are displayed on an oscilloscope screen as anatomic images.

Usually performed with other urologic tests, renal ultrasonography can detect abnormalities or clarify those detected by other tests. Painless and considered safe, this procedure is especially valuable when excretory urography is ruled out—for example, because of hypersensitivity to the contrast medium or the need for serial examinations. Unlike excretory urography, this test is not dependent on renal function and, therefore, can be useful in patients with renal failure.

Ultrasonography is used to determine the size, shape, and position of the kidneys, their internal structures, and perirenal tissues; to evaluate and localize urinary obstruction and abnormal accumulation of fluid; and to assess and diagnose complications following kidney transplantation.

**Structural changes.** Ultrasonography shows cysts as usually fluid-filled, circular structures that don't reflect sound waves. Tumors produce multiple echoes and appear as irregular shapes. Abscesses, with boundaries slightly more irregular than those of cysts, also echo sound waves poorly. A perirenal abscess may displace the kidney anteriorly. Ultrasonography generally fails to detect acute pyelonephritis and glomerulonephritis unless they have scarred and atrophied the renal parenchyma. In such patients, the renal capsule appears irregular and the kidney may appear smaller than normal; also, exaggerated echoes may arise from the parenchyma because of fibrosis. This test can also detect congenital anomalies (horseshoe, ectopic, or duplicated kidneys) and renal hypertrophy. Ultrasonography identifies abnormalities of the adrenal glands, such as tumors, cysts, and adrenal dysfunction. However, a normal adrenal gland is difficult to define ultrasonically because of its small size.

**Fluid accumulation and obstruction.** Renal ultrasonography allows identification of abnormal accumulations of fluid within or around the kidneys from an obstruction. In hydronephrosis, the test may show a large, echo-free, central mass that compresses the renal cortex. Calyceal echoes are usually circularly diffused and the pelvis significantly enlarged. It also detects changes in the shape

## Percutaneous renal biopsy

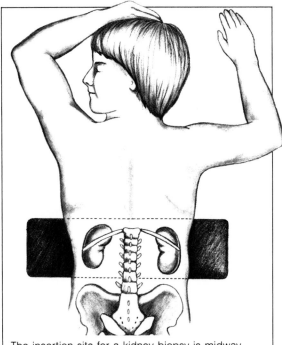

The insertion site for a kidney biopsy is midway between the last rib and the iliac crest. To immobilize the patient's kidney against his back, place a sandbag beneath his abdomen.

After a small incision is made in the anesthetized skin, the patient holds his breath and remains immobile while the Franklin-Silverman (cannula with obturator) needle is inserted. As the patient breathes deeply, entrance into the kidney is indicated by the characteristic needle swing.

of the bladder that result from masses and assesses urine volume. Increased urine volume or residual urine postvoiding may indicate bladder dysfunction.

**Transplant complications.** Following renal transplantation, compensatory hypertrophy of the transplanted kidney is normal, but acute enlargement indicates rejection of the transplant. Ultrasonography also allows evaluation of perirenal structures.

### OTHER TESTS
Other specialized techniques used to evaluate renal structure and function include cystourethroscopy, biopsy, and cystometry.

### Cystourethroscopy
This test combines two endoscopic techniques that allow visualization of the bladder and the urethra. One instrument used in cystourethroscopy is the cystoscope, which has a fiberoptic light source, a magnification system, a right-angled telescopic lens, and an angled beak for smooth passage into the bladder. The other instrument, the urethroscope, is similar but has a straight-ahead lens and is used for examination of the bladder neck and the urethra. Usually a common sheath is in-

serted into the urethra, through which a cystoscope or urethroscope may be passed to obtain the desired view. Other invasive procedures that may be performed through this channel include biopsy of the bladder and prostate, lesion resection, collection of calculi, or passage of a ureteral catheter to the renal pelvis for pyelography. This test is contraindicated in patients with acute forms of urethritis, prostatitis, or cystitis because instrumentation can lead to sepsis. It usually follows KUB and excretory urography.

One of the most common abnormal findings in cystourethroscopy is an enlarged prostate gland in older men. In both males and females, this test commonly detects urethral stricture, calculi, tumors, diverticula, ulcers, and polyps. Cystourethroscopy may also detect congenital bladder wall trabeculation and various congenital anomalies, such as ureteroceles, duplicate ureteral orifices, or urethral valves in children.

### Percutaneous renal biopsy
Percutaneous renal biopsy is needle excision of a core of kidney tissue to obtain a specimen for histologic examination, using light, electron, and immunofluorescent microscopy.

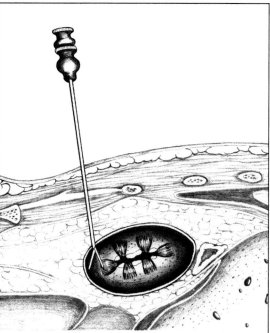

Again, the patient is instructed to hold his breath and remain immobile while the obturator of the needle is removed and the cutting prongs are inserted to full depth.

While the patient holds his breath, the cannula is pushed down over the cutting prongs, and the prongs are withdrawn slightly to allow blood to enter the cannula for later culturing. Finally, the cannula and prongs, with the specimen, are withdrawn.

Such examination is used to differentiate glomerular from tubular renal disease, to monitor the disorder's progress, and to assess therapy.

Percutaneous renal biopsy is contraindicated in patients with renal tumors, severe bleeding disorders, markedly reduced plasma or blood volume, severe hypertension, hydronephrosis, perinephric abscess, advanced renal failure with uremia, or only one kidney. Complications of this test may include bleeding, hematoma, arteriovenous fistula, and infection. Despite these risks, percutaneous renal biopsy is considered safer than open biopsy, usually the preferred method for removing a tissue specimen from a solid lesion. However, recent noninvasive procedures, especially renal ultrasonography and CT scan, have replaced percutaneous renal biopsy in many hospitals.

Histologic examination of renal tissue can reveal malignancy or renal disease. Malignant tumors include Wilms' tumor, which usually occurs in young children, and renal cell carcinoma, prevalent in persons over age 40. Histologic studies may also detect disseminated lupus erythematosus, amyloid infiltration, acute and chronic glomerulonephritis, renal vein thrombosis, and pyelonephritis.

## Cystometry
This test is performed by instillation of normal saline solution or sterile water or by insufflation of gas to evaluate the urination reflex and bladder capacity. Specifically, cystometry assesses the bladder's neuromuscular function by measuring the efficiency of the detrusor muscle reflex, intravesical pressure and capacity, and bladder response to thermal stimulation. (See Chapter 8 for normal and abnormal results of this test.) Cystometry alone can give ambiguous results. Consequently, results of this test require appropriate support by results of other tests, such as excretory urography and voiding cystourethrography.

## The nursing challenge
The more you know about diagnostic tests, the more they enhance nursing management. (See *Review nursing management in diagnostic testing,* page 61.) A thorough working knowledge of diagnostic tests enhances your ability to prepare patients for these tests (intellectually and emotionally, as well as physically), to monitor for possible complications during and after the tests, and to care for these patients after the tests are completed.

## Points to remember

• A wide variety of tests is available to assess the renal system. They include urine and blood studies; clearance and imaging tests; and other specialized tests, including cystourethroscopy, biopsy, and cystometry.
• Urine and blood studies provide information concerning the patient's overall state of health. Urine tests also help evaluate the kidneys' concentrating and diluting ability. Blood tests assess the ability to eliminate waste and maintain homeostasis and to help evaluate glomerular and tubular function.
• Clearance tests for filtration, reabsorption, and secretion permit precise evaluation of renal function.
• Imaging tests—radiography, radionuclide imaging, and ultrasonography—visualize renal abnormalities.
• Other specialized tests include cystourethroscopy, which allows direct visualization of the urethra and bladder and provides a channel for other invasive procedures; biopsy, which permits histologic examination of kidney tissue to aid diagnosis of renal disease; and cystometry, which allows evaluation of the bladder's neuromuscular mechanisms.

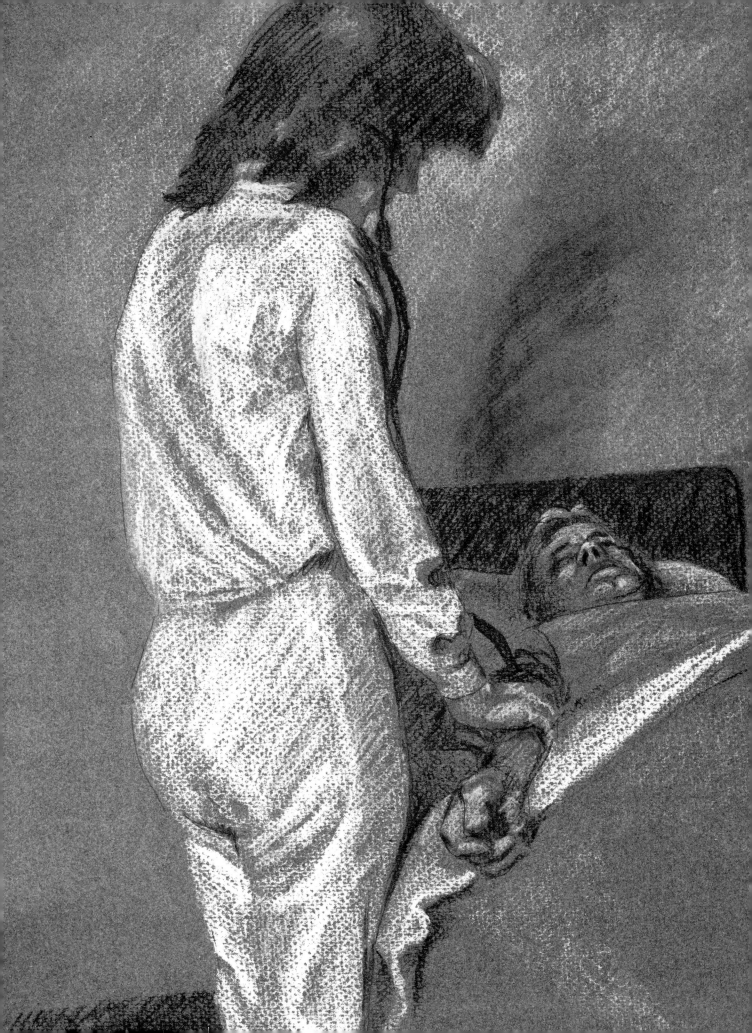

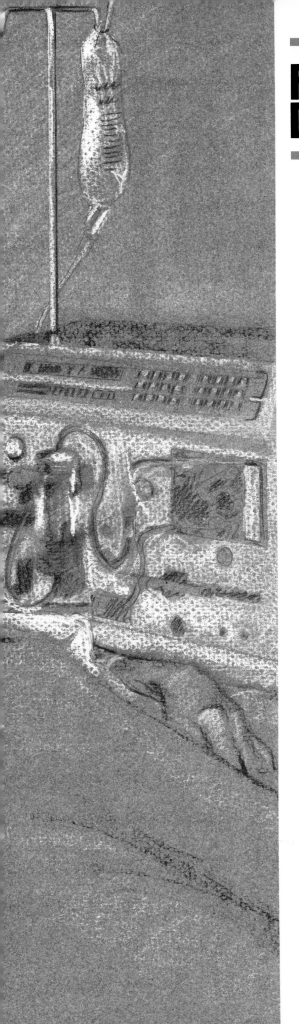

# RENAL DISORDERS

# 4 COMBATING ACUTE RENAL FAILURE

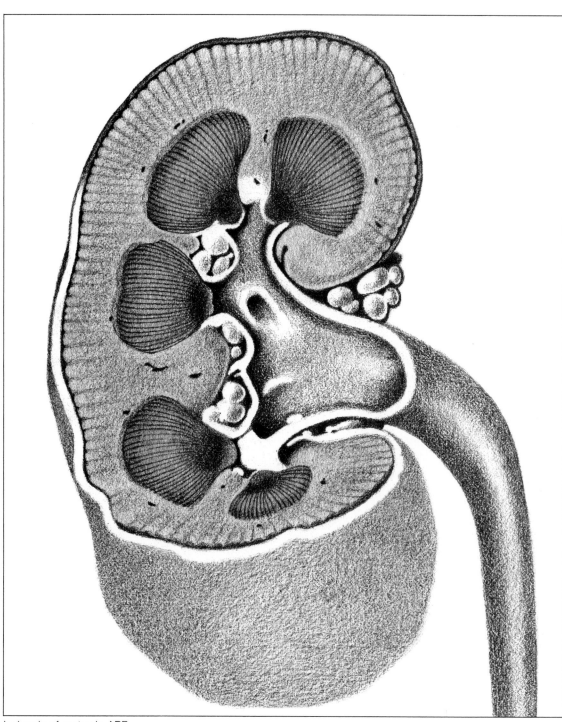

Ischemia of cortex in ARF

During the past 30 years, our improved understanding of the causes and course of acute renal failure (ARF), the use of hemodialysis, and advances in intensive care have cut mortality in ARF from about 90% to 50%. Because early detection and prompt, aggressive treatment can usually reverse this deadly disorder, you're in an excellent position to help reduce ARF mortality even further. First, by performing a thorough and accurate assessment, you can identify patients at risk for ARF. Second, by formulating and implementing an effective care plan, you can help prevent the development, progression, and devastating aftermath of ARF.

## What is acute renal failure?

ARF is the abrupt deterioration of kidney function, which causes metabolic waste and excess water accumulation and a marked decline in urine output. If undetected or inadequately treated, ARF can permanently damage the renal parenchyma and can progress to chronic—and often fatal—renal failure.

## What causes ARF?

The causes of ARF are commonly classified as prerenal, intrarenal (or parenchymal), and postrenal. (See *Causes of acute renal failure,* page 69.) *Prerenal failure* results from conditions that impair renal perfusion, such as congestive heart failure and other cardiovascular disorders, hypovolemia, and renovascular obstruction. *Intrarenal failure* results from disorders that directly affect the renal cortex or medulla, such as acute tubular necrosis (ATN) and acute glomerulonephritis. *Postrenal failure* results from bilateral obstruction of urinary outflow.

## PATHOPHYSIOLOGY

The precise pathophysiology of ARF is unknown, but decreased renal perfusion, nephrotoxic injury, and ischemia can all lead to rapid deterioration of renal function. Decreased perfusion can stem from excessive fluid loss, renal artery stenosis, or impaired cardiac output. To compensate for decreased perfusion and to prevent ischemic damage to the renal parenchyma, two compensatory mechanisms interact. In the first, the renin-angiotensin-aldosterone system works to raise blood pressure. Angiotensin promotes vasoconstriction and aldosterone production by the adrenal gland. The aldosterone expands blood volume by increasing salt and water reabsorption in the distal tubule. The second mechanism, autoregulation, maintains constant renal blood flow by changing blood flow resistance in the afferent and efferent arterioles supplying the glomerulus. When blood flow through the glomerulus is reduced, less water is passed in the filtrate, thereby decreasing the glomerular filtration rate (GFR). If decreased perfusion continues despite compensation, ischemic parenchymal damage results. Renal tubular cells become necrotic, swell, or slough off, resulting in tubular obstruction. Further pathophysiologic processes then follow the same sequence as in ATN.

## Acute tubular necrosis: Five theories

ATN causes about 75% of all ARF cases and is the most common cause of ARF in critically ill patients. ATN clearly damages the tubular segment of the nephron; five theories attempt to explain how this damage occurs.

The *back-leak* theory contends that nephrotoxic injury or ischemia increases tubular epithelium permeability. So the tubules absorb more filtrate from the interstitial fluid, causing decreased urine production and oliguria.

The *tubular obstruction* theory proposes that interstitial edema or casts and epithelial debris cause filtrate accumulation proximal to the obstruction. As tubular hydrostatic pressure rises to the same level as glomerular hydrostatic pressure, the flow of filtrate between the glomerulus and the tubules halts, thereby decreasing urine production. This theory seems unlikely, however, because casts aren't always present in the kidneys, and obstruction doesn't always affect filtration.

The third theory, the *no-reflow phenomenon,* contends that renal capillary obstruction causes oliguric renal failure. Prolonged periods of ischemia supposedly congest the tubules and cause thrombosis of the glomerular capillaries. Ischemic damage to the sodium pump swells endothelial cells, narrowing the capillaries and trapping the blood within them.

A fourth theory reverses the premise of the back-leak theory, suggesting that decreased permeability of the glomerular membrane restricts filtration without reducing renal or glomerular plasma flow.

The fifth theory, the most popular but also the most controversial, proposes that increased vasoconstriction reduces renal perfusion. Because blood is shunted away from the cortex—the site of most glomeruli—into the medulla, the GFR decreases. Two explanations support this theory. First, vasoconstriction results from the direct action of renin and angiotensin on the kidney, rather than from the effects of plasma renin concentrations. Activation of the renin-angiotensin-aldosterone system may result from hypotension or elevated sodium levels in the macula densa. The sympathetic nervous system may also cause arteriolar vasoconstriction through the effects of circulating catecholamines.

Second, decreased vasodilation may occur because renal damage inhibits secretion of prostaglandins.

### Effects of nephrotoxins and ischemia

Histologically, nephrotoxins cause widespread, uniform necrosis of proximal tubular cells and cast formation in distal nephron segments, but they leave the basement membrane of the nephron intact. Ischemia causes patchy necrosis and cast formation throughout the nephron, especially in the proximal tubule. It also damages basement membrane cells, impairing regeneration. Because the status of the basement membrane and its capacity for cellular regeneration is the key factor in the prognosis of ATN, nephrotoxins usually produce reversible damage, whereas ischemia may produce irreversible damage.

### Stages of reversible ATN

Reversible ATN usually progresses through three stages: oliguria, early diuresis, and late diuresis.

Typically, *oliguria* lasts from 7 to 21 days, but longer duration may herald chronic renal failure. Blood urea nitrogen (BUN) levels rise rapidly, exceeding 20 mg/dl. Soon, tubular repair begins, and epithelial and endothelial cells regenerate. However, sometimes oliguria may not occur.

*Early diuresis,* the second stage, can last up to several weeks. During this stage, the kidneys begin producing small amounts of urine. Urine production doubles daily, and the rapid rise in BUN levels halts.

In *late diuresis,* which can last up to 1 year, daily urine output may exceed 1 liter and BUN levels return to normal. During this recovery stage, renal function continues to improve.

### Irreversible ATN: Prognosis poor

Irreversible ATN can begin in various ways, but it always produces the same effects. Tubular epithelium damage impairs tubular function and reduces the GFR, reducing urine output and increasing reabsorption of metabolic wastes, such as urea nitrogen, into the blood. The tubules fail to selectively reabsorb fluids and electrolytes, to concentrate or dilute urine, and to excrete excess fluid. Also, sodium and potassium retention causes electrolyte imbalance. Anuria is rare in ATN; its presence probably represents an obstruction outside the tubular system, such as in the ureter, bladder, or urethra.

### Uremia: Effects on body chemistry and body systems

Uremia, an imbalance between the patient's metabolism and the kidney's ability to excrete waste and to regulate fluid and electrolyte concentration, accompanies kidney failure. Uremia affects body chemistry—altering substances derived from protein metabolism, electrolytes, pH, acid-base balance, and fluid balance—and body systems.

**Effects on body chemistry.** When the kidney is unable to excrete the end products of protein metabolism, these products—urea, the principal end product; creatinine, the end product of creatine; and uric acid, the end product of urine—accumulate in the blood. Urea accumulation is also influenced by dietary protein, gastrointestinal bleeding, the state of hydration, and the rate of protein breakdown and urea synthesis in the liver.

ARF may cause electrolyte changes: hyperkalemia, hypokalemia, hypernatremia, hyponatremia, hypocalcemia, hypermagnesemia, hypomagnesemia, and metabolic acidosis.

• *Hyperkalemia* may result from increased dietary potassium; protein catabolism, which releases intracellular potassium; and sodium deficit, because sodium enhances potassium secretion in the distal tubes. In the diuretic stage of ARF, *hypokalemia* may occur from drugs or from potassium lost through vomiting and diarrhea.

• *Hypernatremia* occurs when the GFR is reduced and the kidney is unable to excrete sodium. Hypernatremia is complicated by increased dietary sodium and usually leads to water retention. In the diuretic phase, *hyponatremia* may occur because of increased urine output.

• *Hypocalcemia* and secondary hyperparathyroidism may occur because of decreased calcium absorption from the intestine. However, the acidotic state of the patient with uremia prevents tetany, which usually accompanies hypocalcemia.

• In the oliguric stage, *hypermagnesemia* may

# Causes of acute renal failure

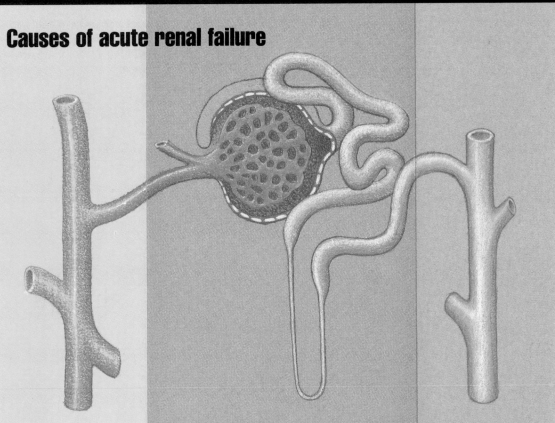

## Prerenal failure

All conditions that lead to prerenal failure impair renal perfusion, resulting in decreased glomerular filtration and increased proximal tubular reabsorption of sodium and water. Causes of prerenal failure include:

**Cardiovascular disorders**
Cardiac tamponade
Cardiogenic shock
Congestive heart failure
Dysrhythmia
Myocardial infarction

**Hypovolemia**
Burns
Dehydration
Diuretic abuse
Hemorrhage
Trauma

**Peripheral vasodilation**
Antihypertensive drugs
Sepsis

**Renovascular obstruction**
Arterial embolism
Arterial or venous
  thrombosis
Tumor

**Severe vasoconstriction**
Disseminated
  intravascular
  coagulation
Eclampsia
Malignant hypertension
Vasculitis

## Intrarenal failure

Parenchymal renal failure, commonly called intrarenal failure, results from damage to the kidneys themselves. Its causes include:

**Acute tubular necrosis**
Ischemic damage to renal parenchyma caused by unrecognized or inadequately treated prerenal failure
*Nephrotoxicity*—analgesics (such as phenacetin), anesthetics (such as methoxyflurane), antibiotics (such as gentamicin), heavy metals (such as lead), iodine-containing radiographic contrast media, organic solvents
*Obstetrical complications*—eclampsia, postpartum renal failure, septic abortion, uterine hemorrhage
*Pigment release*—crush injury, myopathy, sepsis, transfusion reaction

**Other parenchymal disorders**
Acute glomerulonephritis, acute interstitial nephritis, acute pyelonephritis, malignant nephrosclerosis, papillary necrosis, vasculitis

## Postrenal failure

This type of renal failure results from obstruction of urinary flow. Its causes include:

**Bladder obstruction**
Anticholinergic drugs
Autonomic nerve
  dysfunction
Infection
Tumor

**Ureteral obstruction**
Blood clots
Calculi
Edema or inflammation
Necrotic renal papillae
Retroperitoneal fibrosis or
  hemorrhage
Surgery (accidental
  ligation)
Tumors
Uric acid crystals

**Urethral obstruction**
Prostatic hypertrophy or
  tumor
Strictures

result from the kidney's inability to excrete adequate magnesium. Hypermagnesemia may also result from use of magnesium-containing drugs such as antacids. In the diuretic phase or in any stage with persistent vomiting and diarrhea associated with uremia, *hypomagnesemia* may occur.

• *Metabolic acidosis* occurs because of the decreased ability of the kidney to excrete acid, decreased ammonia production by the kidney,

retention of end products of protein metabolism that use available buffers, and decreased ability of the kidney to reabsorb bicarbonate.

**Effects on body systems.** Uremia has a significant effect on most body systems.

• *Hypertension* may occur, probably from activation of the renin-angiotensin-aldosterone system and from fluid overload, which occurs in the oliguric phase of ARF. Hypertension may cause seizures.

## The sodium pump

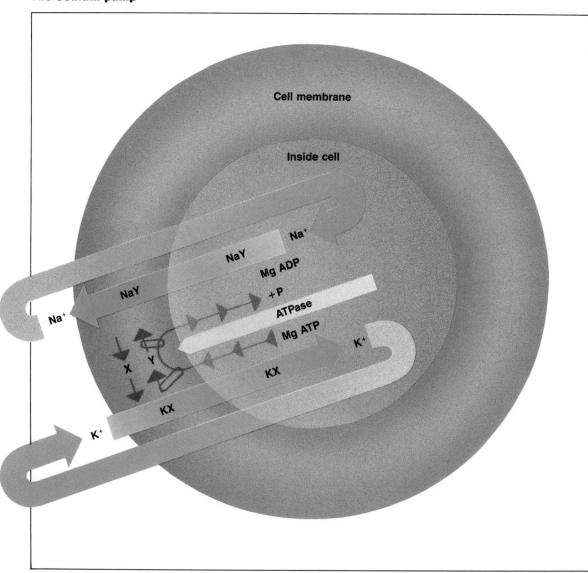

Sodium, the major extracellular cation, helps the kidneys regulate fluid balance. For example, reduced levels of sodium promote water excretion, whereas elevated levels promote water retention. To maintain normal sodium levels and to combat ionic diffusion (the inward movement of sodium ions and the outward movement of potassium ions caused by increased permeability of the cell membrane), an active sodium transport mechanism, called the *sodium pump,* is constantly at work.

Here's how this pump operates. Because sodium and potassium (the major intracellular cation) can't readily penetrate the cell membrane, they combine with a

single lipoprotein carrier—called X in combination with sodium, and Y in combination with potassium. For example, sodium from inside the cell combines with carrier Y to form large quantities of NaY, which diffuses toward the cell's outer surface. Energy provided by adenosine triphosphate (ATP) and adenosine triphosphatase (ATPase) causes release of sodium outside the cells, and Y is transformed to X. Then, carrier X joins potassium, forming KX. As KX within the membrane diffuses inward, ATP and ATPase provide energy to split K from X. K then enters the cell, X undergoes reconversion to Y, and the cycle continues.

• *Systemic edema, congestive heart failure,* and *pulmonary edema* may occur from fluid overload.

• *Uremic pericarditis* and *uremic pneumonitis* may occur from fluid overload.

• *Bleeding tendencies,* such as GI bleeding, may occur, probably from a platelet defect or deficit.

• *Anorexia, nausea,* and *vomiting* may occur, probably from electrolyte imbalance, ammonia intoxication, or acidosis.

• *Behavior changes* or *changes in level of consciousness* may occur from increased serum levels of metabolic toxins.

• *Peripheral neuropathy,* particularly in the legs, and *involuntary muscle twitching,* such as restless leg syndrome, may occur from toxin buildup.

• *Skin changes,* such as dryness, scaliness, and itching, may occur from toxin buildup. Also, the anemia associated with uremia causes gray, chalky skin. Anemia combined with melanin deposits from retained pigments causes a tannish-yellow coloration. In untreated uremia, urea crystallizes from sweat and covers the skin—particularly the face, chest, and abdomen—with uremic frost, a white, powdery material.

• *Hypothermia, susceptibility to infection,* and *reduced wound-healing ability* may result from unknown causes.

## MEDICAL MANAGEMENT

In ARF, diagnostic tests have two major purposes: to classify the type of failure and to determine its cause. The goal of treatment is to correct the cause and to provide support until the tubular epithelial cells regenerate and normal renal function returns.

### Routine tests: BUN and creatinine

Regardless of the cause of ARF, BUN and serum creatinine levels always rise. Nevertheless, elevated BUN levels don't reliably confirm ARF because they reflect both protein intake *and* renal excretory capacity. As a result, ingestion of large amounts of protein and increased protein catabolism (as in burns, fever, or sepsis) can also produce elevated BUN levels.

Serum creatinine provides a more sensitive measure of renal damage than BUN because renal impairment is virtually the sole cause of creatinine level elevation. Because creatinine is easily excreted by the kidneys with little or no tubular reabsorption, its levels are directly related to the GFR. Elevated creatinine levels usually indicate severe damage to 50% or more of the nephrons.

After completion of BUN and creatinine measurements, diagnostic studies attempt to establish if ARF results from prerenal or postrenal causes, which are usually reversible.

### Tests for prerenal failure

*Urinalysis,* perhaps the most valuable test in prerenal failure, may show cellular debris and sediments composed of hyaline or fine granular casts. It usually reveals high urine osmolality (greater than 500 mOsm/liter), sodium levels below 20 mEq/liter, and specific gravity of 1.020 or higher as the kidneys conserve water and sodium to compensate for decreased perfusion. Urine pH may fall below 5.5 because of metabolic acidosis.

*Serum potassium levels* may be depressed from excessive vomiting, diarrhea, or insufficient food intake.

Two other tests help detect the cause of decreased renal perfusion. *Renal angiography* can reveal obstruction or dysplasia of the renal artery. *Hemodynamic monitoring* can demonstrate decreased central venous and pulmonary pressures from hypovolemia.

### Tests for postrenal failure

In postrenal failure, which results from bilateral obstruction of urinary outflow, *urinalysis* reveals sodium levels exceeding 40 mEq/liter but the absence of sediment. Bladder catheterization is performed to determine if the obstruction is urethral. Next, radiographic and sonographic tests help identify the cause of obstruction. *Kidney-ureter-bladder (KUB) radiography* can reveal enlarged kidneys, widened or blocked ureters, or the presence of calculi. *Computerized tomography scan* frequently follows KUB radiography, providing more accurate visualization of the obstruction. *Renal ultrasonography* allows identification of abnormal fluid accumulation within or around the kidneys that may arise from obstruction. It can also detect changes in bladder shape that result from obstruction. *Retrograde ureteropyelography* helps detect obstruction in the calyxes, pelvis, or ureter of the collecting system.

### Tests for intrarenal failure

After excluding prerenal and postrenal failure, diagnostic tests attempt to confirm intrarenal failure. *Urinalysis* reveals cellular casts and large numbers of tubular epithelial cells in the sediment. Urine osmolality is typically less than 350 mOsm/liter, and urine sodium levels exceed 20 mEq/liter. Both urea and creatinine clearance values are depressed.

The *complete blood count* demonstrates reduced hemoglobin and hematocrit levels due to impaired erythropoiesis, hemodilution from fluid overload, or GI bleeding. Transient leukocytosis may develop from stress or tissue damage, but persistent leukocytosis suggests infection. Decreased platelet count may result from impaired bone marrow function.

*Serum electrolyte studies* can reveal various abnormalities. Reduced sodium levels may reflect dilution from fluid retention or may result from extrarenal sodium loss. Elevated potassium levels stem from impaired renal excretion, tissue destruction, blood transfusion, diet, or drugs. Elevated phosphate levels stem from impaired renal excretion and tissue destruction. Blood pH will be low, reflecting metabolic acidosis caused by the kidney's inability to excrete hydrogen ions and by retention of organic acids.

If results of blood and urine tests are inconclusive, *renal biopsy* can help detect the cause of ARF. If oliguria lasts longer than 4 to 6 weeks, biopsy may be necessary to identify the progression of renal failure.

### Treatment
Treatment aims to correct the underlying cause of ARF and to promote regeneration of tubular epithelial cells and the return of normal tubular function. Supportive measures should help to correct uremia, to maintain fluid and electrolyte balance, to provide adequate nutrition, and to prevent complications.

### Prerenal failure: Hydration and diuresis
In prerenal failure, treatment includes replacement fluids to improve hydration and renal perfusion, and diuretics to increase urine output. In oliguria resulting from hypovolemia, I.V. infusion of ½ to 1 liter of normal saline solution over 1 hour usually improves urine output, blood pressure, and central venous pressure. Within a few days, urine output and BUN levels return to normal.

After adequate hydration has been achieved, diuretics may be given to increase urine output. Loop diuretics, such as furosemide and ethacrynic acid, decrease filtrate reabsorption and enhance water excretion. Mannitol, an osmotic diuretic, expands extracellular volume; increases serum osmolality; and is thought to increase glomerular hydrostatic pressure, to inhibit tubular reabsorption of

water and electrolytes during hypoperfusion, and to reduce renin secretion.

If diuretics fail to significantly improve urine output, fluid replacements should be reduced to 500 ml/day to prevent fluid overload. If diuretics cause excessively high serum osmolality, they should be discontinued to prevent cerebral edema.

### Postrenal failure: Removing obstruction
In postrenal failure, treatment usually involves catheterization, to drain urine, and either a surgical or nonsurgical procedure, such as extracorporeal shock wave lithotripsy, to remove the obstructing calculi. Once urine can flow freely, BUN levels rapidly fall to normal. However, postobstruction diuresis causes heavy fluid and electrolyte losses, which, if unreplaced, lead to dehydration and electrolyte imbalance. To prevent hypovolemic and electrolytic imbalance, it's typically necessary to replace about 75% of the previous hour's urine output, along with 720 ml/day (30 ml/hour) for insensible loss.

### Intrarenal failure: Dialysis, nutrients, and drugs
In intrarenal failure, treatment includes dialysis to control uremia, supplemental nutrients to prevent malnutrition, and drugs to combat infection or to prevent complications.

**Peritoneal dialysis.** This form of dialysis removes blood impurities by instilling dialysate solution into the peritoneal cavity via a catheter. (See *Renal mechanisms and dialysis,* pages 74 and 75.) Usually, peritoneal dialysis decreases BUN levels. However, in some patients with rapidly rising BUN levels, peritoneal dialysis works too slowly, and BUN levels may continue to rise despite ongoing dialysis. This procedure can also cause severe complications, such as peritonitis, hypokalemia, hyperglycemia from glucose dialysate solutions, and hypervolemia or hypovolemia. (See *Managing complications of peritoneal dialysis,* pages 82 and 83.)

**Hemodialysis.** This dialysis technique removes blood from the body, circulates it through a dialyzer to remove toxic wastes, and then returns the blood to the body. (See *Renal mechanisms and dialysis,* pages 74 and 75.) Various sites can be used for this lifesaving procedure. (See *Hemodialysis access sites,* pages 78 and 79.)

Hemodialysis is usually performed three or four times weekly to keep BUN levels below

100 mg/dl, to control hydration, and to correct hyperkalemia. In patients with persistent fever, bleeding, or increased protein catabolism, dialysis may be performed daily.

**Continuous slow ultrafiltration (CSUF).** Although this technique doesn't replace dialysis, which is necessary to lower serum levels of accumulating toxic wastes, it does effectively reduce excess fluid, electrolytes, urea, and creatinine. Because isolated ultrafiltration—performed before, during, or after dialysis—removes fluid rapidly (as much as 1 liter/hour), it can cause hemodynamic instability. CSUF, in contrast, removes 150 to 200 ml/hour, over a period of 24 to 48 hours, through an extracorporeal shunt without producing abrupt changes in cardiac output or mean arterial pressure. Equally important, CSUF eliminates the need to restrict fluid intake because it continuously removes excess fluid. Consequently, it allows larger and safer dilution of medications and, if necessary, I.V. hyperalimentation (IVH) in full volumes to meet the patient's nutritional needs.

**Regulating fluid and electrolyte balance.** If CSUF is unavailable, restricted fluid intake and frequent serum tests are necessary to prevent overhydration and electrolyte imbalance.

Because insensible fluid loss averages 800 ml/day, while fluid gain from fat and protein metabolism averages 400 ml/day, fluid replacement is usually restricted to 400 ml/day. Additional replacement fluids can be given to compensate for nasogastric drainage, fever, vomiting, diarrhea, or surgical wound drainage. Later, as the kidneys start to produce urine, urine volume must be replaced as well.

Obtaining accurate daily weight is essential in determining daily fluid allowance. Once daily fluid allowance has been established, all drugs, dietary intake, and other treatment must be controlled within the allowable amount. If blood transfusions must be given, packed cells are preferred over whole blood to avoid infusing excess fluid. If the patient is receiving IVH, dialysis treatments may need to be given more often to handle the extra fluid.

To manage electrolyte balance, serum electrolyte and BUN levels need to be measured at least twice daily. Typically, electrolyte losses are measured and replaced, but maintenance electrolytes are rarely given.

*Hyperkalemia,* the most perilous electrolyte imbalance, prevents normal sodium/potassium exchange. This imbalance is common in ARF. It requires vigorous treatment when serum levels reach 6 mEq/liter (normal plasma value is 3.5 to 5.0 mEq/liter). When potassium rises to hyperkalemic levels, the patient may develop weakness, malaise, nausea, diarrhea, muscle irritability, or intestinal colic. But the most reliable indication of hyperkalemia is the characteristic EKG pattern: tall, peaked T waves; widening QRS segment; and disappearing P waves.

I.V. infusion of sodium bicarbonate or insulin and glucose rapidly lowers potassium levels by effectively forcing potassium back into the cell, but these treatments correct the imbalance only temporarily and may have some rebound effects. Sodium polystyrene sulfonate (Kayexalate), given orally or by retention enema along with sorbitol (to aid expulsion), can correct hyperkalemia overnight by exchanging sodium for potassium in the large intestine. However, if these methods fail to reduce serum potassium levels, hemodialysis may be necessary.

*Hyponatremia* requires stringent fluid restriction to prevent sodium dilution in excessive retained fluid. Severe cases of hyponatremia may require infusion of hypertonic saline solution to prevent seizures. *Hypernatremia* requires increased fluid intake to dilute serum sodium and return it to normal levels.

*Hypocalcemia* usually requires aluminum hydroxide preparations to bind phosphorus in the intestine and to effectively control the calcium:phosphorus ratio. Rarely, it requires calcium supplements.

## Nutrition in ARF

Nutritional management of ARF has improved markedly over the past 20 years—mainly as a result of increased use of feeding tubes, the development of IVH, and improved dialysis techniques. Its aim, though, is virtually unchanged: to restrict intake of sodium, potassium, and protein and to provide adequate calories and essential amino acids.

If the patient is anorectic, small and frequent meals can provide adequate nutrients. If the patient can't tolerate oral intake, feedings instilled through nasogastric, gastrostomy, or jejunostomy tubes can also provide adequate nutrients. However, if gastrointestinal disease or surgery precludes oral or tube feedings, IVH can provide nutrients in amounts that exceed the patient's energy expenditure, thereby achieving anabolism. Because the IVH solution has about six times *(continued on page 76)*

# Renal mechanisms and dialysis

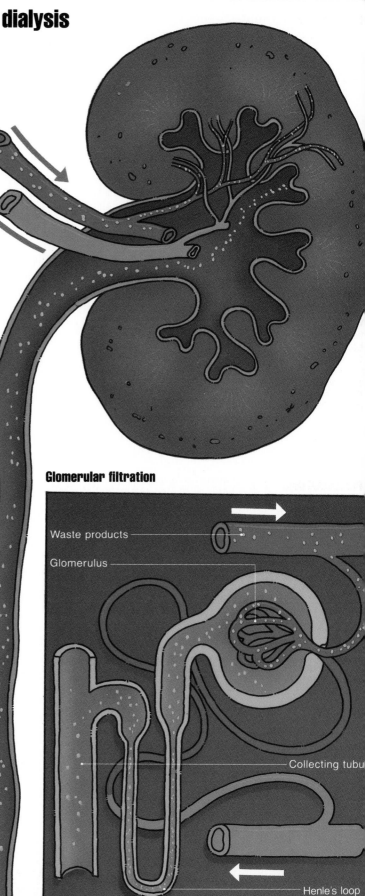

The kidneys remove excess water and waste products and maintain fluid, electrolyte, and acid-base balance.

*Filtration* results from the pressure gradient between the blood in glomerular capillaries and the surrounding interstitial space of Bowman's capsule. Higher glomerular pressure pushes fluid out of the capillaries into Bowman's capsule. During filtration, the semipermeable glomerular membrane acts as a molecular sieve—letting water, electrolytes, glucose, and waste products out, but retaining larger proteins and red blood cells.

*Reabsorption* selectively retains useful substances: water, glucose, sodium, bicarbonate, calcium, and amino acids are almost completely reabsorbed; nitrogenous wastes (urea, creatinine), toxins, dyes, and other compounds are largely excreted.

**Hemodialysis.** When kidney function fails, an external dialyzing system can remove toxic wastes. As blood is pumped through the dialyzer, pressure and concentration gradients between the blood and the dialysis solution remove toxic wastes and excess water. Because the blood contains toxic wastes and higher concentrations of hydrogen ions and other electrolytes, these solutes diffuse across the membrane into the solution. Any solute that's more concentrated in the dialysis solution (glucose or bicarbonate) diffuses into the blood. Thus, hemodialysis removes excess water and toxins, reverses acidosis, and corrects electrolyte abnormalities.

**Peritoneal dialysis.** The peritoneum, the membranous lining of the peritoneal cavity, surrounds the abdominal organs and contacts the rich capillary network of the intestinal walls and mesentery. Its enormous surface area (about 22,000 cm²), which approaches that of the glomerular membranes, makes it an effective dialyzing membrane.

**Glomerular filtration**

Waste products

Glomerulus

Collecting tubu

Henle's loop

## Hemodialysis

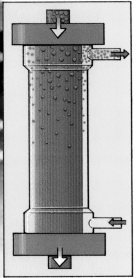

Within the dialyzer, blood flows through hollow fibers, plates, or coils of semipermeable material while a special dialysis solution is pumped around the other side under hydrostatic pressure.

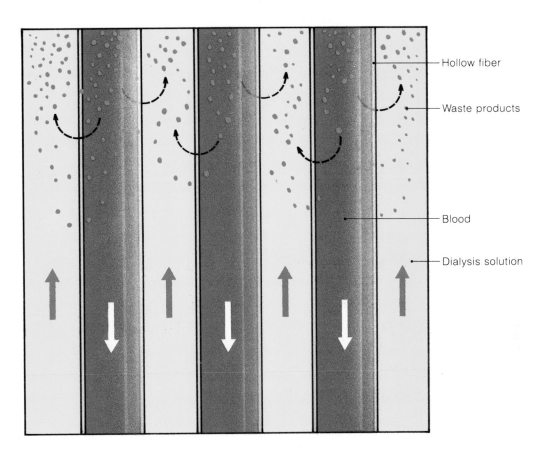

- Hollow fiber
- Waste products
- Blood
- Dialysis solution

## Peritoneal dialysis

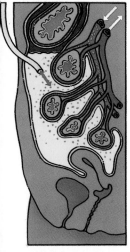

In peritoneal dialysis, a hypertonic dialyzing solution is instilled into the peritoneal cavity. By *osmosis*, water moves from the blood into the dialysis solution; by *diffusion*, excessive concentrations of toxins also move across the membrane. After an appropriate dwell time, the dialysis solution is drained, taking toxins with it.

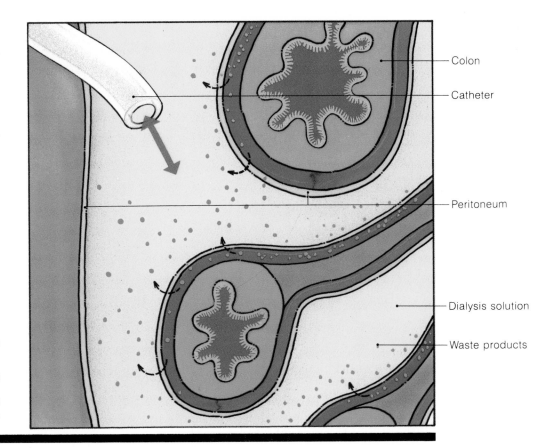

- Colon
- Catheter
- Peritoneum
- Dialysis solution
- Waste products

the solute concentration of blood, it requires delivery into a high-flow central vein to avoid injuring peripheral vasculature. Usually, this solution is delivered to the superior vena cava through an indwelling subclavian vein catheter inserted by the infraclavicular approach or, less often, by the supraclavicular, internal jugular, or antecubital fossa approach. Because the high glucose concentration of the IVH solution provides a good medium for bacterial and yeast growth and the central venous line gives systemic access, contamination and sepsis are always a risk. The high glucose concentration of the IVH solution requires monitoring of serum glucose to detect the body's ability to handle it. Insulin may need to be administered if serum glucose levels rise. Also, the large volume of instilled solution may require additional hemodialysis treatments to eliminate excess fluid.

### Preventing complications of ARF

Because azotemia can mask obvious signs of infection such as fever, the white blood cell (WBC) count is an important diagnostic tool in ARF. But because the WBC count decreases greatly during hemodialysis (from blood stagnation in the dialyzer or leukocyte migration to the lungs), serum samples should always be drawn 1 to 2 hours after dialysis treatment. Other diagnostic tests, such as the chest X-ray, can help detect pneumonia.

If infection does occur, aggressive antibiotic therapy is necessary. However, because hemodialysis removes most antibiotics from the blood, new loading doses are required after each treatment.

To prevent stress ulcers and uremic gastroenteropathy, aluminum hydroxide gels should be administered. Cimetidine helps prevent or control GI bleeding.

### NURSING MANAGEMENT

In ARF, a complete history and physical examination are a must for correct diagnosis and treatment. But both of these assessment steps take considerable time—time that the patient may not be able to spare at admission because of rapidly progressive uremia and deteriorating renal function. As a result, you may have to gather history information from the patient's family or complete your history after the patient's condition stabilizes.

### Take the patient history

Start with the chief complaint, which usually involves altered urination. If the patient says he's voiding "nothing," define if he's voiding less than usual or nothing at all. Oliguria is common in ARF; true anuria is rare and usually associated with obstruction.

**Define the pattern of urination.** Ask the patient to describe any changes in the pattern of urination. Remember, nonoliguric renal failure doesn't reduce urine volume. Also remember that urinating small amounts frequently, a feeling of fullness after bladder emptying, or the inability to control urination can indicate infection or obstruction.

Ask about urine color. Dark amber urine may indicate prerenal failure related to depletion of fluid volume. Clear, colorless urine represents very diluted urine. Red- or brown-tinged urine suggests glomerular disease.

Next, ask the patient about pain. If present, ask about its onset, quality, and location. Painful spasms during urination may indicate renal calculi; a burning sensation may indicate a lower urinary tract infection. Abdominal pain or distention may suggest a tumor.

Check the family history for disorders that can cause renal failure or affect therapy. Congenital renal anomalies, for example, could cause decreased perfusion or obstruction. Diabetes, hypertension, and cardiovascular disease may lead to kidney damage. Renal calculi recur in some families. High uric acid levels associated with gout may cause crystal formation, leading to tubular obstruction.

**Review the medical history.** Ask about previous kidney dysfunction. A history of prostate disease, colon disease, malignancies, renal calculi, urethral strictures, progressive voiding difficulties, or bladder disorders suggests postrenal failure. Also ask about hypertension, atherosclerosis, myocardial infarction, or other cardiovascular diseases, all of which can lead to renal damage. Likewise, diabetes mellitus, systemic lupus erythematosus, sickle cell anemia, or acute pyelonephritis can damage the kidneys and lead to renal failure.

Determine if the patient has suffered a recent infection or sore throat. Beta-hemolytic streptococci commonly attack the glomeruli, causing acute glomerulonephritis. Ask about pulmonary symptoms. For example, if the patient complains of spitting blood, suspect Goodpasture's syndrome with its accompanying glomerulonephritis. If the patient is pregnant, check carefully for signs of toxemia, which can cause oliguria and, if untreated, renal shutdown.

**Review surgery and trauma.** Major abdominal surgery or trauma accompanied by pro-

# Comparing hemodialysis and peritoneal dialysis

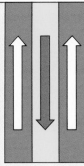

## Hemodialysis

### Advantages
• Takes only 3 to 5 hours per treatment
• Requires only three treatments weekly
• In emergency, I.V. administration avoids surgical access route

### Disadvantages
• Requires surgical creation of vascular access between circulation and dialysis machine
• Requires complex water treatment, expensive dialysis equipment, and highly trained personnel
• Requires larger doses of heparin
• Confines patient to special treatment unit
• Contraindicated in shock and hypotension. Must be used cautiously in infants, small children, and patients with cardiovascular disease
• May cause dysrhythmia, septicemia, air emboli, rapid fluid and electrolyte imbalance (disequilibrium syndrome), hemolytic anemia, metastatic calcification, hepatitis, hypotension, hypertension, itching, pain (generalized or in chest), hemorrhage from heparin toxicity, leg cramps, nausea, vomiting, headache

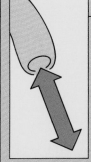

## Peritoneal dialysis

### Advantages
• Can be performed immediately
• Requires less complex equipment and less specialized personnel than hemodialysis
• Requires small amounts of heparin or none at all
• Causes no blood loss and minimal cardiovascular stress; doesn't require venipuncture
• Can be performed by patient anywhere without assistance
• Allows patient independence without long interruptions in daily activities
• Rarely causes disequilibrium syndrome
• May be used for patients with unstable cardiovascular status. Gives better results than hemodialysis in children and diabetic patients with renal failure
• Allows for more liberal diet
• Costs less

### Disadvantages
• Requires 48 to 72 hours for significant response to treatment. May require more than three treatments weekly
• Severe protein loss necessitates high-protein diet (up to 100 g/day).
• High risk of peritonitis: repeated bouts may cause scarring, preventing further treatments with peritoneal dialysis
• Urea clearance less than with hemodialysis
• Requires abdomen free from recent surgery, adhesions, or infection
• May cause dysrhythmia; hyperglycemia; bacterial or chemical peritonitis; pain (abdominal, low back, shoulder); shortness of breath or dyspnea; atelectasis; pneumonia; severe protein loss; fluid overload or loss; constipation; catheter site inflammation, infection, or leakage

---

longed shock can reduce renal perfusion, leading to ischemia and ARF. Massive crush injuries release the pigment myoglobin into the bloodstream, causing tubular obstruction and cast formation. Surgical clamping of the aorta can cause postoperative oliguria. Accidental ligation of the ureters can occur during vaginal or pelvic surgery. Transfusion reaction can cause hemolysis and ARF. Severe allergic reaction to radiographic contrast media can also cause ARF.

**Consider the patient's occupation and lifestyle.** Ask about the patient's workplace to detect exposure to heavy metals or toxic industrial solvents. If he lives or has traveled in the south or southwest, ask about recent snakebites. If you suspect that the patient abuses drugs, ask about sniffing glue, carbon tetrachloride, or other toxins that can cause ARF. Consider that homosexual males with multiple partners may contract acquired immune deficiency syndrome (AIDS). Because AIDS suppresses the immune response and leaves the body vulnerable to infection, it can lead to renal hypoperfusion, ischemia, and ARF. And, to help you plan total care, ask about the patient's support system—family, friends, and social or religious organizations.

**Review the drug history.** Ask about use of prescription and over-the-counter drugs. Prolonged use of nephrotoxic antibiotics, such as tetracyclines and aminoglycosides, can lead to ARF. Diuretic abuse can lead to hypovolemia, hyperkalemia, and ARF. Appetite-suppressing drugs or prolonged weight-reduction diets can lead to renal dysfunction.

### Head-to-toe physical examination
Begin the physical examination by taking vital signs. Fever may indicate infection or sepsis, but it's often masked by azotemia. Mild tachy-
*(continued on page 80)*

# Hemodialysis access sites

| Site and method | Insertion procedure | Advantages and disadvantages |
|---|---|---|
| **Femoral vein catheterization** 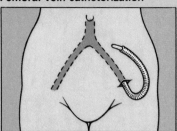 | Using the Seldinger technique, the doctor inserts an introducer needle into the right or left femoral vein. He then inserts a guide wire through the introducer needle and removes the needle. Using the guide wire, he threads a catheter into the vein. The doctor may use a single catheter with a Y hub. Or, if he uses two catheters, he'll insert the second catheter for outflow ½" (1.3 cm) distal to the inflow catheter. | *Advantage:* <br>• Quick emergency access <br>*Disadvantages:* <br>• Immobile patient <br>• Risk of infection and femoral artery puncture |
| **Subclavian vein catheterization** 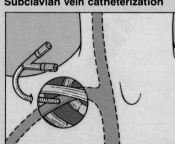 | Using the Seldinger technique, the doctor inserts an introducer needle into the subclavian vein. He then inserts a guide wire through the introducer needle and removes the needle. Using the guide wire, he threads a 5" to 12" (12.7 to 30.5 cm) plastic or Teflon catheter (with Y-connector) into the vein. | *Advantages:* <br>• Quick emergency access <br>• Mobile patient <br>• Less risk of infection than with femoral vein catheterization <br>*Disadvantages:* <br>• Risk of pneumothorax on insertion <br>• Contraindicated in pulmonary hypertension |
| **Arteriovenous shunt** 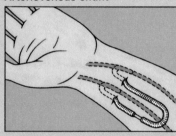 | After making an incision in the patient's wrist or ankle, the doctor inserts one 6" to 10" (15.2 to 25.4 cm) transparent Silastic cannula into an artery and another into a vein. He tunnels the cannulas out through stab wounds and connects them with a 1" (2.5 cm) piece of Teflon tubing. | *Advantages:* <br>• Arterial blood pressure pumps blood <br>• No repeated catheterization or venipuncture <br>*Disadvantages:* <br>• Restricted activity of affected arm or leg <br>• Increased risk of clotting and infection <br>• Chance of accidental separation causing hemorrhage or death |
| **Arteriovenous fistula** 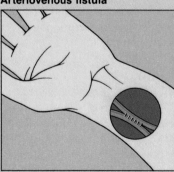 | After making an incision in the patient's wrist, the doctor makes a small incision in the side of an artery and another incision in the side of a vein. He sutures the edges of these incisions together to create a common opening 3 to 7 mm long. | *Advantages:* <br>• Arterial blood pressure pumps blood <br>• Minimal risk of infection or clotting <br>• Less need for revision than with shunt <br>• Unrestricted use of affected arm or leg <br>*Disadvantages:* <br>• Contraindicated in patients with small veins <br>• Possible numbness, tingling, and coldness below fistula site from arterial insufficiency in atherosclerotic or diabetic patients |
| **Arteriovenous vein graft** 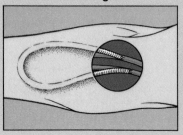 | The doctor makes an incision in the patient's forearm, upper arm, or thigh. Then he tunnels the natural or synthetic graft subcutaneously. He sutures the distal end of the graft to an artery. He sutures the proximal end to a vein. | *Advantages:* <br>• Arterial blood pressure pumps blood <br>• Unrestricted use of grafted arm or leg <br>*Disadvantages:* <br>• Risk of clotting from hypotension and steal syndrome <br>• Risk of infecting tissues surrounding graft |

## Nursing considerations

Use temporarily (about 1 week).
• To prevent clotting, start hemodialysis immediately after insertion.
• After treatment, flush the catheters and fill them with heparinized normal saline solution. Cap and cover them with a sterile dressing.
• Don't allow the patient to walk or sit up in bed. He may dislodge the catheter, damage the vein, or obstruct the blood flow.

Use temporarily (1 to 2 weeks).
• With a Y-connector, use venipuncture equipment, which alternately clamps arterial and venous tubes.
• If the catheter is used only for outflow, insert an over-the-needle catheter into the antecubital vein in the arm opposite the catheter to accommodate venous return.
• Prevent clotting, and flush the catheter as for femoral vein catheterization.

Use temporarily or permanently (average 7 to 10 months).
• Have the patient keep the affected arm or leg straight and elevated for 2 or 3 hours after insertion. For a leg shunt, have the patient use crutches for 3 weeks. Caution him to restrict activity in the arm or leg.
• Assess the shunt site often for good arterial flow. Palpate for thrills and auscultate for bruits.
• Inspect frequently for signs of infection.
• Check blood color in the shunt. Bright red indicates normal flow; dark red to purple indicates a clot is forming; purple-red to black (with separation of purple cells and clear serum) indicates a clotted shunt.
• Instruct the patient to keep the shunt clean and dry. Prohibit bathing for 2 to 3 weeks after insertion. Tell the patient to protect the shunt with plastic once bathing is allowed.
• Don't use the affected arm or leg for blood pressure readings or venipunctures.
• Prohibit tight jewelry or clothing over the shunt site.

Use permanently (average 3 to 4 years).
• Keep the affected arm elevated immediately after fistula surgery.
• Remove dressings after 2 days; clean the suture line with povidone-iodine solution. Apply new sterile dressings daily for 10 to 14 days, until the sutures are removed.
• The fistula may require 6 weeks to mature so that blood vessels are enlarged and walls thickened. But, if necessary, you may perform hemodialysis within 1 week after surgery.
• Assess for blood flow as for the arteriovenous shunt.
• Wash the affected arm daily with antibacterial soap.
• Don't use the affected arm for blood pressure readings or for venipunctures, except for venipunctures when performing hemodialysis.
• Prohibit tight jewelry or clothing over the fistula site.

Use permanently (average 2 years).
• Keep the affected arm or leg elevated immediately after grafting.
• Remove dressings after 2 days; clean the suture line with povidone-iodine solution. Apply new sterile dressings daily for 10 to 14 days, until the sutures are removed.
• Assess for blood flow as for the arteriovenous shunt or fistula. Observe the same restrictions regarding blood pressure readings, venipunctures, and wearing of jewelry and clothing. (To prolong graft life, perform venipuncture using a single-needle, double-lumen catheter.)

## Tips for infusing glucose-insulin solutions

If supportive treatments fail to correct severe hyperkalemia, glucose-insulin infusion can reduce serum potassium levels. If the doctor orders this infusion, keep these pointers in mind.
• Initially infuse 200 to 300 ml of a 50% glucose solution containing 30 to 50 units of regular insulin. After 30 and 60 minutes, decrease the infusion rate, and draw serum samples to determine potassium levels. The infusion should reduce potassium levels by 1 to 2 mEq/liter/12 to 24 hours.
• If the doctor also orders sodium bicarbonate (usually two to four ampuls), add this drug to the glucose-insulin solution for infusion. Sodium bicarbonate raises blood pH, which causes cellular exchange of potassium and hydrogen and promotes potassium excretion.
• Be alert for signs of fluid overload, especially edema.
• Remember that glucose-insulin therapy produces only temporary improvement. Dialysis or the administration of sodium polystyrene sulfonate (Kayexalate) is necessary to correct hyperkalemia.

cardia with normal or slightly elevated blood pressure may indicate fluid overload; marked tachycardia signals shock. An irregular pulse suggests electrolyte imbalance, possibly hyperkalemia. Kussmaul's respirations may result from severe acidosis or right heart failure.

Next, weigh the patient to establish a baseline for evaluating fluid status. Then ask him to lie flat in bed. If he is unable to do so without respiratory distress, suspect fluid overload. If he changes position frequently to relieve flank pain, suspect renal obstruction.

**Assess neurologic status.** Check the patient's level of consciousness. Is he oriented to date, time, and place, or does he appear lethargic and confused? Electrolyte imbalance and accumulation of uremic toxins can cause decreased awareness, poor concentration, memory loss, and headaches.

**Assess the eyes.** Check the retina for small infarctions, hemorrhage, or cotton-wool patches, especially in patients with hypertension. Also check for papilledema, which suggests fluid overload, and sunken eyeballs, which suggests hypovolemia.

**Assess the skin.** First, examine skin color. A gray, chalky appearance can result from low erythropoietin levels; a tannish-yellow appearance, from retained pigments; and fine, white, powdery deposits on the face, chest, and abdomen (uremic frost), from persistent uremia. Then check for bruises from clotting abnormalities. Check skin turgor to assess hydration. Skin that doesn't assume its normal shape immediately after pinching, or dry, itchy skin may indicate hypovolemia. Dry mucous membranes may also indicate hypovolemia. Next, evaluate skin temperature. Hot, dry skin can indicate infection, and cold, clammy skin can indicate hypotension and shock.

Check all dependent areas for edema (see *Testing for peripheral edema*). Check the ambulatory patient's legs and ankles and the bedridden patient's sacral area. Diffuse edema with jugular vein distention indicates fluid overload.

**Assess cardiovascular status.** Auscultate for abnormal heart sounds. Listen carefully for $S_3$, which may signify fluid overload. Also auscultate for friction rub—a result of uremic pericarditis. Next, check heart rhythm. An irregular rhythm may result from electrolyte imbalance, especially hyperkalemia.

**Assess respiratory status.** First, check for labored breathing. Then listen for crackles and wheezes, which may indicate pulmonary edema from fluid overload.

**Assess GI status.** Check the abdomen for ascites—the result of fluid overload or urinary obstruction. Observe for signs of GI bleeding, and listen for bowel sounds to detect ileus.

**Assess genitourinary status.** Check for signs of bladder distention, flank pain, or tumors, which may indicate areas of obstruction.

**Assess the musculoskeletal system.** Observe for flaccid or twitching muscles, which can indicate electrolyte imbalance, commonly hyperkalemia.

### Formulate nursing diagnoses

By integrating the information from the patient's history, physical examination, and laboratory studies, you can develop nursing diagnoses and formulate a flexible care plan. In ARF, typical nursing diagnoses include:

**Altered fluid balance related to hypovolemic shock or fluid overload.** Your goal is to restore and maintain fluid balance. Monitor vital signs, especially blood pressure, to assess renal perfusion. Replace or restrict I.V. or oral fluids, as ordered. Fluid intake should be balanced with output. The allowable daily fluid intake should equal the previous day's output plus 400 ml to replace insensible fluid loss. When fluid restriction is severe, spread the amount of fluid allowed over the entire day. To quench the patient's thirst, offer him ice chips. Measure and accurately record intake and output; be sure to include the ice chips as well as wound and nasogastric drainage and diarrhea. Weigh the patient daily to help determine fluid balance. If he's receiving dialysis treatments, be alert for signs of excessive fluid loss—hypotension and weight loss.

Consider your interventions successful if the patient's blood pressure remains within normal limits; urinary output is 30 to 100 ml/hour; and, in hypovolemia, daily weight increases to normal levels or, in fluid overload, daily weight decreases.

**Altered cardiac output related to hypovolemic shock, fluid overload, or dysrhythmia.** Your goal is to restore and maintain adequate cardiac output. Monitor vital signs, especially heart rate and blood pressure. Frequently check the EKG to detect dysrhythmia, and give oxygen as necessary. Treat dysrhythmias immediately, as ordered. Medicate chest pain, as needed. Assess heart and lung sounds at the beginning and end of each shift; notify the doctor of any change from normal, such as onset of friction rub or $S_3$. Check peripheral pulses to determine adequate tissue perfusion. Monitor intraarterial and intracardiac

## Testing for peripheral edema

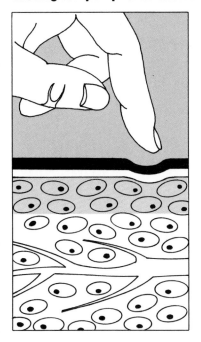

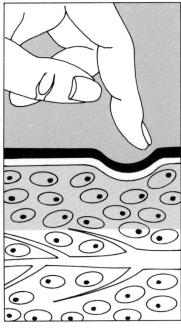

Edema—the buildup of excess sodium and water in interstitial spaces—can signal renal dysfunction. Suspect edema in any swollen area, especially the legs.

To test for edema, press a finger against the suspected edematous area for 5 seconds. Then quickly remove your finger. If edema's present, the skin won't rebound to its original contour right away. Instead, you'll notice a small depression, or pit, in the skin. Measure pitting with a scale approved by your hospital. If you're using the widely accepted four-point scale, record barely perceptible pitting (shown at left) as +1. Record deep pitting (at right), which takes over 30 seconds to rebound, as +4.

pressures, as indicated. If the patient shows signs of hypovolemic shock, give fluids or vasopressors, as required, and place him in Trendelenburg's position, if necessary. If hypovolemia and cardiogenic shock have been ruled out as potential causes of altered cardiac output, suspect septic shock.

Consider your interventions effective if the EKG reveals no dysrhythmia, the patient's blood pressure remains within normal limits, he shows no signs of dehydration, his peripheral pulses are strong, and his cardiac output remains within normal limits.

**Ineffective breathing patterns related to fluid overload, pain, or infusion of peritoneal dialysate.** Your goal is to restore unassisted and comfortable breathing.

Raise the head of the bed so the patient can more easily expand his chest. Give oxygen, as ordered, and encourage deep breathing and coughing every 2 to 4 hours. Frequently turn the patient, and percuss the chest to aerate the lungs and to loosen secretions. If a peritoneal catheter has been inserted, the patient may have incisional pain when trying to deep breathe and cough. If so, give pain medications, as necessary, to promote comfort before deep-breathing exercises. Teach the patient to splint his incision for effective coughing.

Provide dialysis treatment, as ordered, to remove excess fluid and accumulating toxins, thereby improving ventilation. If the patient is receiving peritoneal dialysis, check the out-

flow tubing on the peritoneal dialysis setup for kinks or poor connections to ensure proper drainage so the patient won't become overhydrated. If the patient has difficulty breathing after peritoneal dialysate instillation, check with the doctor about instilling smaller volumes more frequently.

Evaluate your interventions. They were successful if the patient is breathing comfortably without assistance, he is able to splint his incision to cough and breathe deeply, and dialysis improves ventilation.

**Altered urinary elimination pattern related to fluid imbalance, shock, or obstruction.** Your goal is to restore a normal urinary elimination pattern. If the patient's hypovolemic, administer I.V. fluids and drugs, as ordered, to increase renal perfusion and to restore function. Monitor vital signs, especially blood pressure, and measure and record intake, output, and daily weight to assess fluid status. If the patient is hypervolemic or uremic, perform either hemodialysis or peritoneal dialysis, as ordered, to decrease fluid overload. If necessary, prepare the patient for surgery to remove the obstruction.

Consider your interventions successful if the patient shows a normal urinary elimination pattern, his blood pressure remains within normal limits, and he has gained no weight or is expected to lose 1 kg/day.

**Alteration in electrolyte balance: Hyperkalemia related to renal failure.** Your goal is to prevent or correct potassium imbalance and

# Managing complications of peritoneal dialysis

During peritoneal dialysis, 2 to 4 liters of dialysate solution are instilled into the peritoneal cavity over 5 to 10 minutes. The dialysate is left in the peritoneal cavity long enough to allow excess fluid, electrolytes, and accumulated wastes to move through the peritoneal membrane into the dialysate—anywhere from 10 minutes to 4 hours. At the end of the prescribed dwelling time, dialysate is removed into the drainage bag, and the entire cycle is repeated using new solution. During peritoneal dialysis, keep these special considerations in mind.

• To reduce the risk of peritonitis, use strict aseptic technique. Change the catheter dressing every 24 hours or whenever it becomes wet or soiled.

• To prevent respiratory distress, monitor the patient's respiratory status, and promote lung expansion through turning, coughing, and deep-breathing exercises. If respiratory distress is severe, drain the peritoneal cavity of dialyzing fluid and notify the doctor.

• If 4.25% dextrose solution is being instilled, watch for excessive fluid loss and hyperglycemia—severe hyperglycemia may require insulin injection or addition of insulin to the dialysate.

• Check serum potassium levels since hypokalemia may require addition of potassium to the dialysate solution to prevent further losses.

to maintain normal cardiac rhythm. Monitor serum potassium levels, and watch for signs and symptoms of hyperkalemia: tachycardia, malaise, anorexia, and muscle weakness. Alert the doctor to elevated serum potassium levels. If they rise above 6 mEq/liter, infuse sodium bicarbonate or glucose-insulin solution, and administer a sodium polystyrene sulfonate enema, as ordered. Restrict potassium intake and, if necessary, provide hemodialysis or peritoneal dialysis to promote removal of excess potassium.

Consider your interventions successful if potassium levels remain within normal limits or, if hyperkalemia develops, drug therapy or dialysis corrects it.

**Inadequate nutrition related to nausea, vomiting, or dietary restriction.** Your goal is to maintain nutritional balance. Provide a high-calorie, low-protein, low-sodium, and low-potassium diet with vitamin supplements. Give the anorectic patient small, frequent meals. To combat nausea, provide high-calorie, low-protein snacks between meals. Monitor blood

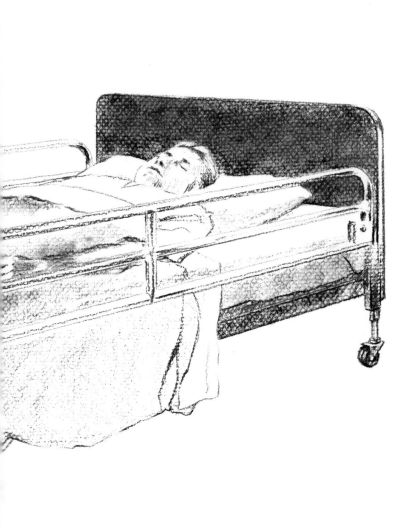

• Carefully monitor fluid balance, blood pressure, and pulse. Notify the doctor if the patient retains 500 ml or more of fluid for three cycles in a row, or if he loses 1 liter or more of fluid for three cycles in a row. Weigh the patient daily when his peritoneal cavity is empty.

• If inflow and outflow are slow or absent, check the tubing for kinks. You can also try raising the I.V. pole or repositioning the patient to increase the inflow rate. Applying manual pressure to the lateral aspects of the patient's abdomen may help increase drainage. If these maneuvers fail to improve the flow rate, notify the doctor.

• Always examine outflow fluid (effluent) for color and clarity. Normally, it's clear and pale yellow, but pink-tinged effluent is common during the first three to four cycles. However, if the effluent remains pink-tinged or becomes grossly bloody, suspect bleeding into the peritoneal cavity, and notify the doctor.

• If the patient feels pain during the procedure, determine when it occurs, its quality and duration, and whether it radiates to other body parts, and then notify the doctor. Remember, patient discomfort at the start of the procedure is normal. Pain during infusion usually results from a cold or acidic dialysate solution. Pain may also result from rapid inflow; slowing the inflow rate may reduce the pain. Severe, diffuse pain with rebound tenderness (and cloudy effluent) may indicate peritoneal infection. Pain that radiates to the shoulder often results from air accumulation under the diaphragm. Perineal or rectal pain can result from improper catheter placement.

chemistry studies, especially of potassium, albumin, and protein, to evaluate nutritional status. If the patient can't ingest an adequate amount of nutrients, notify the doctor. If the patient can't tolerate oral feedings, give nasogastric or jejunostomy feedings or IVH in order to ensure an anabolic state.

Evaluate your interventions. Consider them successful if the patient receives adequate nutrients by oral, tube, or IVH feedings and if potassium, protein, and albumin levels remain within normal limits.

**Potential for sepsis related to immune system compromise.** Your goal is to prevent sepsis by recognizing infection and treating it aggressively. Collect blood samples for culture, and obtain a chest X-ray. Use meticulous aseptic technique when performing catheterization and dressing changes. Use of intermittent catheterization instead of an indwelling (Foley) catheter has been shown to reduce the risk of catheter-related infection. Also use aseptic technique when assisting with insertion of a hyperalimentation line; a peritoneal

## Special considerations for effective hemodialysis

Although hemodialysis is usually performed in a special unit, it can be performed at bedside, especially if the patient is acutely ill. If you need to prepare the patient and the hemodialysis equipment, keep these special considerations in mind.
• Use strict aseptic technique while preparing the machine to avoid pyogenic reactions.
• Immediately report any machine malfunction or equipment defect.
• Don't handle shunt tubing unnecessarily. However, be sure to inspect the shunt carefully for patency by observing its color, inspecting for clots and serum and cell separation, and checking the temperature of the Silastic tubing. Assess the shunt insertion site for signs of infection, such as bloody or serosanguineous drainage, inflammation, and tenderness, which may indicate the body's rejection of the shunt.
• Check also to see if the shunt insertion tips have become exposed. If the ends of the shunt are split, cut off the deteriorated portion behind the split to prevent leakage.
*During hemodialysis:*
• Make sure you complete each step in this procedure accurately. Overlooking a single step or performing it incorrectly can cause unnecessary blood loss or inefficient treatment due to poor clearances or inadequate fluid removal.
• Carefully monitor vital signs. Take blood pressure at least hourly and, if needed, every 15 minutes.
• Periodically check blood lines to make sure connections are secure.
• Periodically perform tests for clotting time on the patient's blood and on samples from the dialyzer.
• Continue giving needed drugs during dialysis unless the drug would be removed in the dialysate; if so, give after dialysis.

## Managing hemodialysis complications

| Complications | Possible causes | Nursing considerations |
|---|---|---|
| Internal hemorrhage | Excessive heparinization | Reduce the heparin dose, or use minimal or regional heparinization. Observe the patient for signs of internal bleeding; apprehension; restlessness; pale, cold, clammy skin; excessive thirst; hypotension, rapid, weak, and thready pulse; increased respirations; and decreased temperature. If ordered, perform a blood transfusion. |
| External hemorrhage | Line disconnection | Observe blood lines for leakage. Keep clamps ready in case any line disconnects, and keep a blood pressure cuff nearby to use as a tourniquet. |
| Hepatitis | Transfusion with infected blood | Use aseptic technique when performing blood transfusion and dialysis; wear gloves, particularly if you have an open wound; and cap all needles. Test the patient for hepatitis every 4 weeks. If the patient develops hepatitis, keep him in isolation during hemodialysis. |
| Dialysis disequilibrium syndrome (headache, fatigue, muscle agitation, twitching, and confusion, possibly leading to grand mal seizure) | Rapid shift of fluid and electrolyte levels | Reduce blood flow, and inform the doctor immediately. He may order diazepam or phenytoin sodium, or he may discontinue dialysis. |
| Hypotension | Septic shock, decreased cardiac output, or reduced blood volume from extracorporeal circulation | Place the patient in Trendelenburg's position. Infuse normal saline solution, as necessary, to restore blood volume. If ordered, administer mannitol, plasma, or albumin. Check blood pressure every 10 minutes until it stabilizes. |
| Dysrhythmia or angina | Rapid shift of fluid and electrolyte levels, reduced blood volume from extracorporeal circulation, or reduced hematocrit level | As ordered, give sodium polystyrene sulfonate (Kayexalate) for hyperkalemia, blood transfusions for decreased blood volume, or antiarrhythmics. |
| Muscle cramping | Rapid shift of fluid and electrolyte levels | If ordered, administer normal saline solution infused with 100 ml 25% mannitol, 10 ml 23% sodium chloride, or 50 ml dextrose 50%. |
| Lower back pain | Too rapid blood flow rate at start of hemodialysis | Reduce the blood flow rate. |
| Air embolism | Insufficient blood flow, empty I.V. bag, or loose connections | Monitor the blood flow rate carefully, clamp the I.V. line before the bag empties, and make sure tubing connections are secure. If the patient develops cyanosis, hypotension, or weak, rapid pulse, turn him onto his left side and lower the head of the bed. This position will help keep on the right side of his heart any air that's entered, so that the pulmonary artery can absorb air bubbles. Notify the doctor immediately. |

dialysis catheter; or any other invasive device, such as a Swan-Ganz catheter. Since azotemia can mask fever, look for other signs of infection, such as warm, tender, reddened areas and purulent drainage. Report any evidence of infection immediately so aggressive therapy can begin. Give antibiotics, as ordered, to combat infection. Watch for signs and symptoms of septic shock, such as oliguria, sudden fever, chills, nausea, vomiting, diarrhea, restlessness, irritability, tachycardia, tachypnea, and hypotension. Institute and plan for pulmonary care to prevent pneumonia. This plan should include coughing and deep-breathing exercises, incentive spirometry, and chest physiotherapy to help mobilize secretions, to keep airways patent, and to decrease the risk of infection. Assess lung sounds to determine signs of pneumonia.

Consider your interventions successful if the patient is afebrile and free of infection; blood cultures and chest X-ray are normal; and the patient shows no signs of access site infection, septic shock, or pneumonia.

**Activity intolerance related to waste product accumulation, fluid overload, or decreased hematocrit levels.** Your goal is to increase the patient's activity tolerance. Monitor fluid balance and electrolyte, BUN, creatinine, and hematocrit levels. During and after hemodialysis or peritoneal dialysis, be especially alert for electrolyte or fluid imbalance. Administer blood or anabolic steroids, as ordered, to help increase hematocrit levels. Monitor nutritional status by measuring serum protein levels. When administering blood, watch for signs of transfusion reaction, such as chills, rash, or pruritus. If you observe any evidence of reaction, stop the blood infusion and notify the doctor. Encourage the patient to eat small, frequent meals, or provide supplemental feedings. Perform passive range-of-motion (ROM) exercises, or promote active ROM exercises. Encourage early ambulation.

Consider your interventions successful if the patient eats sufficiently and exercises and if fluid status and blood chemistry studies are within normal limits.

**Altered mentation related to waste product accumulation.** Your goal is to restore normal thought processes. Explain all procedures in terms the patient can understand, and monitor BUN and serum creatinine levels. Use a radio, TV, or clock to keep him oriented to date, place, and time. If the patient is confused or having seizures, keep the bed's side rails raised and padded, and apply restraints. Also,

leave a light on in his room because darkness may intensify confusion. During a seizure, maintain a patent airway, and protect the patient from harm. If the patient is comatose, keep the bed's side rails raised, and be sure to provide mild stimulation.

Consider your interventions successful if the patient is aware of his surroundings and responds appropriately.

**Fear related to the disorder and expected life-style changes.** Your goal is to allay the patient's fears and to promote adjustment to necessary life-style changes. Teach the patient about ARF: its pathophysiology, causes, course, treatment, and prognosis. Explain all procedures, such as implantation of a peritoneal catheter, before implementing them. Allow the patient time to express his fears about his illness and its impact on his life-style.

Consider your interventions successful if the patient understands and expresses his fears about the disorder, its treatment, and its effect on his life-style.

**Impaired skin integrity related to waste product accumulation.** Your goals are to relieve patient discomfort and to prevent skin breakdown. Give frequent skin care using a bland soap without perfumes or drying agents. Use oil along with lotions such as lanolin. Observe the skin for rashes or signs of breakdown. If the patient has terminal uremia, he may have uremic frost—urea crystals on his skin—so frequently wash off the crystals with water. Since the crystals are water-soluble, soap is not necessary. Evaluate your interventions. Mark them successful if the patient's skin is free from breakdown and infection and the patient is free from itching.

**Impaired physical mobility related to prolonged bed rest.** Your goal is to maintain optimal mobility and to prevent muscle atrophy. Perform passive ROM exercises three or four times a day, or promote active ROM exercises. Turn the patient frequently. Encourage him to participate in the activities of daily living, and promote early ambulation, if possible.

Consider your interventions successful if the patient complies with the exercise program and participates in daily activities.

### The nursing challenge
Managing ARF takes perseverance and patience. Avoiding irreversible parenchymal damage and promoting recovery require ongoing assessment, meticulous attention to fluid and nutritional status, and continuous emotional support for the patient.

**Points to remember**

- Acute renal failure (ARF) affects both kidneys simultaneously. It can result from prerenal, intrarenal, or postrenal causes.
- Acute tubular necrosis (ATN) accounts for about 75% of all cases of ARF. Nephrotoxin-induced ATN usually causes reversible damage, whereas ischemia-induced ATN usually causes irreversible damage.
- The creatinine clearance test provides the most accurate measure of renal function.
- Peritoneal dialysis and acute hemodialysis are the primary treatments for ARF.
- An accurate patient history and a complete physical examination provide valuable information for formulating nursing diagnosis and implementing an effective care plan.

# 5 MANAGING CHRONIC RENAL FAILURE

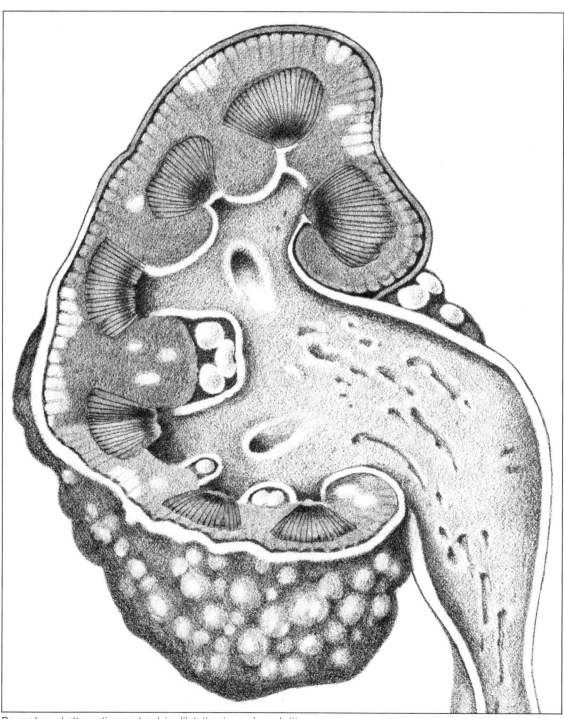

Parenchymal attenuation and pelvic dilatation in pyelonephritis

Thanks to dialysis and kidney transplants, people with chronic renal failure are surviving longer than ever before. That, however, may be a mixed blessing both for the patient and for you. After all, chronic renal failure is still an irreversible and progressive disease—it can be controlled for a time but it can't be cured. Eventually, it causes deterioration of all body systems. And, as it follows its inexorable course, it confronts the patient with periodic crises, psychosocial difficulties, frequent hospitalizations, and the prospect of impending death.

Effective care of the patient with chronic renal failure poses a critical test of your nursing skills. For example, you'll need to refine your assessment skills to detect signs of cardiovascular complications, such as pericardial friction rub and paradoxical pulse. You'll need to provide meticulous skin and mouth care, to carefully monitor the patient's fluid and nutritional status, and to prevent infection. To promote patient compliance with prescribed treatment, you'll have to provide thorough patient teaching about dietary restrictions, drug regimens, and dialysis options, and provide needed emotional support.

To meet these challenging responsibilities, you'll need a thorough understanding of the causes, signs, and treatment of chronic renal failure.

### Who gets chronic renal failure?
Almost anyone. The disorder strikes men and women equally and can occur at any age. In the United States it affects about 8 million people, causing about 60,000 deaths annually.

### PATHOPHYSIOLOGY
Chronic renal failure results from extensive, irreversible damage to nephrons. Inflammation anywhere in the renal system can cause such damage. This can result from bacteria, viruses, fungi, nephrotoxins, immune complex formation, or autoimmune reactions. (See *Causes of chronic renal failure,* page 89.) Because inflammation can stimulate antibody formation and immune complexes can initiate inflammation, chronic renal failure often results from a combined immune-inflammatory reaction. These processes ultimately affect the glomerulus, resulting in glomerulonephritis of the tubules and surrounding interstitial tissue, causing tubular-interstitial nephritis. In both of these disorders, pathologic changes can affect the nephrons, the surrounding blood vessels, and the interstitium.

### Glomerulonephritis: Chief cause of chronic renal failure
In glomerulonephritis, morphologic changes can occur in the capillary endothelium: mesangium (which supports the glomerular capillaries); glomerular basement membrane; visceral epithelium of the tuft; and parietal epithelium of Bowman's capsule. (See *Glomerular changes in immune-inflammatory disorders,* page 91.) These changes result from an immune-inflammatory reaction in the glomerulus, which, in turn, results from ischemia caused by renal arterial disease (for example, stenosis) or from the presence of immune complexes in the glomeruli.

Immune complexes can affect the glomeruli in two ways. First, circulating antigens that enter the body from outside sources (exogenous antigens), or antigens that are generated from exogenous material within the body, react with plasma antibodies to form large immune complexes in the vascular bed. These complexes can become lodged in the glomeruli, where they provoke an immune-inflammatory response.

Second, antibodies can form immune complexes with a component of the glomerulus itself, such as the glomerular basement membrane (as in Goodpasture's syndrome), or with exogenous antigens planted in the glomerulus (as in nephrotoxin-induced glomerulonephritis).

The extent and degree of glomerular involvement depend on the type and duration of the immune-inflammatory reactions. In certain types of glomerulonephritis, morphologic changes may initially be segmental, involving only some regions of the glomerulus, and focal, affecting only some glomeruli. Typically, as the disease progresses, these changes become global, involving the entire glomerulus, and more diffuse, affecting most glomeruli. In poststreptococcal glomerulonephritis, diffuse morphologic changes appear from the onset; in focal sclerosing glomerulonephritis, these changes remain focal.

Glomerulonephritis produces varying degrees of hematuria from damage to the glomerular capillary, proteinuria from loss of epithelial foot processes with increased glomerular permeability to protein (particularly albumin), and oliguria from a loss of functional nephrons. It also causes edema from increased sodium and water retention or hypoalbuminemia, and hypertension from increased blood volume or enhanced secretion of renin and aldosterone.

## Varying clinical patterns

Signs of glomerulonephritis can occur in many combinations, any of which can eventually lead to chronic renal failure.

**Acute glomerulonephritis.** This disorder has an abrupt onset, producing hematuria and hypertension. Typically, it follows untreated streptococcal infection of the respiratory tract, staphylococcal infections (bacterial endocarditis), viral diseases, transfusion reactions, or polyarteritis nodosa. This disorder can also result from chronic sclerosing glomerulonephritis, diabetes mellitus, and Alport's syndrome—diseases that result in glomerular sclerosis and replacement by hyaline material. Systemically, the manifestations of sclerosing nephropathy are those of uremia.

**Chronic glomerulonephritis.** This slowly progressive disorder can result from amyloidosis, Alport's syndrome, diabetes mellitus, systemic lupus erythematosus, and diffuse membranous glomerulonephritis. In all cases, circulating immune complexes are deposited in the glomerulus, causing diffuse morphologic changes that obstruct glomerular blood flow. The resultant effects include a decreased glomerular filtration rate (GFR), with fluid and sodium accumulation in the extracellular space, and hypertension.

**Rapidly progressive glomerulonephritis.** This disorder can progress to renal failure. It results from poststreptococcal glomerulonephritis, Goodpasture's syndrome, lupus erythematosus, and polyarteritis nodosa. Its chief pathologic characteristic is the presence of crescent-shaped structures within the glomerular urinary space—the result of epithelial cell proliferation, fibrosis, and leukocyte infiltration. Diffuse nephron obstruction causes rapid loss of renal function and progression to renal failure.

**Nephrotic syndrome.** Characterized by heavy proteinuria (greater than 3.5 g/24 hours), hypoalbuminemia, edema, and hyperlipidemia, this syndrome can result from diverse disorders, such as membranous, membranoproliferative, and chronic glomerulonephritis; hereditary diseases, such as diabetes mellitus and Alport's syndrome; systemic diseases, such as lupus erythematosus and amyloidosis; vascular diseases, such as renal vein thrombosis; and nephrotoxicity caused by gold salts and mercurial diuretics. In nephrotic syndrome, pathologic changes include glomerular basement membrane thickening, loss of epithelial foot processes, cellular proliferation, and loss of glomerular architectural structure.

## Tubular-interstitial nephritis

Pathologic changes in the tubules of the nephron and interstitium result in tubular-interstitial nephritis. These changes produce the characteristic effects of chronic renal failure: nocturia, urinary sodium and potassium loss, decreased ability to excrete acids, and various defects in tubular reabsorption or secretion.

Like glomerulonephritis, tubular-interstitial nephritis often results in reduced numbers of functional nephrons and impaired renal function.

**Chronic pyelonephritis.** Frequently, this type of nephritis results from upper urinary tract obstruction. But it can also be associated with hydronephrosis. It affects the renal medulla, damaging the tubular cells or causing inflammation. The resultant cellular dysfunction in the distal tubules and collecting ducts leads to defects in concentrating urine, excreting acids, and maintaining sodium balance. In addition, hypertension, fibrosis and scarring of the interstitium, calyces, and pelvis frequently occur.

**Interstitial nephritis.** This condition—the inflammation of the interstitial tissue enveloping the nephrons and renal vessels—can result from nephrotoxic damage to the interstitium, pyelonephritis, glomerulonephritis, hereditary diseases, or ischemic vascular diseases. Typically, it results in interstitial fibrosis, papillary necrosis, and tubular atrophy leading to uremia.

## Nephrotoxic disorders

Although many nephrotoxins (heavy metals, chemicals, and certain drugs) cause acute renal failure, which is reversible, they may also cause partial irreversible kidney damage, resulting in chronic renal failure. Heavy metals and chemicals can cause glomerulonephritis, tubular necrosis, interstitial nephritis, and, eventually, renal failure. Drugs, such as penicillins, sulfonamides, and aminoglycosides, can cause vasculitis, necrosis, and tubular dysfunction; prolonged use of phenacetin-containing analgesics can cause interstitial nephritis and papillary necrosis. Radiographic contrast media used in intravenous pyelography can cause renal failure in a dehydrated patient. Certain disorders, such as diabetes mellitus and myeloma, can render the kidneys

## Causes of chronic renal failure

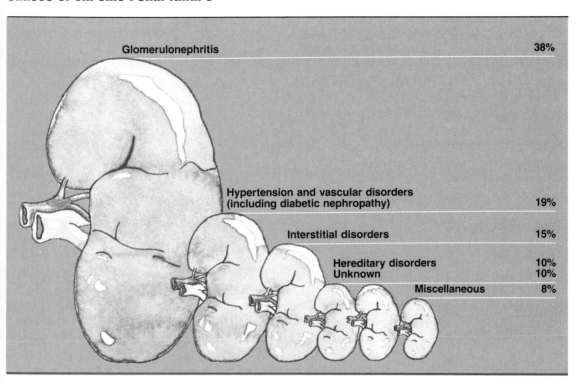

Glomerulonephritis — 38%

Hypertension and vascular disorders (including diabetic nephropathy) — 19%

Interstitial disorders — 15%

Hereditary disorders — 10%
Unknown — 10%

Miscellaneous — 8%

more susceptible to nephrotoxic damage.

Nephrotoxic disorders produce acidosis, hyperkalemia, and anemia associated with tubular dysfunction, as well as varying degrees of uremia, edema, and hypertension associated with glomerular dysfunction and renal insufficiency.

### Obstructive disorders

Partial or complete lower or upper urinary tract obstruction can also produce an immune-inflammatory response in the kidney that leads to chronic renal failure.

**Lower urinary tract obstruction.** Urethral stenosis or strictures, benign or malignant prostatic hypertrophy, and bladder neck obstruction can cause incomplete bladder emptying, urine stasis, cystitis, and urine backflow into the ureters (vesicoureteral reflux). These disorders can lead to acute pyelonephritis and possible renal tubular dysfunction.

**Upper urinary tract obstruction.** Ureteral scarring, retroperitoneal fibrosis, calculi, sloughed papillae, or abdominal neoplasms can cause upper urinary tract obstruction. Urine flow from the affected kidney then becomes partly or totally blocked, causing *hydronephrosis.* This condition is characterized by fluid accumulation and stasis within the renal tubules, increased intratubular pressure,

reduced blood flow and ischemia, decreased GFR, and damaged tubular epithelium and interstitium. Despite these effects, renal dysfunction may not be apparent unless hydronephrosis affects both kidneys. Bilateral hydronephrosis causes anuria, uremia, and rapid onset of renal failure.

**Neoplasms.** Although renal tumors make up only 1% to 3% of all tumors, about 85% of them are malignant. *Wilms' tumor,* the most common intraabdominal malignant tumor in children, contains epithelial and mesodermal cells, grows rapidly, and metastasizes early. This typically unilateral tumor produces abdominal enlargement, hypertension, and vomiting. In contrast, *renal cell carcinoma* usually occurs in older adults, grows slowly, and is well encapsulated. *Transitional cell carcinoma,* a rare neoplasm, occurs in adults and involves the renal calyces and pelvis.

These tumors may not cause any overt symptoms until later stages, when their first sign may be the abrupt onset of visible hematuria in the absence of other urinary tract disorders.

*Extrarenal tumors* can also affect renal function. Abdominal neoplasms can obstruct urine flow from the kidneys and cause infection and inflammation. Metastasizing *bronchogenic carcinoma* may affect the glomerulus, causing an immune-inflammatory reaction and glomerulonephritis. Also, multiple myeloma may cause deposition of amyloid, with subsequent reduction of the GFR.

**Hypertensive and vascular disorders**
Although hypertension commonly results from many primary kidney diseases, it's also an important cause of nephrosclerosis and chronic renal failure.

Normally, the kidneys play an important role in regulating arterial pressure, especially when blood volume and extracellular fluid volume fall markedly. Reduced arterial pressure leads to an increased sympathetic stimulation of the afferent renal arterioles' smooth muscle, reducing renal perfusion and, consequently, the GFR. As blood flow to the glomeruli diminishes, an enzyme, renin, is released from the juxtaglomerular cells. (See *Understanding renovascular hypertension,* pages 92 and 93.)

Renin acts on its blood substrate (angiotensinogen), initiating a series of reactions leading to the formation of angiotensin II. This vasoactive substance then acts on the smooth muscle cells in the walls of the systemic arterioles, causing vasoconstriction, which leads to increased arterial pressure. It also stimulates release of aldosterone from the adrenal cortex. This hormone acts on the distal renal tubules to promote sodium and water reabsorption.

As intravascular fluid volume expands, mean arterial pressure increases, thereby reducing sympathetic stimulation of the afferent renal arterioles' smooth muscle and increasing blood flow through these vessels. This brings about decreased renin release by a negative feedback mechanism. Thus, normally reduced renal perfusion initiates a homeostatic mechanism, leading to increased extracellular volume and increased arterial pressure.

The primary causes of renal arterial narrowing include atherosclerosis, vasculitis, embolism, and thrombosis.

**Atherosclerosis.** Formation of hyaline deposits, atherosclerotic plaques, or fibrous tissue in the renal arterial and capillary walls is the most common cause of renal vascular disease. When atherosclerosis results from hyaline deposition (as in primary hypertension, diabetes mellitus, and scleroderma), the resulting morphologic renal changes are called *nephrosclerosis*. This disorder commonly produces moderate hypertension and leads to sclerosis, glomerular destruction, tubular atrophy, a reduced GFR, reduced kidney size, and chronic renal failure.

*Malignant nephrosclerosis*, associated with severe hypertension, is characterized by vasculitis, focal fibroid necrosis of the arterial walls and glomerular tuft, and severe arteriolar ischemia with additional activation of the renin-angiotensin-aldosterone system. These changes frequently result in widespread necrosis, thrombus formation, ischemic tubular atrophy, and partial renal infarction, resulting in greatly diminished renal function.

Atherosclerosis resulting from plaque deposition and hyperplasia of muscle cells in the walls of the aorta, main renal artery, and its branches is the primary cause of renal artery stenosis. This reduces blood flow to the affected kidney, and it activates the renin-angiotensin-aldosterone system to raise arterial pressure.

**Vasculitis.** As a result of endothelial inflammation, the renal arterioles and capillaries narrow, resulting in reduced perfusion, ischemia, hypertension, and renal infarction. If it affects medium-sized renal arteries, the areas fed by these arteries may be infarcted; if it primarily affects the arterioles, focal glomerular injury develops. This nephropathy can result from immune-inflammatory reactions (polyarteritis nodosa, hypersensitivity angiitis) or trauma and can progress rapidly to renal failure.

**Thrombosis.** Thrombus formation and embolization can occur anywhere in the body. Since the kidneys receive about one fourth of the blood pumped from the heart, emboli derived from intracardiac thrombi resulting from bacterial endocarditis or mitral stenosis occasionally lodge in the renal arteries and cause infarction. Thrombi can form in the renal arteries as a result of arteriosclerotic disease; vasculitis; or intravascular coagulation defects resulting from septicemia, toxemia of pregnancy, or severe dehydration.

**Congenital disorders: Onsets vary**
Congenital defects in renal structure or function can result in chronic renal failure. These defects may affect one or both kidneys, but their effects can arise either at an early age or not until midlife.

One such defect is *renal agenesis*—the congenital absence of one or both kidneys. Obviously, bilateral renal agenesis is fatal, but unilateral agenesis can allow normal renal function. However, the functioning kidney

## Glomerular changes in immune-inflammatory disorders

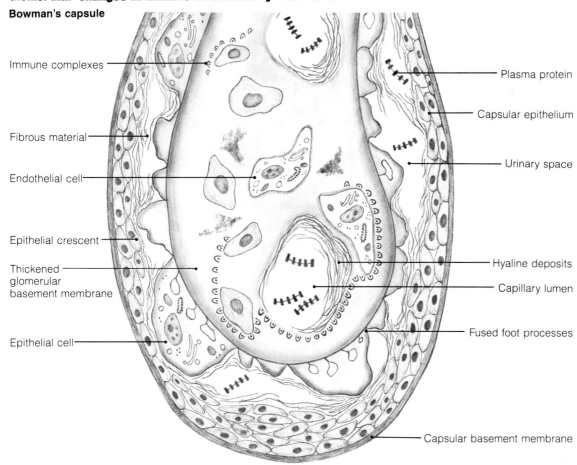

**Bowman's capsule**

Immune complexes

Fibrous material

Endothelial cell

Epithelial crescent

Thickened glomerular basement membrane

Epithelial cell

Plasma protein

Capsular epithelium

Urinary space

Hyaline deposits

Capillary lumen

Fused foot processes

Capsular basement membrane

The glomerulus includes the glomerular tuft (the capillary bed between the afferent and efferent arterioles), the urinary space, and Bowman's capsule. In immune-inflammatory disorders, the glomerulus undergoes various pathologic changes, such as proliferation of endothelial, epithelial, and mesangial cells in the glomerular tuft, and of epithelial cells in Bowman's capsule. Leukocytes and immune complexes infiltrate the glomerulus, and the basement membrane thickens. Glomerular sclerosis and fusion of foot processes (podocytes) in the visceral epithelium also occur.

tends to have structural anomalies, such as cysts or dysplasia. Other defects, such as supernumerary or malpositioned kidneys, do not necessarily produce renal dysfunction.

In kidneys that are malformed (for example, horseshoe kidney) or that have structurally nonfunctional tissue, renal reserve can be reduced and the tubular-interstitial region predisposed to inflammation resulting from obstruction or urine stasis.

*Cysts* form primarily in the medulla, although they may form anywhere in the nephron. Because these cysts communicate with the glomeruli or tubules, they may fill with glomerular filtrate, swell, and compress adjacent vessels. As a result, the nephrons and interstitium are deprived of oxygen. Local inflammation follows, causing destruction or impairment of renal cells. Destruction of renal cells further reduces renal reserve, whereas cell dysfunction produces defects in tubular reabsorption and secretion. Trapped filtrate in the cysts and sluggish renal tubular flow further predispose the interstitium to infection and inflammation.

*Aplastic kidneys* do not contain functional nephrons. Like bilateral renal agenesis, bilateral renal aplasia is fatal. In many aplastic kidney defects, renal function is not lost, but renal reserve is decreased because of the aplastic tissue in the kidney. Renal function may be deranged because of the relative or absolute lack of certain proteins or enzymes caused by a particular defect.

### Rarely, genetic disorders

Genetically transmitted disorders directly or indirectly cause kidney dysfunction. Generally, they affect the glomeruli or tubules. Bilateral renal dysfunction associated with these defects may appear at birth or develop later and can result in chronic renal failure.

**Glomerular dysfunction.** Diseases predominantly affecting the glomeruli include Alport's syndrome, Fabry's disease, primary amyloidosis, and diabetes mellitus. They produce progressive pathology—glomerular basement membrane thickening, immune complex or amyloid deposition in the glomerulus, altered permeability, and glomerular sclerosis with hyaline deposition. They frequently lead to tubular atrophy and interstitial fibrosis.

# Understanding renovascular hypertension

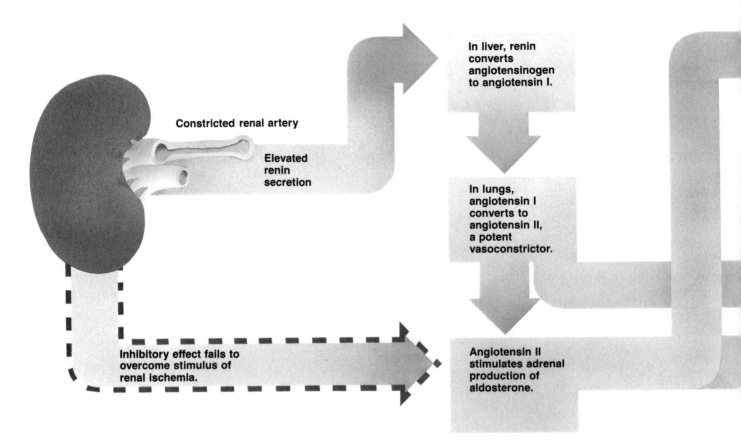

**In liver, renin converts angiotensinogen to angiotensin I.**

**Constricted renal artery**

**Elevated renin secretion**

**In lungs, angiotensin I converts to angiotensin II, a potent vasoconstrictor.**

**Inhibitory effect fails to overcome stimulus of renal ischemia.**

**Angiotensin II stimulates adrenal production of aldosterone.**

Renovascular hypertension results from reduced renal perfusion, which, in turn, can result from obstruction or atherosclerotic narrowing of the renal artery. The ensuing renal ischemia abnormally stimulates the renin-angiotensin-aldosterone system, causing increased fluid volume and arterial blood pressure, which leads to hypertension.

Hematuria and mild proteinuria, initially in the nonnephrotic range (less than 3.5 g of protein/24 hours), reflect glomerular injury. Sclerosis is associated with mild hypertension that may aggravate preexisting glomerular injury, leading to further glomerular damage, destruction of nephrons, further reduction of renal reserve, and renal insufficiency.

**Tubular dysfunction.** Hereditary diseases causing major tubular dysfunction include Fanconi's syndrome, sickle cell disease, congenital hyperuricemia, and congenital renal tubular acidosis. These inherited defects primarily affect distal renal tubule secretion; Fanconi's syndrome includes proximal tubular reabsorption defects.

In congenital hyperuricemia and congenital renal tubular acidosis, the defective transport apparatus for secreting and excreting uric acid and hydrogen ions in the distal tubules causes these substances to accumulate in the blood, in turn causing hyperuricemia and acidosis. With rising plasma uric acid levels, urate crystals may deposit in the tubules, *vasa recta,* and medullary interstitium, reducing renal blood flow and causing hypertension, tubular ischemia, and chronic inflammation of the medullary interstitium.

In sickle cell disease, thrombosis in the *vasa recta* leads to distal tubular ischemia resulting in impaired urinary acidification and excessive urinary potassium excretion, papillary necrosis, hematuria, and progressive renal failure.

## The "intact nephron"

The kidney's remarkable ability to maintain homeostasis despite 75% to 80% function loss is partially explained by the "intact nephron" (or Bricker) hypothesis. Bricker observed that, in renal disease, two types of nephrons coexist: nonfunctional nephrons destroyed by disease and functioning nephrons that remain disease-free and hypertrophy to do the work of the destroyed nephrons.

## End-stage renal disease

Hypertrophy of the disease-free nephrons maintains homeostasis until late renal failure. Eventually, as more and more nephrons are destroyed, the kidneys lose all regulatory ability. Regardless of the cause of renal failure, deteriorating renal function produces devastating effects on every body system.

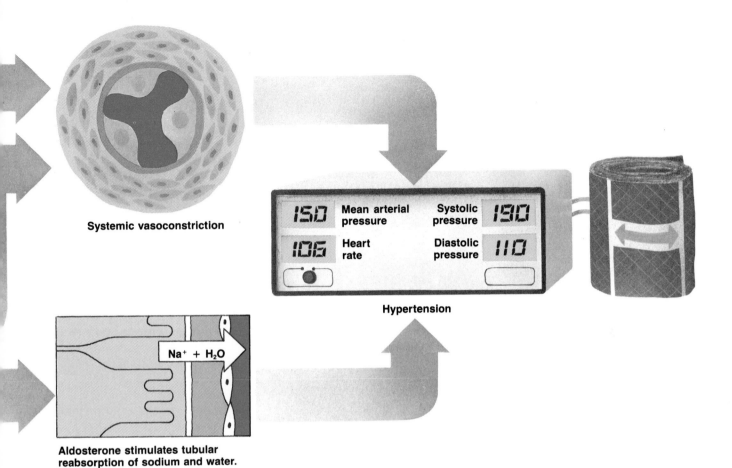

**Systemic vasoconstriction**

| 150 | Mean arterial pressure | Systolic pressure | 190 |
| 106 | Heart rate | Diastolic pressure | 110 |

**Hypertension**

$Na^+ + H_2O$

**Aldosterone stimulates tubular reabsorption of sodium and water.**

## MEDICAL MANAGEMENT

Because chronic renal failure affects every body system, diagnostic tests and treatment are necessarily complex and comprehensive.

### Diagnostic tests: A complete workup

The complete diagnostic workup includes routine blood and urine studies, renal function tests, X-rays of the kidneys and lower urinary tract, and, depending on the patient's signs and symptoms, studies of renal or urinary tract structure.

Creatinine clearance, blood urea nitrogen (BUN), and serum creatinine tests are frequently used to evaluate chronic renal failure. Because creatinine filters freely at the glomerulus and the tubules do not reabsorb or secrete it, creatinine clearance is considered an accurate estimate of GFR. After age 40, creatinine clearance slowly declines, and by age 80, it may be 50% of that in the normal young adult.

Typically, chronic renal failure progresses in the following stages:
• *decreased renal reserve,* in which BUN and serum creatinine levels are normal, and the patient is asymptomatic

• *renal insufficiency*, in which more than 75% of the nephrons have been destroyed, the GFR is 25% of normal, BUN and serum creatinine levels begin to rise above normal, and nocturia and polyuria occur because of loss of normal urine concentrating ability
• *end-stage renal disease* (ESRD), or uremia, in which 90% of the nephrons have been destroyed, the GFR is 10% of normal or less, BUN and serum creatinine levels rise sharply and rapidly with further small decreases in nephron mass, the patient becomes oliguric, and every organ system is affected.

Patients with chronic renal failure usually have mild thrombocytopenia. Purpura may result from a minor injury, and bleeding from body orifices or mucous membranes may occur. Other blood test results in chronic renal failure show a prolonged bleeding time, decreased platelet adhesiveness, abnormal prothrombin consumption time, and elevated serum potassium levels.

The hematocrit level usually falls slowly over several months, stabilizing at 20% to 25%. To compensate for this, levels of the enzyme 2,3-diphosphoglycerate (2,3-DPG) increase, which causes hemoglobin to liberate oxygen to the tissues more readily.

The chest X-ray helps evaluate heart size and may indicate long-standing hypertension. Congestive changes in the lung fields should also be assessed.

Palpation may reveal large, irregular, tender masses in the abdominal cavity, indicating polycystic kidney disease. Abdominal bruits, severe hypertension, cardiac enlargement, and advanced hypertensive retinopathy may indicate bilateral renal artery stenosis.

Hyperkalemia is a major complication of advanced renal failure. EKG changes are the single most important indication of severe hyperkalemia. These changes include tall, tented T-waves; loss of P waves; ST segment depression; prolonged PR interval (first-degree AV block); and broadened QRS complex, leading to cardiac fibrillation and arrest.

### Treatment conserves renal function

Even though renal failure adversely affects all body systems, it can often be managed conservatively with diet and fluid restrictions and drugs until the GFR falls to 10% or 15% of normal. Then, maintenance dialysis or kidney transplantation is necessary to sustain life.

Effective treatment requires careful management of hydration, control of metabolic acidosis, control of cardiovascular abnormalities, correction of potassium imbalance, and treatment of anemia.

**Hydration.** The patient with chronic renal failure may be dehydrated or overhydrated, depending on underlying pathology and severity of renal failure. Overhydration is managed by limiting sodium and water intake and by ultrafiltration during dialysis to reduce the risk of cardiopulmonary complications while promoting the patient's comfort. Uremic pneumonitis, one manifestation of fluid overload, usually disappears following fluid removal during two or three dialyses. Frequent chest X-rays are necessary to detect changes in pneumonitis. Antibiotics may prevent bacterial infection in the "wet" uremic lung.

To prevent nocturnal dehydration, the patient's fluid intake should be distributed over 24 hours. The 24-hour sodium and fluid intake is individualized based on weight change, serum sodium concentration, urine volume, and maintenance of maximum GFR. A general rule to determine the daily fluid allowance is to restrict fluid intake to 500 ml (insensible fluid losses) plus an amount equal to the previous 24-hour urinary output. This corresponds to a fluid gain of approximately 1 lb/24

hours, which can be easily removed during dialysis.

**Metabolic acidosis.** Clinically evident acidosis or a plasma bicarbonate level of less than 15 mEq/liter requires treatment, possibly with an oral alkalizing agent such as Shohl's solution (Bicitra), intravenous sodium bicarbonate, or dialysis. In severe acidosis with Kussmaul's respirations, intravenous sodium bicarbonate may be administered slowly; if given too rapidly, it may precipitate hypocalcemic tetany.

The degree of calcium ionization is determined by the pH; the more acid the plasma, the more ionized calcium is present. If acidosis is rapidly corrected, the plasma-ionized calcium level decreases as the calcium ions bind with bicarbonate and proteins. Ten to thirty g of calcium gluconate, slowly given intravenously when the sodium bicarbonate is administered, may prevent hypocalcemic tetany.

Dialysis corrects acidosis by removing hydrogen ions and by adding acetate, a bicarbonate precursor that buffers acids.

**Hypertension.** The most common cardiovascular problem in chronic renal failure is hypertension. To help control it, a beta-adrenergic inhibitor, such as propranolol, a vasodilator, such as methyldopa, or a renin-angiotensin inhibitor, such as captopril, may be given. When all other methods fail, bilateral nephrectomy may be required to remove the source of renin production.

**Potassium imbalance.** Hyperkalemia may be prevented by closely monitoring the patient's potassium intake in medications and food. Serial serum potassium levels and serial EKGs should be available as guides in looking for and treating potassium intoxication.

Because hyperkalemia produces few warning signs, the hyperkalemic patient often presents as a medical emergency when cardiac toxicity has set in, leading to ventricular asystole or fibrillation. Emergency treatment consists of intravenous sodium bicarbonate, calcium, and hypertonic glucose and insulin, and a cation-exchange resin.

Serum potassium levels decrease within minutes after administration of adequate sodium bicarbonate. Two to three ampules (44 to 132 mEq) of sodium bicarbonate help correct acidosis and shift potassium back into the cells. Even in nonacidotic patients, sodium bicarbonate effectively reduces serum potassium levels. However, large amounts of sodium may precipitate congestive heart failure or lead to a hyperosmolar state.

Intravenous calcium (10 to 30 ml of 10% calcium gluconate intravenously over a 1- to 5-minute period) counteracts the damaging effect of elevated potassium levels on the heart. However, calcium itself may induce cardiac dysrhythmias and should be given with EKG monitoring. Calcium does not decrease serum potassium concentration.

Intravenous hypertonic glucose and insulin (200 to 500 ml of 10% glucose or lesser amounts of 20% to 50% glucose) may be infused rapidly. Ten units of regular insulin may be added to the infusion or given subcutaneously. As glucose is transported across the cell membrane, potassium moves into the cell, lowering serum potassium levels. Also, a cation-exchange resin such as sodium polystyrene sulfonate (Kayexalate), given orally or as a retention enema, helps remove potassium from the body.

Kayexalate is usually administered with sorbitol to induce mild diarrhea and to move Kayexalate fairly rapidly through the system. Beneficial effects occur in 30 to 60 minutes when given rectally and in 1 to 2 hours when given orally.

Kayexalate has an exchange capacity of approximately 1 mEq of potassium/g. The sodium content is approximately 100 mg/g of the drug. During the resin's action in the intestine, sodium is released mole for mole with potassium uptake.

A single dose (15 g) of Kayexalate contains 60 mEq of sodium. The cation-exchange process is about 33% efficient; therefore, about 20 mEq of sodium is actually exchanged. As the resin passes along the intestine or is retained in the colon after enema administration, the sodium ions are partially released and replaced by potassium ions. This takes place mainly in the large intestine, which excretes more potassium than does the small intestine.

Kayexalate therapy can remove enough potassium to cause serious potassium deficiency (hypokalemia), so monitoring serum potassium levels frequently is imperative. However, serum levels do not necessarily reflect intracellular potassium levels; therefore, the duration of Kayexalate treatment must be determined individually for each patient, depending on clinical condition and EKG results. Marked hypokalemia may be indicated by severe muscle weakness.

Kayexalate therapy must be administered with special caution to patients who cannot tolerate small increases in sodium loads (which may result in congestive heart failure, hypertension, or marked edema). Also, because Kayexalate therapy causes loss of small amounts of other cations—such as magnesium and calcium—the patient must be monitored for other electrolyte imbalances.

**Anemia.** Because of potential problems, blood transfusions are not given in chronic renal failure until anemia produces overt symptoms—dyspnea, fatigue, tachycardia, and palpitations. Disadvantages of blood transfusions include suppression of hematopoiesis, transfusion dependence to maintain the patient's hematocrit level, the danger of transfusion reactions, transmission of blood-borne diseases (such as hepatitis), and formation of cytotoxic antibodies.

Cytotoxic antibodies form in response to an antigen contained in virtually all body tissues except red blood cells (RBCs). If a patient receives a whole blood transfusion, antibodies form against the white blood cells (WBCs) and platelets.

When the patient eventually receives a kidney transplant, a hyperacute rejection reaction may occur because of the presence of preformed antibodies from previous blood transfusions against the transplanted organ. Leukocyte-poor blood or frozen blood is used to mitigate this problem. Leukocyte-poor blood has been centrifuged to remove platelets and WBCs, which contain the antigen causing the cytotoxic reaction. Frozen blood also lacks platelets and WBCs, which are removed when the frozen blood is deglycerolized. In either case, the patient receives blood with greatly decreased antigenicity, and few cytotoxic antibodies form.

The patient with an iron or folate deficiency requires treatment with iron or folate supplements. To prevent gastrointestinal irritation, iron is customarily given with meals unless the patient is receiving phosphate-binding medication, which would bind most of the iron, preventing its absorption. Iron may be given as ferrous fumerate, sulfate, or ferrocholinate, or parenterally as iron dextran (Imferon). For maximum benefit, folic acid should be given after dialysis, because hemodialysis removes folic acid given before or during treatment.

Erythropoietin has been used to treat anemia in chronic renal failure. However, it is not currently FDA-approved and is now too costly to be practical.

Androgen therapy has been used with some

## Equivalent dosages of phosphate-binding preparations

| Preparation | Basic dose | Elemental aluminum content | Dose equivalent to 30 ml Amphojel |
|---|---|---|---|
| Amphojel liquid | 30 ml | 665 mg | |
| Amphojel (5-grain tablet) | 1 tablet | 104 mg | 6.4 tablets |
| Amphojel (10-grain tablet) | 1 tablet | 208 mg | 3.2 tablets |
| Alu-Cap | 1 capsule | 126 mg | 5.3 capsules |
| Phos-Lo cookie | 1 cookie | 416 mg | 1.6 cookies |
| Basaljel tablet | 1 tablet | 173 mg | 4.0 tablets |
| Basaljel capsule | 1 capsule | 173 mg | 4.0 capsules |
| Basaljel liquid | 30 ml | 852 mg | 23.5 ml |
| Extra-strength Basaljel liquid | 30 ml | 2,080 mg | 9.6 ml |

success to increase the hematocrit level of patients with chronic renal failure. For example, testosterone or nandrolone decanoate (Deca-Durabolin) is usually administered at weekly intervals. However, these drugs may cause acne, hirsutism in women, and priapism in men.

### GI problems

If the patient has diarrhea, an antidiarrheal agent, such as diphenoxylate hydrochloride (Lomotil), may be given. Since it contains atropine, the dosage must be monitored carefully. If the patient is constipated, a bulk-forming laxative (Metamucil) or a stool softener (Colace, Doxidan) may be given.

Laxatives containing magnesium (such as Milk of Magnesia) should be avoided because of the possibility of hypermagnesemia—the diseased kidneys can't adequately remove magnesium.

### Osteodystrophy and calcification

Renal osteodystrophy and metastatic calcification must be treated by lowering serum phosphate levels. Phosphate-binding medications, such as aluminum carbonate or aluminum hydroxide gels, are commonly used. The medication must be taken at mealtimes so that both food and phosphate binder are present in the GI tract at the same time. The aluminum in the gels binds with phosphates in food to form the insoluble compound aluminum

phosphate. The compound is excreted unchanged in the feces, thus preventing phosphate absorption from the GI tract. This decreases the plasma phosphate level and raises the plasma calcium level.

Phosphate-binding medications should be given with a stool softener since they may cause constipation. They're available in gel, tablet, capsule, and cookie form, so if the patient finds one form unpalatable, he may find another acceptable. (See *Equivalent dosages of phosphate-binding preparations.*)

Vitamin D supplements may enhance intestinal absorption of calcium to increase the plasma calcium level. Vitamin D is available as dihydrotachysterol or calcitriol, a readily usable form that does not need to be activated by the kidney. However, plasma phosphate levels must be within a normal range before starting vitamin D; otherwise, metastatic calcifications may occur. The patient must also be monitored for hypercalcemia when vitamin D is given.

With plasma phosphate at or near normal levels, oral calcium lactate or calcium carbonate may be used to raise the low plasma calcium level.

A subtotal parathyroidectomy (removal of three and a half of the four parathyroid glands) may be indicated if the patient has severe hyperparathyroidism with osteolysis. Bone remineralization occurs slowly after this operation.

## Dietary guidelines in renal failure

| Recommended nutrients and ions | During initial renal failure | During maintenance dialysis |
|---|---|---|
| High-biologic-value protein | 20 to 40 g | In hemodialysis: 1 g/kg body weight (adult), 1.5 g/kg body weight (child) In peritoneal dialysis: Usually unrestricted |
| Low-biologic-value protein | 10 g or less | 15 g or less |
| Carbohydrates | Unrestricted | Unrestricted |
| Fat | Unrestricted | Unrestricted |
| Calories | Adult: 45 to 50 kcal/kg Child: 80 kcal/kg | Adult: 45 to 50 kcal/kg Child: 80 kcal/kg |
| Sodium | Individualized | Individualized (500 to 2,000 mg) |
| Potassium | Individualized (40 to 70 mEq) | Individualized (40 to 70 mEq) |
| Calcium | RDA (800 to 1,200 mg) | RDA (800 to 1,200 mg) |
| Phosphate | Unrestricted in diet (controlled by drugs) | Unrestricted in diet (controlled by drugs) |

### Diet and dialysis

Diet planning for the dialysis patient must achieve several goals. The diet must:
• provide adequate caloric intake to achieve ideal body weight
• provide adequate protein to maintain positive nitrogen balance (for example, use of high-biologic-value protein and essential amino acids)
• control sodium to prevent hypotension, hypertension, or excessive thirst
• control potassium to prevent hyperkalemia or hypokalemia
• control phosphorus to augment phosphate-binding drugs
• control fluids to prevent hypertension or edema
• provide vitamin and mineral supplements, as needed.
The diet must also be practical, palatable, and acceptable to the patient.

Use of low-biologic-value proteins provides few essential amino acids and furnishes more urea nitrogen than high-biologic-value proteins during metabolism, which increases the BUN level. (See *Dietary guidelines in renal failure.*)

### Renal dialysis: Two approaches

Dialysis provides vital filtration and detoxifying functions that have been lost in patients with ESRD. It does not duplicate kidney function entirely since normal kidneys perform many functions that dialysis cannot provide. Two types of dialysis are currently in use: peritoneal dialysis and hemodialysis, both with similar principles and outcomes but with considerably different mechanisms.

The three physical principles of dialysis are diffusion, osmosis, and hydrostatic pressure. *Diffusion* is the movement of particles from an area of greater to an area of lesser particle concentration; the difference in concentrations is the concentration gradient. In dialysis, high concentrations of uremic toxins and electrolytes in the plasma diffuse across a semipermeable membrane into a dialysis solution (dialysate), where concentrations are lower.

*Osmosis* is the passive transport of water across a semipermeable membrane from an area of low particle concentration to an area of high particle concentration (or from high water concentration to low water concentration.) In dialysis, excess water leaves the patient's plasma and enters the dialysate.

*Hydrostatic pressure* is exerted by the weight of a column of water in its container. This pressure may be positive or negative. For example, if the container has semipermeable walls, positive hydrostatic pressure inside the container would expel the fluid through the walls; conversely, if a negative hydrostatic pressure exists outside the container, the fluid would be pulled through the walls of the container. Positive and negative hydrostatic pressures are used during hemodialysis to move excess water rapidly from the patient's plasma. This rapid removal of water is called ultrafiltration.

### Peritoneal dialysis

In peritoneal dialysis, the dialysate is instilled into the peritoneal cavity, allowed to dwell there for a specified time, then drained from the peritoneal cavity. The patient's own peritoneal membrane serves as a semipermeable dialyzing membrane across which solutes move by diffusion and water moves by osmosis. Thus, excessive concentrations of electrolytes and uremic toxins diffuse from the plasma, and excessive water moves by osmosis from the plasma.

In this procedure, a catheter is inserted in the peritoneal cavity through a small incision in the midline of the abdomen below the umbilicus. Since the peritoneal catheter provides a permanent portal of entry to the peritoneum, peritonitis is an ever-present danger. Scrupulous sterile technique is required when connecting and disconnecting the dialysate tubing and when changing the dressing around the catheter.

Peritoneal dialysis may be performed manually, by an automatic cycler machine, or as continuous ambulatory peritoneal dialysis (CAPD). Manual dialysis requires the nurse, the patient, or a family member to run dialysate through the catheter into the peritoneal cavity, to allow the proper amount to infuse, to time the duration of the dwell, and then to allow the infusion to drain out of the peritoneal cavity. The process is repeated for 6 to 8 hours and is performed five to six times a week.

The cycler machine requires sterile connection technique; it then automatically performs the rest of the procedure until it's disconnected from the peritoneal catheter.

CAPD is performed by the patient himself. He instills 2 liters of dialysate from a plastic bag attached to the catheter with special tubing into the peritoneal cavity. He can roll up the empty plastic bag and place it in a shirt pocket until time for drainage 6 to 8 hours later. Then he drains the "spent" solution into the unrolled bag and attaches and instills a bag of new dialysate. He repeats the process to ensure continuous dialysis 24 hours a day, 7 days a week.

Potential complications of peritoneal dialysis include peritonitis from bacteria entering the peritoneal cavity through or around the catheter; catheter blockage from clots, lodgment

## Peritoneal dialysis catheters

Peritoneal dialysis requires insertion of a Tenckhoff, Gore-Tex, or column-disk catheter into the peritoneum, usually under local anesthetic.

### Tenckhoff

To implant the *Tenckhoff catheter,* the doctor inserts the first 6¾" (17 cm) of the device into the patient's abdomen. The next 2¾" (7-cm) segment, which the doctor tunnels subcutaneously, has a Dacron cuff at each end. Within a few days after insertion, the patient's tissues grow closely around these Dacron cuffs, forming a tight barrier against bacterial invasion. The remaining 3⅞" (10 cm) of the catheter extends outside the abdomen. The external tip of the catheter is equipped with a metal adapter so it can be connected to dialysate tubing.

### Gore-Tex

To insert the *Gore-Tex* catheter, the doctor positions its flanged collar just below the dermis so that the device extends through the abdominal wall. The distal end of the cuff should not extend into the peritoneum because this may cause adhesions.

### CDPC

To secure the *column-disk peritoneal catheter* (CDPC), the doctor rolls up the flexible disk section of the implant, inserts it into the peritoneal cavity, and retracts it against the abdominal wall. The implant's first cuff rests just outside the peritoneal membrane; its second cuff rests just beneath the skin. Because the CDPC does not float freely in the peritoneal cavity, it increases patient comfort during dialysis since the inflowing dialysate isn't directed at sensitive organs.

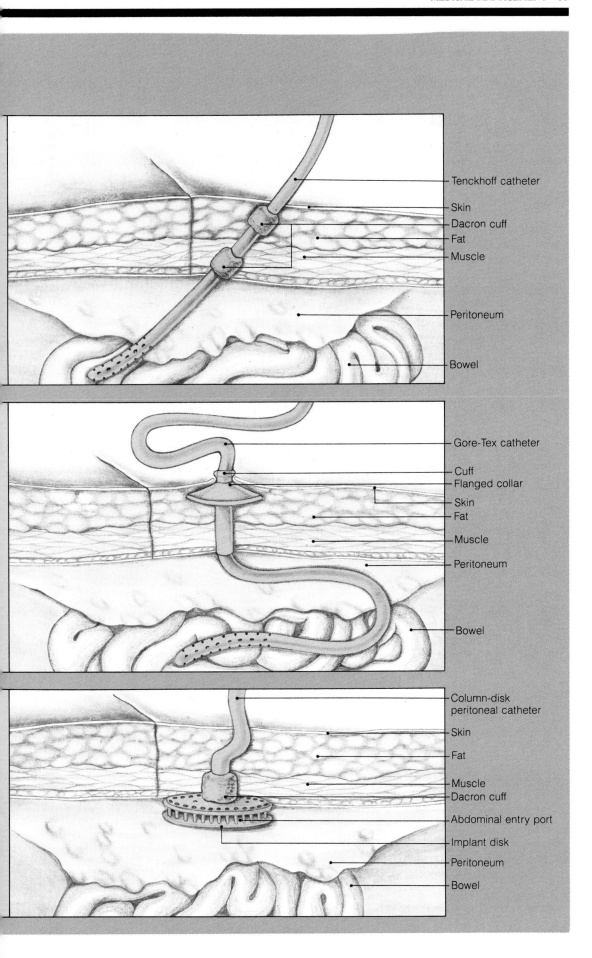

Tenckhoff catheter
Skin
Dacron cuff
Fat
Muscle
Peritoneum
Bowel

Gore-Tex catheter
Cuff
Flanged collar
Skin
Fat
Muscle
Peritoneum
Bowel

Column-disk peritoneal catheter
Skin
Fat
Muscle
Dacron cuff
Abdominal entry port
Implant disk
Peritoneum
Bowel

against the abdominal wall, kinking, or constipation; and hypotension and hypovolemia due to removal of excessive fluid from the plasma. (See *Peritoneal dialysis catheters,* pages 98 and 99.)

### Hemodialysis

In this procedure, waste-laden blood is routed from the patient's body, via a shunt or fistula, through an artificial kidney machine (dialyzer), then back to the circulation. Inside the dialyzer, the blood is kept separate from the dialysate by a semipermeable membrane. Excessive electrolytes and uremic toxins diffuse from the blood compartment into the dialysate. Fresh dialysate and fresh blood from the patient are continuously pumped through the dialyzer to maintain a high concentration gradient between the two compartments and to allow rapid solute removal. Excessive water is removed from the blood by applying a positive hydrostatic pressure to the blood compartment and a negative hydrostatic pressure to the dialysate compartment (ultrafiltration). Heparin is added to the blood to prevent clotting. The procedure takes 3 to 4 hours and is repeated three times a week.

Potential complications include hypotension, shock, nausea, and vomiting from too rapid fluid removal and hypovolemia; blood loss due to a torn dialyzer membrane or accidental disconnection of blood lines; bleeding from heparin administration; and dialysis disequilibrium syndrome (headache, restlessness, confusion, nausea, vomiting, and seizures) resulting from urea nitrogen being removed from the blood more rapidly than from the central nervous system (CNS). This creates an osmotic gradient that shifts water into the CNS, resulting in cerebral edema.

Hemodialysis requires permanent access to the patient's bloodstream through an external shunt or an internal arteriovenous fistula. (See Chapter 4.)

In an *external shunt,* a Silastic catheter is inserted through skin incisions into a large artery and a large vein in the patient's wrist or ankle. When he's not receiving hemodialysis, the two cannulae are connected to each other, and blood flows through the tubes. During dialysis, the cannulae are clamped, separated, and connected to the blood lines leading to and from the dialyzer. They are then unclamped, and blood is pumped from the arterial side to the dialyzer and then returned to the patient through the venous side.

Potential complications related to external shunts include infection around the skin insertion sites, blood clotting inside the shunt, accidental or intentional separation of the cannulae (as in a suicide attempt), and exsanguination.

An *internal arteriovenous fistula* is created in the patient's forearm by anastomosing a large artery to a large vein. The force of arterial blood flowing into the veins eventually causes them to enlarge. Large-gauge needles are inserted into the enlarged veins (or fistula) to obtain blood flow for dialysis. One needle moves blood from the patient to the dialyzer; the other returns blood from the dialyzer to the patient. The internal fistula produces fewer complications than the external shunt.

A Hemasite shunt can make dialysis less painful for patients with damaged blood vessels or a fear of needles. This shunt, no bigger than a shirt button, is made of the same material used in artificial heart valves. It's permanently implanted in a patient's arm or leg and has two holes leading to plastic tubes, which connect to a vein and an artery. During dialysis, the patient is connected to the machine by placing a two-pronged plug in the shunt. This device is presently under trial in some centers.

### Chronic renal failure and transplantation

A kidney transplant does not cure renal failure; it is an additional treatment method. The kidney may be donated by a recipient's relative or it may be taken from a cadaver. Regardless of the source, the donor's and recipient's tissues must match as closely as possible to prevent transplant rejection by the recipient's body.

Preoperative care includes physical and emotional preparation. The patient, his family, and the living donor must understand the goals of the surgery, the potential complications, and the requirements of immediate and long-term care. The patient must be prepared for the possibility of, and treatment for, transplant rejection and must have a thorough medical evaluation before surgery. He may be dialyzed immediately before surgery to ensure optimal fluid, electrolyte, and acid-base balances and low levels of uremic toxins in his body.

The donated kidney is implanted in the iliac fossa. (See *Renal transplantation,* pages 102 and 103.) The patient's own kidneys are usually not removed unless they are infected, greatly enlarged, or causing medically uncontrollable hypertension. The transplanted kidney's renal artery is anastomosed to the recipient's hypogastric artery; the renal vein to the iliac vein; and the ureter to the bladder by ureteroneocystostomy. After transplantation, postoperative care consists of maintaining the indwelling (Foley) catheter's patency with continuous irrigation, maintaining fluid and electrolyte balance, observing for complications, and preparing the patient for discharge.

### Histocompatibility tests
The major obstacle to a renal transplant's success is the body's ability to recognize and reject foreign tissue, thereby making the transplanted kidney nonfunctional. Four tests are currently used to ensure compatibility between a kidney donor and recipient: ABO blood typing, white cell cross matching, human leokocyte antigen (HLA) typing, and mixed lymphocyte culture.

*ABO blood typing* ensures RBC compatibility between donor and recipient lest the transplanted kidney immediately be rejected.

*White cell cross matching* identifies preformed, circulating cytotoxic antibodies in the recipient. Such antibodies may have been formed following blood transfusions, pregnancies, infections, or previous transplants. The presence of antibodies against the donor lymphocytes would cause immediate transplant rejection. The test involves mixing the recipient's serum with donor lymphocytes and observing for cell agglutination or lysis (positive reaction). A negative cross matching is essential for transplantation.

*Lymphocytotoxicity (HLA) testing* identifies the donor's and recipient's specific HLAs. Lymphocytes from the donor and recipient are exposed to antiserums with a known antibody composition. The lymphocytes undergo lysis if they have a cell surface antigen recognized by the serum's antibodies. Thus, specific antigens against which the specific antibody is reacting can be identified. With this test, the genetic makeups of the donor and recipient are compared to select the most compatible pair for transplantation. (See *The HLA system.*)

*Mixed lymphocyte culture testing* determines the degree of incompatibility between the donor and recipient without defining the exact antigens responsible. It involves mixing together donor and recipient lymphocytes and measuring the degree to which the lymphocytes enlarge and multiply. The greater the response, the more incompatible the donor and recipient.

### Transplant rejection
The singular purpose of tests to match donor and recipient is to prevent a reaction that destroys the transplanted organ (rejection).

Two types of lymphocytes are involved in the rejection phenomenon: B-lymphocytes and T-lymphocytes. B-lymphocytes form antibodies when they recognize foreign antigens (a transplanted kidney) in the body. This reaction, *humoral immunity,* also activates the complement and kinin systems to deposit platelets and fibrin at the reaction site. T-lymphocytes mature in the thymus and activate *cell-mediated immunity*. These lymphocytes release chemical factors (lymphokines) that directly destroy cells carrying the specific antigens. The sensitized lymphocytes also convert other T-lymphocytes to "killer" cells, ultimately causing necrosis of the transplanted kidney.

Four forms of transplant rejection have been identified: hyperacute, accelerated, acute, and chronic.

**Hyperacute rejection.** This involves a humoral immune response between antigens in the transplanted kidney and preformed, circulating antibodies in the recipient's serum. Within minutes after the transplant's completed, rejection occurs. The kidney darkens and becomes necrotic as antibodies, complement, and fibrin are deposited, resulting in thrombosis. Because hyperacute rejection has no treatment, a negative cross matching before transplantation is essential to prevent its occurrence.

**Accelerated rejection.** Occuring 24 to 36 hours after transplantation, this type of rejection has the same pathologic basis as hyperacute rejection. During transplantation, the level of circulating antibodies in the recipient's serum isn't high enough to cause rejection. However, within a few hours, these levels begin to rise and ultimately cause rejection. Accelerated rejection has no successful treatment, nor can it always be prevented by pretransplant cross matching.

**Acute rejection.** This is a cell-mediated immune response that occurs a week to a few months after transplantation. T-lymphocytes gradually become sensitized with antigens from the foreign transplanted tissue and trigger kidney necrosis. Signs and symptoms of acute rejection vary but may include oliguria or anuria; fever over 100° F. (37.8° C.); a

### The HLA system
This diagram shows a typical pattern of human leukocyte antigen (HLA) inheritance in a family group. Each letter represents an antigen pair, or haplotype. Each person inherits one HLA chromosomal region from each parent. Each HLA region contains an antigen pair so that each offspring shares one antigen pair with each parent. Only four different combinations are possible from one set of parents; the statistical chance of each child bearing the same HLA type is one in four.

An identical HLA match between kidney donor and recipient offers the best chance for transplant success.

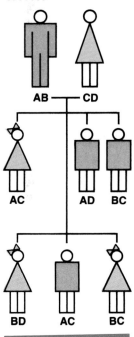

## Renal transplantation

Before transplantation, the donor kidney is flipped over to position the renal artery anteriorly and the renal vein posteriorly so that the vein can be anastomosed first. The common, internal, or external iliac arteries and veins may be used. A submucosal tunnel is created for the ureter, which is then implanted into the bladder or connected to the stump of the recipient's own ureter. The submucosal tunnel acts as a one-way valve to prevent urine reflux into the transplanted kidney.

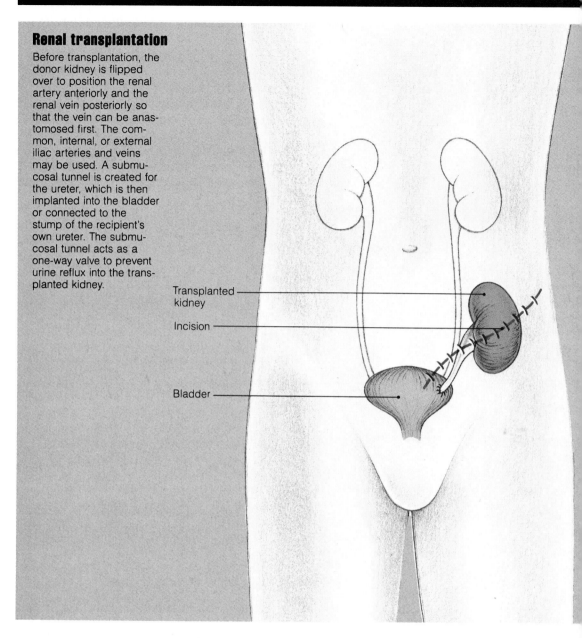

Transplanted kidney

Incision

Bladder

soft, tender, swollen transplanted kidney; hypertension or weight gain from fluid retention; malaise; changes in BUN, serum creatinine, creatinine clearance, and serum electrolyte levels; urine component changes; and slow dye uptake and excretion on renogram.

**Chronic rejection.** Occurring several months to a few years after transplantation, this type of rejection is probably a combination of humoral and cell-mediated immune responses. T-lymphocytes enhance B-lymphocyte antibody production, causing progressive deterioration of transplant function. BUN and serum creatinine levels increase gradually. Electrolyte imbalance, proteinuria, weight gain, hypertension, and edema are concomitant problems. Chronic rejection has no successful treatment, and the transplanted kidney's function

is eventually lost. (See *Mechanism of transplant rejection,* page 104.)

### Immunosuppressive therapy promotes acceptance

Immunosuppressive therapy aims to prevent the body from recognizing the transplanted kidney as foreign, thereby allowing it to be accepted. Several immunosuppressive therapies—including corticosteroids, purine analogues, radiation, antilymphocyte globulin (ALG), and cyclosporine—have been used with varying degrees of success.

**Corticosteroids.** Prednisone or other corticosteroids suppress the body's inflammatory response to foreign material by preventing leukocyte infiltration into tissues. In addition, they decrease antibody production and inhibit

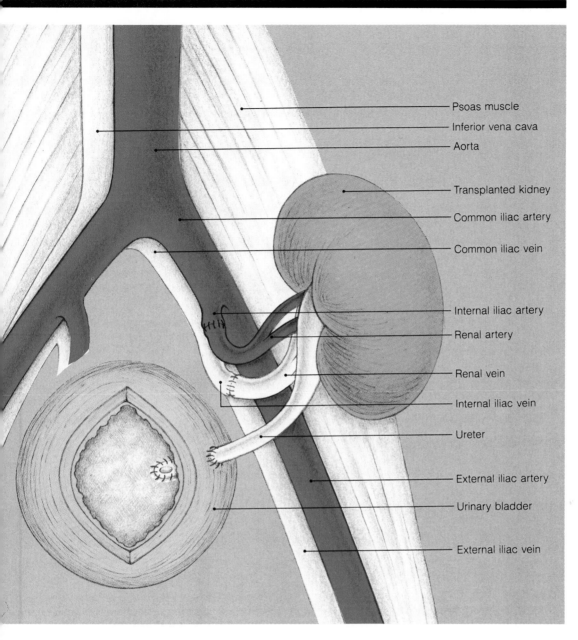

Psoas muscle
Inferior vena cava
Aorta
Transplanted kidney
Common iliac artery
Common iliac vein
Internal iliac artery
Renal artery
Renal vein
Internal iliac vein
Ureter
External iliac artery
Urinary bladder
External iliac vein

antigen-antibody complexing. During the initial postoperative period, patients receive large doses of I.V. methylprednisolone that are gradually replaced by daily maintenance doses of oral prednisone (10 to 20 mg/day). However, additional large doses of methylprednisolone may be given to reverse threatened rejection.

Prolonged administration of corticosteroids may produce numerous undesirable side effects, such as predisposition to viral, fungal, and bacterial infections; gastrointestinal ulceration and bleeding; diabetes mellitus; cushingoid appearance; acne; delayed wound healing; aseptic necrosis of the femoral head; cataracts; steroid psychosis; pancreatitis; increased appetite; and hypertension from salt and water retention.

**Purine analogues.** Azathioprine, the most frequently used purine analogue, alters the immune response by interfering with purine synthesis, thus decreasing antibody production. The usual daily dosage is 2 mg/kg of body weight. Bone marrow suppression, a possible side effect, may result in leukopenia and thrombocytopenia. If serious side effects occur, the dosage may be decreased, temporarily discontinued, or replaced with cyclophosphamide.

**Radiation therapy.** This therapy slows lymphocyte migration to the transplant site and inhibits antibody formation. Local radiation to the graft site—up to a limit of 1,500 to 2,000 rads—is most commonly performed.

**Antilymphocyte globulin.** Still gaining acceptance as an immunosuppressive agent,

# Mechanism of transplant rejection

The transplanted (donor) kidney (at top) releases antigens and stimulates lymphocytes to produce humoral antibodies and cytotoxic (sensitized) lymphocytes. These then attack the transplanted kidney.

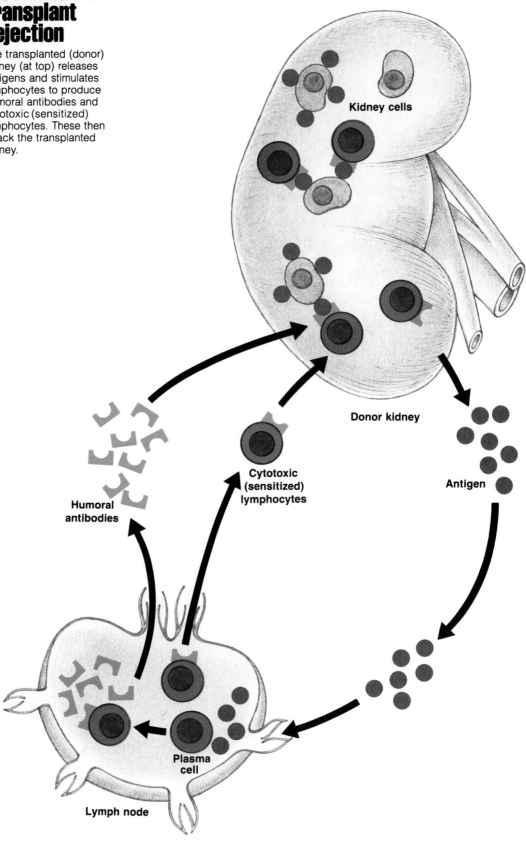

Kidney cells

Donor kidney

Antigen

Humoral antibodies

Cytotoxic (sensitized) lymphocytes

Plasma cell

Lymph node

ALG is made by injecting human leukocytes into a horse, cow, or rabbit. The animal forms antibodies to the human cells, and its serum is then refined to produce the immunoglobulin ALG. After transplantion, ALG is given intravenously through a central venous line. T-lymphocytes become coated with the ALG and are susceptible to phagocytic destruction by cells from the reticuloendothelial system. Common side effects include sensitization to the animal's serum, fever, and thrombocytopenia.

**Cyclosporine.** The newest therapy for organ transplant rejection, cyclosporine (Cyclosporin A) is manufactured from a metabolite of the fungus, *Tolypocladium inflatum,* that has immunosuppressive properties. Cyclosporine, a selective immunosuppressive agent, acts on T-lymphocytes, which are partially responsible for transplant rejection. The cyclosporine dosage is determined by blood level measurements and may be given orally or intravenously. Side effects include hypertension, lymphoma formation, infection, nephrotoxicity, hirsutism, muscle cramps, nausea, diarrhea, anorexia, and paresthesias.

## NURSING MANAGEMENT
What's most likely to impress you about the patient with chronic renal failure is the number and diversity of his problems. Management of this challenging patient demands a systematic process of assessing, diagnosing, planning, implementing, and evaluating. Applying the nursing process successfully ensures that no problem will go unnoticed or untreated.

### History taking: Gathering the first clues
Begin assessment by investigating the patient's chief complaint. Then obtain a health, family, and psychosocial history to help pinpoint the cause of chronic renal failure. A history of proteinuria, hematuria, or hypertension suggests some type of chronic glomerulonephritis.

Inquire about previous medical examinations for life insurance or for military service to help determine the duration of the underlying disease. Acute nephritis or Bright's disease contracted during childhood may indicate chronic glomerulonephritis. Micturition difficulties in childhood may indicate lower urinary tract abnormality with obstructive uropathy. In older men, symptoms of prostatism may suggest prostatic outlet obstruction as a possible cause of chronic renal failure.

A family history of nephropathy and deafness suggests sickle cell anemia. If your patient is black, ask about sickle cell anemia. Recurrent urinary tract infections may indicate chronic pyelonephritis, obstructive uropathy, hydronephrosis, vesicoureteral reflux, or renal calculi.

Ask about the patient's drug history. Does he habitually abuse analgesics? If so, he may have papillary necrosis with renal colic. Renal colic also suggests primary renal calculi or calculi secondary to hyperparathyroidism, hypercalcemia, or gout. Use of such drugs as methysergide may cause chronic renal failure, whereas diuretics, sulfonamides, and methicillin may cause superimposed acute injury. Heavy metal poisoning may also cause chronic renal failure.

Hemoptysis suggests Goodpasture's syndrome and rapidly progressive glomerulonephritis. Multisystem involvement suggests a collagen disease, such as systemic lupus erythematosus or polyarteritis nodosa. Long-standing, insulin-dependent diabetes mellitus strongly suggests diabetic glomerulosclerosis. Skin tightness and dysphagia suggest scleroderma. Bone pain and weakness, especially in older patients with renal failure, suggest multiple myeloma. Recurrent joint pain and swelling suggest gouty arthritis and, possibly, coexistent gouty nephropathy.

### Physical examination: Approaching body systems one-by-one
Regardless of the primary cause, the clinical signs of chronic renal failure—and its end-stage uremia—are typically widespread, requiring systematic physical examination.

**Inspect the skin.** In uremia, the skin is typically pallid, grayish bronze, dry, and scaly. The discoloration results from retained pigments; the pallor, from anemia. Decreased oil gland activity and sweat gland size diminish perspiration, causing dryness. Dryness and irritating calcium phosphate deposits, in turn, cause severe itching. The patient is compelled to scratch, and his skin may become excoriated and infected. Because of abnormal clotting activity and heightened capillary fragility in uremia, minor blows to the skin may cause ecchymoses and purpura.

**Assess fluid status and acid-base balance.** The patient with chronic renal failure may be dehydrated or overhydrated, depending on the cause and degree of renal failure. Monitor intake and output, and assess the skin for poor turgor or peripheral edema. Substantial urinary fluid loss in late renal failure may be caused by polycystic kidneys. Creatinine clearance of less than 4 or 5 ml/minute usually signals fluid overload. Other symptoms may include headache, dizziness, and shortness of breath.

When metabolic acidosis complicates renal failure, the patient compensates by hyperventilating (Kussmaul's breathing) to remove excess $CO_2$.

Acidosis results from the kidney's inability to excrete hydrogen ions and to produce sufficient ammonia, from retention of acid end products of protein metabolism, and from loss of bicarbonate in the urine. In severe acidosis, lethargy and coma develop; however, an altered level of consciousness may also result from the underlying disease, such as diabetic acidosis. Decreased plasma bicarbonate levels and low arterial blood pH characterize acidosis. Because bone helps buffer excess hydrogen ions, acidosis contributes to renal osteodystrophy.

**Evaluate cardiovascular status.** Hypertension is the most common threat to the cardiovascular system from chronic renal failure. Other renal-related cardiovascular problems include additional electrolyte imbalances (hyperkalemia, hypermagnesemia, hypocalcemia); and serious pathologic changes (myocardial and arterial calcification, cardiomyopathy, pericarditis, pericardial effusion, and cardiac tamponade). (See *Detecting cardiovascular complications,* page 109.)

Hypertension results from fluid and sodium overload or from malfunction of the renin-angiotensin system. In fluid and sodium overload, the kidney fails to excrete sodium and water, causing circulatory overload and elevated blood pressure. Reducing sodium and fluid intake or removing fluid during dialysis usually helps control blood pressure.

However, hypertension resulting from malfunction of the renin-angiotensin system doesn't respond well to fluid and sodium restriction or to dialysis. In this case, significant fluid removal during hemodialysis may increase renal ischemia and renin production, aggravating the hypertension.

Assess the patient's blood pressure frequently to monitor hypertension. In mild hypertension, diastolic pressure is 100 mm Hg or less; in moderate hypertension, it's between 100 and 120 mm Hg; in severe hypertension, it's above 120 mm Hg; and in malignant hypertension, it's above 140 mm Hg.

Other signs and symptoms of hypertension include funduscopic changes, such as arteriovenous nicking, exudates, hemorrhages, papilledema, and decreased vessel size.

Causes of hyperkalemia in renal failure include acidosis, excess potassium intake, failure to comply with the dietary regimen, blood transfusions, and bleeding.

Normal serum potassium levels (3.5 to 5.0 mEq/liter) are maintained until the 24-hour urine output falls below 500 ml. When the serum level reaches 7 or 8 mEq/liter, muscle weakness may develop, or severe electrocardiographic changes may rapidly progress to cardiac arrest and death.

Assess the patient's serum potassium level and EKG status regularly. Acidosis increases serum potassium levels because the kidneys (if functional) excrete excess hydrogen ions instead of potassium ions to maintain acid-base balance. Also, increased extracellular hydrogen diffuses into the cells while abundant intracellular potassium diffuses out into the blood.

**Review hematologic status.** Chronic renal failure may cause anemia and platelet defects as well as bleeding and clotting disorders. Anemia may result from decreased RBC production (normally, the kidney produces erythropoietin or its precursor in response to hypoxia—this substance stimulates bone marrow production of RBCs); decreased RBC survival time (due to destruction by elevated uremic toxin levels); or blood loss from gastrointestinal bleeding, dialysis (accidental dialyzer membrane rupture, hemolysis, residual dialyzer blood loss), or frequent blood tests.

Watch for pallor, dyspnea, fatigue, tachycardia, palpitations, and low hemoglobin and hematocrit levels.

**Check pulmonary status.** Pulmonary complications in chronic renal failure include pulmonary edema, pleuritic pain, pleural rub, pleural effusions, uremic pleuritis, and uremic pneumonitis. Observe for tenacious sputum and a depressed cough reflex. Increased susceptibility to infection results from reduced pulmonary macrophage activity in uremia.

**Determine gastrointestinal status.** Widespread inflammation and ulceration of the GI mucosa in uremia may cause stomatitis, uremic fetor (urine and ammonia odor on the breath), esophagitis, gastritis, gastric and duodenal ulcers, small- and large-bowel lesions, proctitis, anorexia, nausea, and vomiting. Monitor the patient's nutritional status, appetite, weight, and electrolyte levels.

Salivary urea may increase to approximately three fourths of the serum level. In renal failure, the enzyme urease (produced by oral bacteria) converts excess salivary urea to ammonia, which, in turn, may produce uremic fetor, gum ulceration, bleeding, metallic taste, and generalized stomatitis. These symptoms usually subside after the patient is placed on dialysis.

Nausea and vomiting associated with uremia resemble the early morning sickness of pregnancy. Typically, these symptoms result from nocturnal dehydration, which increases serum uremic toxin levels.

**Ask about gonadal function.** In advanced renal failure, infertility occurs in both men and women, with amenorrhea and cessation of ovulation in women, impotence in men, and decreased libido in both sexes.

Decreased libido and impotence probably result from both psychological and physiologic factors. Following dialysis, libido tends to improve in both sexes. Ovulation and menstruation may resume in women. Indeed, excessive bleeding may become a problem because of heparinization during dialysis. Successful pregnancy for women with chronic renal failure—before or after regular hemodialysis—is rare.

**Evaluate musculoskeletal status.** Some degree of calcium phosphate imbalance appears in nearly every case of renal failure. Observe for signs of hypocalcemia (levels lower than 9 mg/100 ml), especially involuntary spasms. Test for Chvostek's sign by tapping your finger in front of the patient's ear at the angle of the jaw, over the facial nerve. Contracture of the lateral facial muscles is a positive sign. Also, the patient's upper lip may twitch on the side of the tapping. Test for Trousseau's sign by inflating a blood pressure cuff around the patient's upper arm for 3 minutes. Carpopedal spasm—adduction of the thumb and extension of the phalangeal joints—is a positive sign.

Also observe for signs of hyperphosphatemia (levels greater than 4.5 mg/100 ml); hyperparathyroidism; inadequate vitamin D metabolism; osteodystrophy; calcium deposits in joints, arteries and arterioles, soft tissue, and other areas; and limited mobility.

In many patients, renal osteodystrophy and metastatic calcifications may not be clinically apparent; however, in advanced renal disease, extreme bone disturbances may dominate the illness, causing bone pain, fractures, subperiosteal erosions, and periarticular calcifications. If calcium phosphate levels exceed about 70 mg/100 ml of plasma, extensive calcium phosphate deposits and metastatic calcifications may occur in the brain, eyes, gums, joints, lungs, myocardium, heart valves, blood vessels, and skin.

**Assess neurologic status.** Nervous system changes occur in virtually all uremic patients but vary with the degree of uremia and the part of the nervous system affected—central, peripheral, or autonomic. Changes may occur in mentation, behavior, and sensory and motor function.

Mentation changes include shortened memory and attention span, lack of interest in the environment, confusion, stupor, coma, and convulsions. EEG changes reflect a metabolic encephalopathy.

Behavioral changes depend on the patient's personality and may range from slight irritation to complete withdrawal. Other changes may include psychosis, delusions, decreased or absent libido, agitation, and depression.

Slowing of peripheral nerve conduction results in peripheral neuropathy, marked by symmetrical numbness and burning, beginning in the toes and spreading up the legs; restless legs syndrome; foot drop; and burning feet syndrome.

The restless legs syndrome, one of the earliest signs of peripheral neuropathy, usually develops during the night. It consists of painful cramps and crawling, prickling, and itching sensations in the legs. Moving the legs may relieve the symptoms, thus the term "restless legs." The burning feet syndrome consists of bilateral, painful burning, prickling, and tingling in the feet, which may curtail ambulation and cause insomnia. Bilateral foot drop is the most common motor dysfunction of uremic neuropathy. If dialysis is instituted before motor dysfunction develops, peripheral neuropathy may slowly reverse.

**Assess psychosocial status.** Patients with chronic renal failure use many defense mechanisms to protect their psychological equilibrium. Among them are denial, displacement, projection, regression, intellectualization, isolation of affect, and reaction formation. Remember, these defense mechanisms serve an important purpose for the patient, and dealing with them requires intensive psychological intervention. The patient may refuse to comply with the treatment regimen; he may fail to take his medications, to adhere to his diet, to stay with the dialysis schedule, or to perform proper shunt care.

Assess the patient's psychological status carefully. Look for mood swings, excessive crying, increased demands, withdrawal, neglect of self-care, and role changes within the family. He may express feelings of worthlessness, concern about treatment costs, and worry about decreased libido or impotence or his personal appearance.

**Formulate a care plan**
Develop a specific, individualized care plan for your patient. You'll probably have to try more than one approach to make him comfortable, because treatment is primarily symptomatic. Persist in your efforts, and consistently respond to the patient's complaints. Above all, try to establish a trusting relationship to facilitate interventions for nursing diagnoses like the following:

**Knowledge deficit related to dialysis techniques.** Your goal in this diagnosis is to help the patient choose the type of dialysis appropriate for him and then to manage that dialysis successfully.

Begin by encouraging him to become independent of the dialysis center and its more restrictive dialysis procedures. Teach the patient about basic renal anatomy and physiology and the principles of dialysis. Also tell the patient about the advantages and disadvantages of each type of dialysis, and work with him to select the type that's appropriate for his life-style and type of renal failure.

Teach the patient about the possible complications of dialysis procedures. For example, peritonitis is the most frequent complication of peritoneal dialysis, resulting from contamination of the dialysate or catheter. (See *Sterile connection device helps prevent peritonitis,* page 111.) Complications of hemodialysis include air embolism, hypovolemia and hypotension (from excessive fluid removal), hemolysis, and exsanguination (from ruptured bloodlines).

Consider your interventions successful if the patient:
• understands the purpose of dialysis
• confidently and correctly performs his own dialysis treatment
• recognizes complications of dialysis that require medical treatment.

**Potential for impaired skin integrity related to effects of chronic renal failure.** To maintain skin integrity, assess skin color, texture, turgor, and vascularity periodically. Look for bruises, purpura, and signs of infection. Inspect the conjunctiva, mouth, and nails for pallor and the dependent areas and periorbital spaces for edema.

Warn the patient to avoid falls or even minor skin trauma. If he's bedridden, pad the side rails. Turn him frequently and pad bony prominences to prevent decubiti. Also provide an egg-crate mattress or flotation pad to relieve pressure.

If the patient develops uremic frost (a white powdery substance on the skin, composed mainly of urates), remove it with soap and water. However, uremic frost is rare with modern therapy.

Relentless itching and scratching predispose the patient to infection and make him irritable, restless, and frustrated. Correction of elevated phosphate levels and dialysis may partially relieve the itching. You can also help by keeping the patient's skin clean. Try to relieve itching and dryness by using nonirritating soap, sodium bicarbonate in bath water, oatmeal baths, bath oil, or lotion. Apply ointments or creams for comfort. Provide an antipruritic medication, such as trimeprazine tartrate (Temaril) or cyproheptadine hydrochloride (Periactin) to control itching. During intense itching, have the patient rub lotion into the skin instead of scratching. Trim his nails to prevent excoriation from scratching. Explain to the patient that toxic substances in his blood are causing the skin irritation.

Consider your interventions effective if the patient:
• maintains good skin integrity
• expresses relief of itching and frustration
• understands how uremia irritates skin.

**Potential for alteration in blood pressure (hypertension) related to sodium and water retention and renin-angiotensin system dysfunction.** Periodically monitor blood pressure with the patient supine, sitting, and standing. Record blood pressure on a flow sheet, monitoring the influence of drugs, diet, weight, and other stressors. Describe for the patient the actions and side effects of ordered drugs. Warn him about orthostatic hypotension, and advise him to move slowly from lying to standing positions.

If ultrafiltration is used for fluid removal during hemodialysis, withhold all antihypertensive medications for 8 to 10 hours before dialysis. Antihypertensives prevent the vascular system from reacting normally to decreased blood volume caused by ultrafiltration; therefore, shock may develop. These drugs also prevent removal of adequate fluid during dialysis.

# Detecting cardiovascular complications

Pericarditis occurs in up to 50% of patients with chronic renal failure and, if untreated, may lead to life-threatening hemorrhagic effusion and cardiac tamponade. Normally, 10 to 15 ml of fluid are present between the visceral and parietal pericardial layers. This fluid allows the layers to glide smoothly over each other during heart movements. In renal failure, however, uremic toxins irritate and inflame the pericardial sac, causing the layers to rub together. You can hear this *pericardial friction rub,* a harsh grating sound, during auscultation of the precordium as the heart moves. Also, be alert for other signs and symptoms of pericarditis, such as low-grade fever, hypotension, and chest pain that worsens with deep inspiration and eases when the patient sits up and leans forward.

Pericardial effusion, the major complication of pericarditis, can produce signs of heart failure (dyspnea, orthopnea, and tachycardia), substernal pain, and a feeling of fullness in the chest.

To detect this complication, check for absence of a preexisting pericardial friction rub caused by enlargement of the pericardial space by fluid accumulation, which also restricts cardiac filling and reduces cardiac output.

Check also for paradoxical pulse. In paradoxical pulse, the fall in arterial pressure exceeds the 10-mm Hg decline that's normal during inspiration. Paradoxical pulse may be a sign of cardiac tamponade, which may occur if pericardial fluid accumulates rapidly. Because this condition requires immediate treatment, be alert for its characteristic signs: increased venous pressure, bulging neck veins, narrowing pulse pressure, profound hypotension, weak peripheral pulses, and muffled heart sounds.

**Myocardium**  **Visceral pericardium**  **Parietal pericardium**

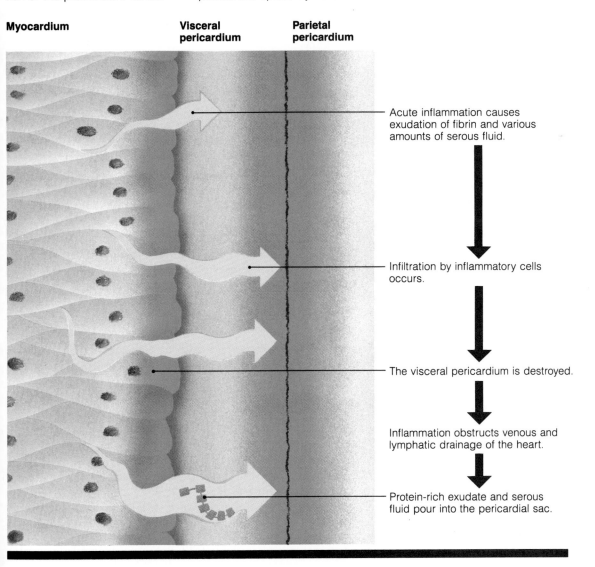

Acute inflammation causes exudation of fibrin and various amounts of serous fluid.

Infiltration by inflammatory cells occurs.

The visceral pericardium is destroyed.

Inflammation obstructs venous and lymphatic drainage of the heart.

Protein-rich exudate and serous fluid pour into the pericardial sac.

## CAPD: Indications and benefits

Continuous ambulatory peritoneal dialysis (CAPD) is a self-care treatment for end-stage renal disease (ESRD). It's especially useful for patients who have experienced complications of hemodialysis. In fact, it may be necessary for diabetic patients with ESRD, since the excellent control of blood pressure and uremia and the satisfactory control of serum glucose levels achieved by intraperitoneal administration of insulin may ameliorate diabetic complications.

CAPD helps promote the patient's independence and a return to a near-normal life-style. Besides freeing the patient from confining hemodialysis treatments, it removes the need for frequent venipunctures and restrictions on diet and fluid intake. In addition, CAPD helps maintain hematocrit levels and helps regulate plasma volume.

Closely monitor fluid status, and instruct the patient to keep track of intake and output.

Have him consider foods that are liquid at room temperature as fluid intake. Advise the patient to control thirst and fluid intake by sucking on a lemon or hard candy or by taking medications with applesauce instead of water. Instruct him to report signs of fluid overload, such as periorbital, sacral, or peripheral edema; headaches; seizures; or blurred vision.

Use an ophthalmoscope to inspect for funduscopic changes, such as arteriovenous nicking, exudates, hemorrhages, decreased vessel size, and papilledema.

Consider your interventions effective if the patient:
• acknowledges his feelings about the disease
• actively seeks help from available resources to cope with the disease
• maintains an acceptable blood pressure
• maintains fluid balance.

**Potential for electrolyte imbalance related to metabolic acidosis, excessive oral intake of potassium, bleeding, or decreased potassium excretion.** Monitor serum potassium levels; notify the doctor if levels exceed 5.5 mEq/liter. Also observe for EKG changes indicating hyperkalemia and for weakness and malaise. Inform the patient how potassium levels relate to diminished kidney function. Emphasize the importance of following the prescribed diet and avoiding foods high in potassium. Typically, dietary potassium intake is based on urine output and serum potassium levels. If the patient is also on a salt-restricted diet, advise him not to use salt substitutes containing potassium or ammonium as the cation.

Administer blood transfusions during dialysis to remove excess potassium. Use washed packed cells because whole blood transfusions may increase the serum potassium levels. Provide emergency treatment for lethal hyperkalemia (serum potassium levels greater than 7 mEq/liter).

Because metabolic acidosis may precipitate or aggravate hyperkalemia, monitor pH.

However, treatment for metabolic acidosis with sodium bicarbonate may decrease calcium levels. Watch for twitching, muscle spasms, and other signs of hypocalcemia with rapid correction of acidosis. Give intravenous calcium gluconate slowly to prevent hypocalcemic tetany. Monitor EKG during calcium administration. Calcium acts synergistically with digitalis and may trigger sustained cardiac contractions. Administer a cation-exchange resin (Kayexalate), as ordered. Monitor for hypokalemia from overzealous treatment. Prepare for dialysis as soon as possible.

Consider your interventions effective if the patient:
• maintains serum electrolytes and arterial pH within normal limits
• understands the importance of compliance with dietary regimen.

**Potential for decreased cardiac output related to pericarditis, pericardial effusion, and pericardial tamponade secondary to uremia.** Pericarditis or pericardial effusion requires intensive dialysis, sometimes daily, until the condition improves. Monitor the patient before, during, and after dialysis for changes in cardiac status. Carefully auscultate for pericardial friction rub (best heard at the left fifth intercostal space during systole). Observe for paradoxical pulse during routine blood pressure measurement; report paradox greater than 10 mm Hg.

Palpate peripheral pulses for rate and quality; note waxing and waning. Periodically monitor for low-grade fever, chest pain, ST segment changes on EKG, and shock with tamponade (profound hypotension; narrow pulse pressure; weak peripheral pulses; cold, poorly perfused extremities; decreasing sensorium; increased venous pressure; bulging neck veins). If tamponade occurs, prepare for emergency pericardial aspiration and cardiopulmonary resuscitation.

Consider your interventions effective if the patient maintains an acceptable blood pressure and strong peripheral pulses.

**Potential for anemia related to uremia or blood loss.** To prevent anemia, give iron and folate supplements, as ordered, preferably 30 to 60 minutes before meals. Avoid giving iron at the same time as phosphate-binding drugs. Give androgens, as ordered, and watch for possible side effects, such as fluid retention, masculinization, hirsutism, and skin infections. Instruct the patient to avoid fatigue. Avoid unnecessary blood specimen collection. Teach the patient about normal platelet function and the changes that occur in uremia. Advise him to prevent bleeding by using a soft toothbrush, avoiding vigorous nose blowing, preventing constipation, and avoiding contact sports.

Administer blood transfusions, as ordered. Potential renal transplant recipients usually are transfused only with blood with decreased antigenic properties. However, recent

# Sterile connection device helps prevent peritonitis

**P**eritonitis, the most common and most serious complication of continuous ambulatory peritoneal dialysis (CAPD), can result from infection with *Staphylococcus epidermidis* or *S. aureus*. Its signs and symptoms include cloudy drainage, fever, abdominal pain and tenderness, diarrhea, and vomiting.

The patient is taught to use strict aseptic technique when performing dialysate exchange, to avoid the risk of peritonitis. Adhering to aseptic technique is easier if the patient uses a portable sterile connection device (SCD), such as the one shown at right. Recently developed, the battery-driven SCD disconnects the used dialysate bag from the patient administration set and automatically makes a sterile, welded connection to the tubing of a new dialysate bag. When used correctly, the peritoneal dialysis system remains closed—and sterile—throughout the procedure.

**Portable SCD unit**

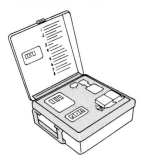

**Making a sterile connection with the SCD**

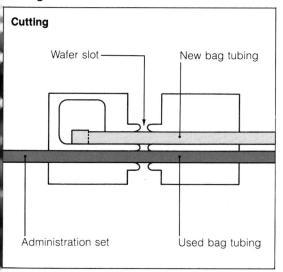

Tubing connecting the administration set and the used dialysate bag is placed in the front slot of the SCD; the new bag tubing is placed in the rear slot. At the push of a button, a welding wafer heats to above 500° F (260° C.) to ensure sterility then automatically melts through both pieces of tubing.

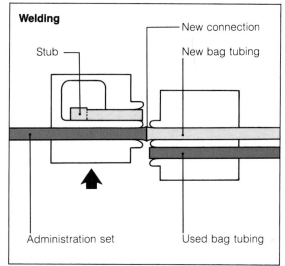

With the wafer still in position, the left tubing holder automatically aligns the administration set tubing with the new bag tubing. The device then simultaneously retracts the wafer and welds the tubes together.

research suggests that whole blood transfusions reduce transplant rejections.

Consider your interventions effective if the patient:
• maintains stable hematocrit levels at 20% to 25%
• understands what causes anemia and how to prevent it.

**Potential for impaired gas exchange related to fluid overload, unstable cardiovascular status, and increased susceptibility to infection in uremia.** Monitor respirations for rate, depth, and quality. Auscultate lung fields for normal and adventitious breath sounds. Observe sputum amount and character. Instruct the patient in deep breathing and coughing exercises. Maintain good oral hygiene. Advise the patient to avoid crowds and exposure to people with upper respiratory infections. Monitor for pulmonary edema. Obtain arterial blood gases, as indicated.

Consider your interventions effective if the patient:
• maintains normal respiratory rate and depth and stable arterial blood gases
• demonstrates no evidence of pulmonary infection (adventitious breath sounds, pulmonary congestion on X-ray, positive sputum culture).

**Potential for inadequate nutrition related to anorexia, nausea and vomiting, altered carbohydrate and protein metabolism, restricted nutrient intake, and GI inflammation.** Monitor BUN, serum creatinine, sodium, and potassium levels to evaluate nutrition. Weigh the patient daily.

Explain to him the prescribed dietary regimen. Schedule fluid intake to allow sufficient fluid consumption at bedtime and to prevent nocturnal dehydration.

If the patient finds food distasteful upon awakening in the morning, encourage him to wait for 2 or 3 hours before trying to eat small servings. If he requests special foods, include them in his dietary regimen. Order an antiemetic, such as prochlorperazine (Compazine) or promethazine hydrochloride (Phenergan), if necessary. Early morning nausea and vomiting often remit after dialysis begins.

Encourage or provide frequent oral hygiene. Advise the patient to brush his teeth several times daily to remove bacteria that produce urease; to use a soft brush and avoid rigorous brushing to prevent gum injury and bleeding; and to use mouthwash, sourballs, lemon juice, or chewing gum to improve taste and alleviate thirst.

A vinegar mouthwash helps neutralize ammonia formed by bacterial action. Moisten dry, cracked lips and mucous membranes with petrolatum jelly or mineral oil. Avoid using glycerine, which has a long-term drying effect. Advise the patient to eat soft, bland, easily digested foods and to avoid spicy and difficult-to-chew foods.

Examine all vomitus and stools for gross or occult blood. Blood urea nitrogen levels rise if blood remains in the GI tract; therefore, provide cleansing enemas to remove blood from the bowel.

Consider your interventions effective if the patient:
• complies with the prescribed diet
• maintains stable weight and acceptable BUN, serum creatinine, sodium, and potassium levels
• demonstrates good oral hygiene.

**Potential for altered musculoskeletal function related to decreased vitamin D, hyperparathyroidism, and decreased phosphate excretion.** Watch for bone, joint, and muscle pain and for increasingly impaired mobility. Monitor serum calcium, phosphate, and alkaline phosphatase levels; be aware of products containing calcium phosphate.

Periodically monitor X-ray films for pathologic fractures, bone demineralization, and joint deposits. Observe for changes in gait, range of motion, and muscle strength. Palpate joints for swelling and tenderness. Help the patient establish and implement an individualized exercise plan to maintain strength and mobility. Avoid immobilization, if possible,

because it increases protein catabolism and bone demineralization.

Give analgesics for pain, as needed. Relate dosage to the degree of renal function loss. Periodically question the patient about hypocalcemia; ask about tetany, carpopedal spasms, seizures, confusion, and numbness and tingling in the fingertips and toes. Monitor the EKG for prolonged QT interval, irritable dysrhythmias, and AV conduction defects secondary to calcium imbalance. Check for positive Chvostek's and Trousseau's signs.

Give medications, as ordered: phosphate-binding medications with meals and snacks, calcium supplements, and vitamin D. Watch for constipation, a possible side effect of phosphate-binding agents. Administer a stool softener or bulk laxative. Watch for hypercalcemia when administering calcium supplements and vitamin D. Develop and implement a teaching program to inform the patient about signs and symptoms of altered calcium metabolism and effective treatment. Allow time for the patient and his family to ask questions. Prepare for dialysis therapy.

Consider your interventions effective if the patient:
• maintains serum calcium, phosphate, and alkaline phosphatase levels within limits defined for each patient.
• shows minimal bone demineralization and no calcium phosphate deposits on X-ray
• successfully complies with his exercise plan
• understands the cause, signs and symptoms, and treatment of calcium phosphate imbalance.

**Impaired physical mobility related to uremia's effects on peripheral nerves.** Consult the physical therapist to assess the patient's muscle strength, gait, and degree of impairment. Then collaborate with him to develop an appropriate exercise plan. Help the patient implement the plan, and encourage him to maintain the prescribed activity level. Protect him from leg and foot trauma. Give analgesics and observe for side effects.

Consider your interventions effective if the patient:
• successfully complies with a prescribed exercise plan
• performs activities of daily living safely and comfortably.

**Alterations in thought processes related to uremia's effects on the nervous system.** Inform the patient and his family about uremia's effects on the nervous system. Help them understand that the patient's behavior may be

## Preserving a cadaver kidney

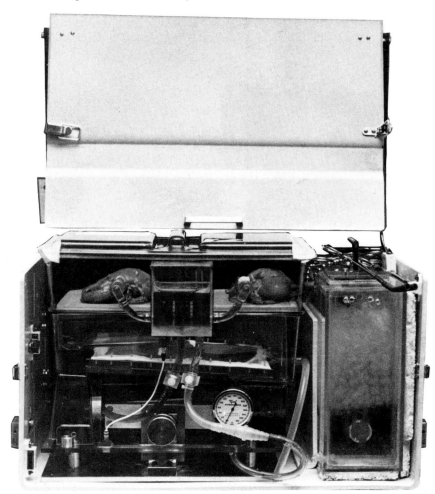

Many kidneys for renal transplant come from cadavers rather than from living, related donors. Most cadavers have suffered fatal head trauma; therefore, their availability can't be predicted. For a cadaver to be used for renal transplant, the donor must be diagnosed as legally brain dead and may be artificially sustained on a ventilator. Also, he must have been under age 55 and free of infection, renal disease, hypertension, and cancer.

If the cadaver meets these conditions, it's tested for compatibility with the renal transplant patient. If the tests prove favorable, a surgeon removes the kidney from the cadaver and places it in a preservation machine, like the one shown here. This machine keeps the kidney healthy by pumping plasma and oxygen into it. A temperature of 43° to 46.5° F. (6° to 8° C.) is maintained inside the machine.

Even with this support, however, a cadaver kidney can be maintained for only 72 hours after it's removed from the donor.

beyond his control. Assess the patient's ability to think and reason before offering instruction or asking him to make decisions. Approach him in a calm, reassuring manner. Minimize environmental stimuli. Avoid fatigue. Note behavior changes, and check for cerebral edema. Take seizure precautions. Administer drugs cautiously since uremia potentiates most drug actions. Avoid opiates or long-acting barbiturates.

Consider your interventions effective if the patient and his family:
• understand how uremia affects the nervous system
• appropriately modify the environment to ensure the patient's comfort and safety.

**Ineffective patient coping related to effects of disease and its treatment on life-style.** Chronic renal failure typically disrupts the core of the patient's life; it changes family roles and often impinges on the patient's career. Added to this psychological stress are the tremendous difficulties of procuring and transplanting the needed organ. (See *Preserv-*

*ing a cadaver kidney.*) Consequently, it's no surprise that helping the patient cope with his disease is one of your most important responsibilities. Begin by encouraging him to express anger and frustration. Help the patient's family understand his behavior. Display a noncritical, listening attitude. Spend scheduled time with the patient to discuss or listen to his concerns. (See *Transplantation: Its psychosocial toll,* page 114.) Assess family roles and strengths, and maximize the strengths. Encourage communication among family members. Suggest possible outside resources for the patient. For example, in 1973, Congress passed the ESRD Medicare Program, which provides for payment of 80% of costs related to dialysis and transplantation for anyone covered by Social Security benefits.

Consider your interventions effective if the patient:
• acknowledges his feelings about the disease
• actively seeks help from available resources to cope with the disease.

**Disturbance in self-concept related to physi-**

# Transplantation: Its psychosocial toll

**Foreign body stage**

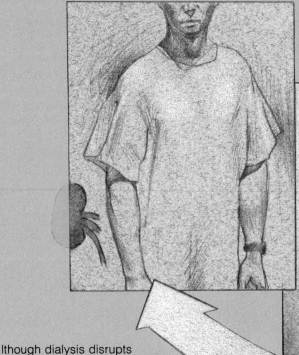

**Partial internalization**

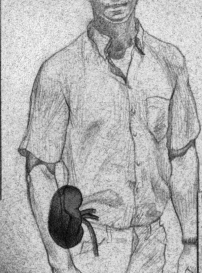

**Regression to foreign body stage**

Although dialysis disrupts a patient's life-style and constantly reminds him of his illness, it promotes dependence on machines, medical staff, and family members and provides positive feelings of security and comfort. Unfortunately, this dependence fosters fears about having a kidney transplant. To help the patient cope with his fears and stresses, you'll need to understand their origins. Consider, for example, the patient who decides to become a transplant candidate. Because weeks, months, or even years may pass before a suitable donor can be found, the patient will have to deal with the stress of continued dialysis as well as the uncertainty of the transplant and of its outcome. Worst of all, the patient's stress may actually increase his risk of transplant rejection.

After transplantation, the patient depends totally on the staff of the intensive care or renal transplant unit. He may continue to show dependent behavior for about 2 weeks after surgery because of his insecurity about the success of the transplant.

If signs of rejection (oliguria, edema, fever, high blood pressure, weight gain, swelling and tenderness of the graft) occur during hospitalization, a return to dialysis, even if temporary, is extremely difficult for the patient to accept. He feels threatened by his vulnerability. Because his self-esteem is often tied to the performance of his new kidney, he may try to downplay the effects of its loss.

## Stages of acceptance

Even if the patient is discharged with a functioning kidney, he may need up to 2 years to accept the transplant psychologically. Typically, the patient goes through three or four stages. In the *foreign body stage*, he thinks the kidney feels strange and that it's sticking out of his body. He moves about cautiously and overemphasizes the kidney's fragility. Next, in the *partial internalization stage*, the patient talks less about the kidney and starts to show interest in other aspects of his life. In the *complete internalization stage*, the patient accepts the kidney, focusing on it only when others direct conversation to it.

During either internalization stage, *regression* to the foreign body stage can occur. Typically, it follows threat of rejection but may even develop during routine medical follow-up.

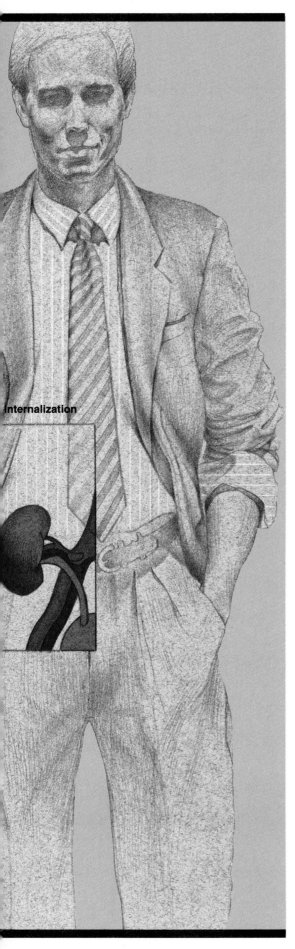

Internalization

**cal effects of uremia and presence of shunt or peritoneal catheter for dialysis.** Explain to the patient how uremia causes physical changes. Encourage him to express his feelings. Teach him how to choose clothing to conceal the shunt.

Consider your interventions effective if the patient:
• demonstrates successful coping mechanisms
• expresses feelings of self-worth and dignity.

**Sexual dysfunction related to effects of uremia and its treatment.** Like many others, you may feel uncomfortable addressing the patient's sexual function. One useful approach is to explore the meaning of sexuality with the patient and his sexual partner. An important issue to pursue is how the couple describes their needs, desires, and feelings about their relationship. The following questions may be helpful: How does the patient express his needs for dependence, independence, intimacy, or isolation? How is the loss of sexual potency related to other areas, such as his job, sports, and hobbies? How does he define himself in light of a changing body image? How does he view his masculine role? Does he have enough trust, sharing, and communication with his partner and the hospital staff to deal with these personal issues? A psychiatric nurse specialist may help explore these areas. By sharing their problems with a careful listener, the couple may work out many of their difficulties. When discussing sexuality, it helps to change the focus from "performing" to "being," to help the couple recognize the human need for touch, tenderness, and respect. You also legitimize their personal style of giving and sharing affection. The strength, companionship, and comfort derived from a healthy love or marital relationship serve the patient well in coping with the demands of his chronic illness.

Consider your interventions effective if the patient maintains a healthy, satisfying sexual relationship with his partner.

## Ongoing evaluation

Continually evaluate your care plan to ensure its success. Establish realistic target dates to achieve each of the expected outcomes, and periodically assess the patient's progress. If he's not achieving desired goals, develop new interventions or make the goals more realistic. And, above all, continually update nursing diagnoses to address the patient's changing problems and to help him best cope with this taxing disease.

## Points to remember

• Chronic renal failure is usually the end result of a gradually progressive loss of renal function.
• Glomerulonephritis is the leading cause of chronic renal failure.
• As kidney function deteriorates, all body systems eventually become involved.
• Renal insufficiency occurs when more than 75% of the nephrons have been destroyed. Uremia occurs when 90% of the nephrons have been destroyed.
• Chronic renal failure may often be managed conservatively with diet, fluid restrictions, and drugs until the glomerular filtration rate decreases to 10% or 15% of normal.
• End-stage renal disease requires maintenance dialysis or a kidney transplant to sustain life.

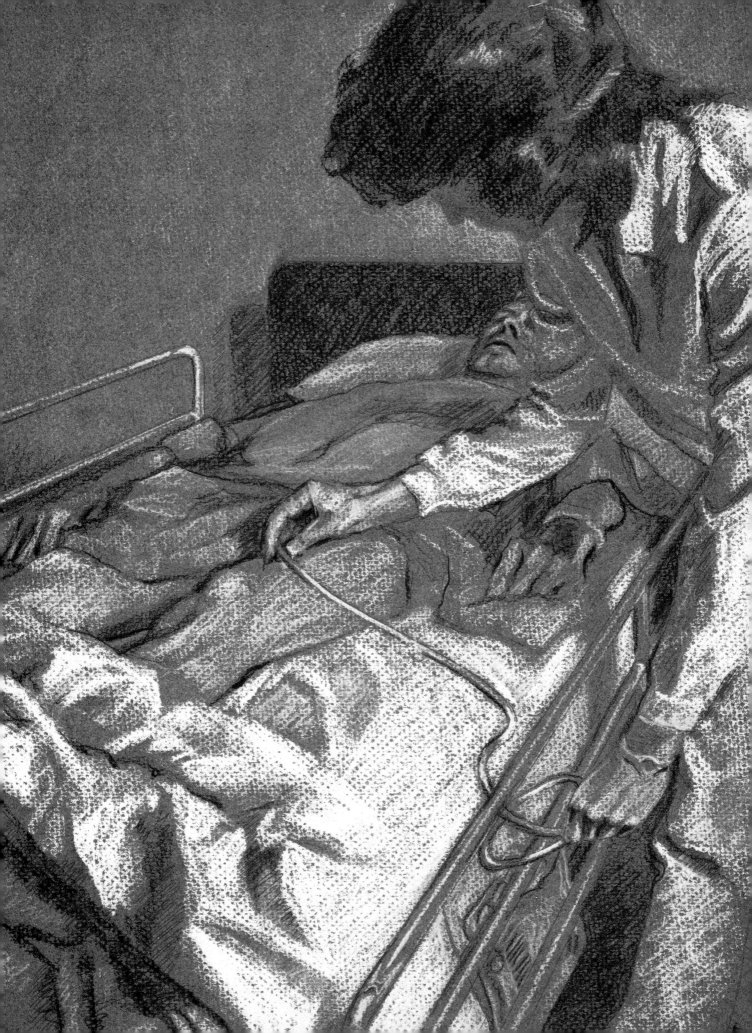

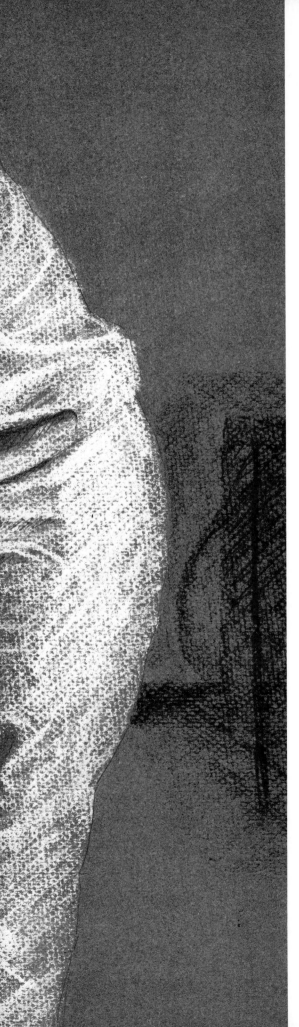

# UROLOGIC DISORDERS

# 6 RELIEVING DISTRESS IN OBSTRUCTION

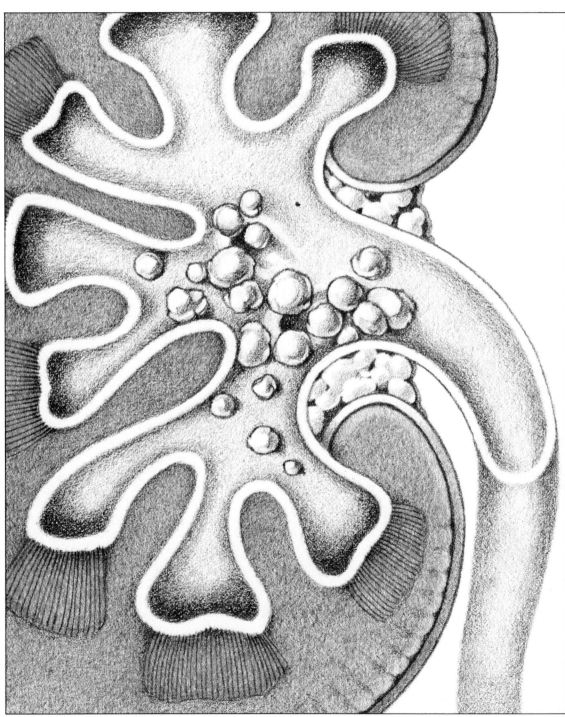

Renal calculi

Whatever their causes, obstructions of the urinary tract pose a serious threat to the kidneys—and, ultimately, to the patient's life. Obstructions may occur at any point in the urinary tract from the urethra (as with prostate enlargement) to the renal pelvis (as with stones, cysts, and tumors). Because urinary tract obstructions commonly produce vague or nonspecific changes—flank pain, hematuria, bacteriuria—you'll need keen assessment skills to distinguish obstructive from other renal or urinary disorders, to plan and execute effective nursing care, and to help the patient preserve as much renal function as possible. Good patient teaching is also essential, since patient compliance in diet and drug therapy is often the most important factor in preventing recurrence.

## Patterns of prevalence

Urinary tract obstructions stemming from calculi or structural or functional abnormalities are fairly common in both sexes and can occur at any age. (See *Causes of urinary tract obstruction,* page 120.) But certain obstructive disorders are more common at certain ages. For example, obstruction in infants usually stems from phimosis, meatal stenosis, neurogenic bladder, and congenital ureteropelvic junction stricture. In older children of both sexes it stems from neurogenic bladder. In male children, obstruction usually occurs from urethral valve obstruction; in female children, from vesicoureteral reflux and ureteropelvic junction obstruction, including congenital strictures. Also, abnormal growth patterns may alter urinary tract structure.

Young adult males are more susceptible to renal calculi, whereas pregnancy is a common cause of obstruction in young adult females. In males over age 50, obstruction frequently results from prostatic enlargement, benign hyperplasia, or prostatic carcinoma; in females over age 50, it commonly results from pelvic tumor. Although urinary obstruction may be surgically corrected, residual abnormality may persist after surgery.

## Causes: Intrinsic and extrinsic

Urinary obstruction divides into intrinsic and extrinsic disorders. Intrinsic disorders stem from obstruction in the urinary tract; extrinsic disorders, from abnormality outside it.

**Intrinsic disorders.** These disorders occur more frequently and may be congenital or acquired. Congenital defects may be obvious in childhood or may not become apparent until years later. Defects amenable to surgical correction include ureteral stricture and urinary meatal stenosis. Such defects most commonly develop at the ureteropelvic and ureterovesical junctions.

Acquired intrinsic defects are more common in adults and include renal, ureteral, or bladder calculi; bladder and kidney tumors (and, more rarely, ureteral tumors); blood clots; renal papillary necrosis; and neurogenic bladder.

Renal papillary necrosis with tissue sloughing may cause unilateral or bilateral obstruction. Papillary necrosis is commonly associated with intrarenal infection and is most likely to occur in diabetic patients, who are more susceptible to infection and renal vascular damage. Neurogenic bladder may result from spina bifida with myelomeningocele or from long-term neuropathy (due to diabetes mellitus) or other neurologic disease. It's often associated with urinary stasis and results in infection leading to end-stage renal disease.

**Extrinsic disorders.** These disorders may obstruct urine flow anywhere in the urinary tract and may cause acute or chronic disorders, though acute disorders are more likely. Extrinsic disorders include abdominal or pelvic problems, such as intestinal masses or uterine tumors or disease; dissection of the aortic bifurcation and ensuing impingement on the ureter; and fibrosis or scarring stemming from inflammation, as in retroperitoneal fibrosis. Iatrogenic causes include ligation, trauma, and acute ureter angulation during lower abdominal or gynecologic surgery.

## PATHOPHYSIOLOGY

Many factors affect the outcome of urinary obstruction and the extent of permanent kidney damage that may result. Probably the most important are how quickly the disorder is detected and resolved and whether associated infection is eradicated and recurrence is avoided. Other significant factors include the patient's general health; the site of obstruction (kidney, ureter, bladder, or urethra); the level of obstruction (upper, at or above the ureterovesical junction, or lower, below the ureterovesical junction); onset (acute or chronic); and cause (mechanical or functional).

## Obstruction invites infection

Normally the urinary tract is sterile. However, obstruction predisposes the patient to urinary

# Causes of urinary tract obstruction

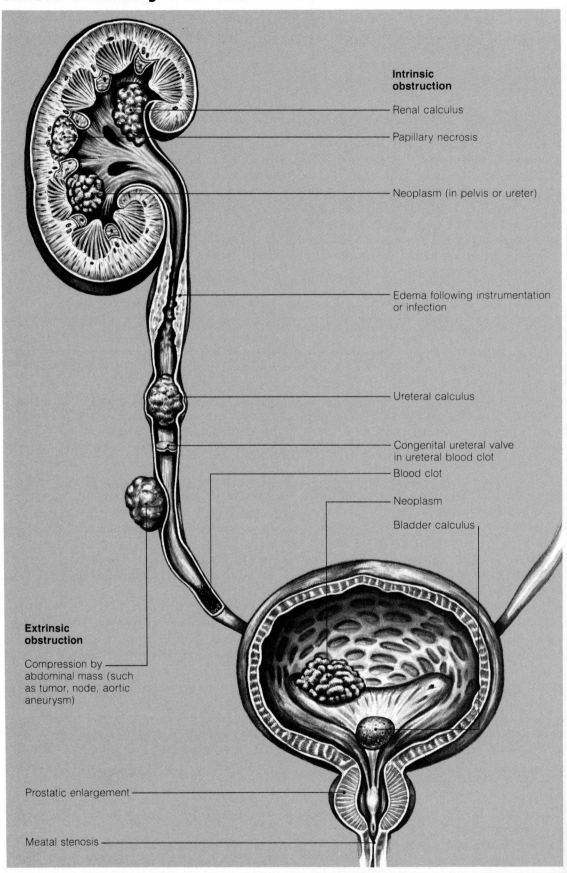

**Intrinsic obstruction**

Renal calculus

Papillary necrosis

Neoplasm (in pelvis or ureter)

Edema following instrumentation or infection

Ureteral calculus

Congenital ureteral valve in ureteral blood clot

Blood clot

Neoplasm

Bladder calculus

**Extrinsic obstruction**

Compression by abdominal mass (such as tumor, node, aortic aneurysm)

Prostatic enlargement

Meatal stenosis

tract infection (UTI) resulting from urine stasis. Obstruction complicated by infection can be difficult to control, particularly if the infection occurs above the obstruction site. Common infecting bacteria include gram-negative organisms, such as *Escherichia coli,* which reach the genitourinary tract from the gastrointestinal tract. Other factors predisposing to infection are systemic immunologic disease or treatment with immunosuppressive drugs.

## Obstruction may involve kidneys
The obstruction site determines whether kidney involvement is unilateral or bilateral. Obstruction above the bladder is usually unilateral. Common obstruction sites above the bladder include the ureteropelvic junction, the midureter, and the ureterovesical junction. Ureteral obstruction usually involves only the kidney served by the involved ureter. Thus, partial or total occlusion of one ureter may not cause oliguria if the other kidney is normal, except in children, in whom the functioning kidney also hypertrophies. In contrast, urethral obstruction (below the bladder) invariably blocks urine flow or increases residual urine. Accumulating residual urine and subsequent bladder dilation may, if undetected or untreated, lead to bilateral kidney involvement.

## Acute and chronic obstruction
Prompt detection and treatment of acute obstruction greatly enhances the patient's chances of preserving renal function. Unfortunately, the onset of chronic obstruction is typically insidious and may be confused with acute obstruction when any undetected obstruction suddenly causes acute symptoms. Chronic onset increases the risk of infection because it causes urine stagnation and urinary backflow, which compress renal tissue and vessels. It's also more likely to cause permanent renal damage.

## Compensation leads to decompensation
The urinary system tries to compensate for obstruction in a variety of ways. Eventually, an obstruction below the bladder initiates a series of physiologic events, which, if untreated, progress up the urinary tract to involve the ureters and, finally, the kidneys. First, to overcome urethral resistance, the bladder neck and muscles hypertrophy. Bladder wall thickness may double, and the pressure generated during a detrusor muscle contraction greatly increases to overcome outlet obstruction. As a result, the overworked muscle begins to decompensate, preventing complete bladder emptying; thus, after the patient voids, insufficient bladder emptying repeatedly stimulates the micturition reflex, causing urinary frequency.

Next, the trigonal area and the interureteric ridge hypertrophy, and coarse, muscular ridges (trabeculae) develop in the usually smooth bladder wall mucosa. During micturition, these trabeculae may push the cellules, small pockets lining the bladder, forcing them between bladder muscle fibers. Eventually, the cellules become saccular and, as the detrusor muscle decompensates, form diverticula. (See *Formation of diverticula,* page 122.) Because bladder diverticula have no muscle, they cannot expel the urine within them into the bladder. Urine stasis in these pockets can easily lead to secondary infection, stone formation, and possibly tumors.

If obstruction persists, the bladder becomes more distended. The thickened, trabeculated bladder wall obstructs urine flow through the ureterovesical junction, elevating intravesical pressure. This increases resistance to urine flow from the ureters, resulting in incomplete ureteral emptying; the ureters hypertrophy in an effort to overcome resistance.

Eventually, the ureters elongate, dilate, and kink. Since ureteral diameter isn't consistent, some ureteral sections narrow more than others, and these points may become stenotic. Unrelieved ureteral obstruction transmits reflux pressure to the renal calyxes and pelvis, resulting in hydronephrosis. Ultimately, increased compression of the renal parenchyma by a grossly distended pelvis depresses renal blood flow and the glomerular filtration rate, resulting in tubular ischemia and tissue atrophy and necrosis.

In tubular ischemia, formed urine leaks into peritubular tissue and is thought to return to the bloodstream via the lymphatics. This urine makes its way back to the peritubular capillaries, eventually impairing glomerular filtration, damaging renal parenchyma, and causing renal failure.

## Mechanical and hormonal effects
Mechanical effects of urinary tract obstruction vary according to the cause and level of the obstruction. For example, an upper urinary tract obstruction, such as a ureteral calculus, results in renal colic: severe, intense pain that radiates over the flank and down the ureteral

# Formation of diverticula

**B**ladder outlet obstruction causes cellules (small pouches) to develop between hypertrophied muscle bundles of the bladder wall. Eventually, as outlet obstruction persists, the detrusor muscle decompensates, and cellules grow into diverticula of various sizes, occasionally exceeding the diameter of the bladder. Diverticula occur more commonly in men than in women because of bladder outlet obstruction resulting from prostatic enlargement.

Diverticula may cause urinary stasis, which can lead to calculus formation or infection or both, or, more rarely, tumors. Diverticular tumors are particularly dangerous because of the ease with which they can spread through thin diverticular walls and invade neighboring structures. Also, diverticula sometimes may herniate through the abdominal wall.

The obstruction that causes diverticula must be removed; if the patient has a persistent infection, the diverticula must be removed as well.

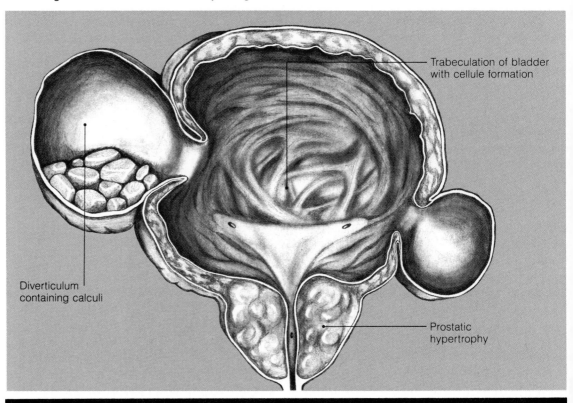

Trabeculation of bladder with cellule formation

Diverticulum containing calculi

Prostatic hypertrophy

path. Pain may also radiate into the vulva or the genitalia and the thighs. Usually, the patient seeks immediate attention; such pain is typically so severe that the patient may present with pallor, diaphoresis, nausea, and vomiting. Along with severe pain, other signs and symptoms include blood or debris (such as necrotic tissue or gravel) in the urine and, if infection is present, chills, fever, and cloudy urine.

An enlarged prostate obstructing the lower urinary tract may cause acute urinary retention—painful bladder spasms associated with bladder distention. Other possible signs and symptoms of lower UTI include lower abdominal fullness, incomplete bladder emptying, diminished force and size of urinary stream, urinary frequency, nocturia, predisposition to bacterial invasion and calculus formation, and, occasionally, overflow incontinence resulting from an overdistended bladder.

When hydronephrosis occurs secondary to obstruction anywhere along the urinary tract, azotemia develops, sometimes followed by uremia. (See *Hydronephrosis: A dangerous complication.*) Signs and symptoms of uremia may include nausea, vomiting, weight loss, weakness, pallor, pruritus, and changes in behavior.

Hormonal effects of urinary obstruction result from decreased renal blood flow and ischemia, which stimulates the renin-angiotensin-aldosterone system and prostaglandin production. Hormone stimulation attempts to increase renal blood flow, causing hypertension and increased sodium retention.

## MEDICAL MANAGEMENT

Effective treatment of urinary obstruction can begin only after detection of its cause. This requires integration of diagnostic tests with the patient history and physical examination results. In the male, the physical includes examination of the penis and rectum; in the female, it includes a pelvic examination. Careful analysis of all subjective and objective data gathered may also reveal the extent of the disorder and its probable causes.

### Diagnostic tests

Catheterization, radiologic tests, ultrasonography, and laboratory tests help determine the location and cause of obstruction.

**Catheterization.** Catheterization is the first step in evaluating suspected urinary tract obstruction. If the catheter drains a large volume of urine, the obstruction level is below the bladder neck. At least a portion of the urine is saved for laboratory tests. Anuria suggests advanced obstruction, unless the obstruction results from a clogged catheter.

**Radiologic tests.** These tests include a variety of contrast studies, scintiscans, and computerized tomography (CT) scans.

*Kidney-ureter-bladder (KUB) radiography (flat-plate abdominal film).* Usually the first step in diagnostic urinary testing, the KUB film surveys the abdomen to determine the position of the kidneys, ureters, and bladder and to reveal gross abnormalities and the presence of radiopaque stones along ureteral paths. This test carries little risk but is contraindicated if the patient is pregnant or has a draining wound.

*Excretory urography (intravenous pyelography).* This is one of the most important structural and functional tests because it allows visualization of renal parenchyma, calyxes, and pelvis and reveals dilation, obstruction, or displacement (shown by delayed dye excretion). It may also be used to determine kidney size and exact kidney position prior to renal biopsy. Sometimes this test is supported by *nephrotomography,* which visualizes selected planes within the kidney to help locate a calculus or a space-occupying lesion.

Excretory urography carries a risk of systemic hypersensitivity to the contrast medium, which may result in transient acute or even

## Hydronephrosis: A dangerous complication

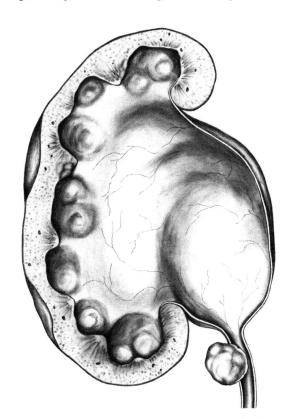

Eventually, urinary tract obstruction can cause hydronephrosis, dilation of the kidneys' collecting system. Hydronephrosis may be unilateral or bilateral, depending on the obstruction site. In early stages, when compression and renal parenchymal atrophy have not yet occurred, hydronephrosis may have little clinical significance unless infection is present. However, without treatment, the dilated pelvis may become large enough to hold several liters of urine, causing renal insufficiency and tissue destruction.

permanent renal failure in some patients (usually those with elevated serum creatinine levels and those predisposed to renal disease because of diabetes mellitus or multiple myeloma). Also, the necessary bowel preparation contributes to existing dehydration and increases the risk of contrast-induced renal failure. When the test is absolutely required in patients likely to be sensitive to the hyperosmotic effects of the contrast medium, administering mannitol and continuous I.V. fluids may hasten dye excretion to minimize tubular damage.

*Computerized tomography.* The abdominal CT scan is becoming increasingly popular and available. Usually performed with injection of a contrast medium, it may be performed without injection of a contrast medium, making it a valuable alternative to excretory urography. This test can distinguish cysts, tumors, calculi, and other masses; pelvic or ureteral dilation; and bladder distention.

*Cystoscopy with retrograde ureteropyelography.* This test allows radiographic examination of the renal collecting system after injection of a contrast medium through a urethral catheter during cystoscopy. It is used to visualize the precise location of a urethral obstruction (such as a stricture) or a bladder neck obstruction (such as an enlarged prostate) and to assess the structure and integrity of the calyxes, renal pelvis, and ureter. Cystoscopic instrumentation through the urethra and into the bladder allows irrigation or use of manipulative procedures, such as litholapaxy or lithotripsy, during cystoscopy to release obstructing elements, eliminating the need for surgery.

*Voiding cystourethrography.* This test can help differentiate mechanical obstruction or urine stasis from neurogenic bladder and other obstructive disorders. It reveals bladder incompetence or urethral stricture, outlet obstructions, and residual urine. In vesicoureteral reflux, the contrast medium passes from the bladder up into the ureters and renal pelves during voiding.

*Renal angiography.* This test permits examination of the renal vasculature and parenchyma after arterial injection of a contrast medium. Rapid-sequence radiographs show the vessels during three filling phases: arterial, nephrographic, and venous. The test is indicated for renal masses, pseudotumors, unilateral or bilateral kidney enlargement, nonfunctioning kidneys in patients with acute renal failure, vascular malformations, and intrarenal calcifications of uncertain origin.

*Radionuclide renography.* This test involves I.V. injection of a radionuclide, followed by scintiphotography. Observation of isotopic uptake and transit allows assessment of renal blood flow, function of the nephrons and collecting system, and renal structure. Depending on the patient's clinical status, this test may include dynamic scans to assess renal perfusion and static scans to assess structure. This test can be used in place of excretory urography if the patient is sensitive to the contrast agent used in that procedure.

In hydronephrosis, the scan shows poor isotope uptake, slow isotope transit through the parenchyma, and isotope accumulation in the renal pelvis.

**Ultrasonography.** In this noninvasive test, high-frequency sound waves (usually 1 to 5 million cycles/second) are transmitted from a transducer through the kidneys and peri-renal structures. The resulting echoes are seen on an oscilloscope screen as anatomic images. This test can confirm or rule out obstruction by allowing assessment of kidney location and size, renal pelvic or ureteral dilation, and bladder distention; it also reveals calculi. Its advantages include minimal patient preparation and lack of significant risk or discomfort. The test is especially valuable when excretory urography is ruled out, for example, in patients with elevated serum creatinine levels. Since the test doesn't depend on renal function, it's also useful in patients with renal failure. Its disadvantage—variations in the reliability of findings—can be minimized by skillful interpretation of results.

**Laboratory tests.** Lab tests include urinalysis, blood chemistry, creatinine clearance, and blood gas analysis.

*Urinalysis.* Direct microscopic observation may show sediment, red blood cells, pus, or bacteria but rarely shows formed elements, such as casts, unless actual tubular or glomerular damage exists. Sometimes, a patient with a calculus will excrete crystals of the same type as the calculus. If analysis reveals blood or pus, a culture is taken to identify the infecting organism. Hematuria may also indicate a calculus or tumor, or it may result from trauma during catheterization.

Urine specific gravity may be low or fixed, reflecting loss of tubular ability to concentrate urine. Alkaline urine may indicate a phosphate calculus.

*Blood chemistry.* This group of blood tests allows evaluation of renal function by assessing electrolyte and acid-base balance and blood urea nitrogen (BUN) and serum creatinine levels. Elevated BUN and creatinine levels indicate azotemia, which may be the first sign of renal dysfunction in an otherwise asymptomatic patient. In renal failure, serum phosphorus levels rise because the kidneys can't excrete phosphorus. And serum calcium levels decrease because of the body's attempt to maintain the normally inverse relationship between calcium and phosphorus. Meanwhile, serum bicarbonate levels decrease as base reserves are used to buffer nonexcreted hydrogen ions. Renal ability to conserve and regenerate bicarbonate is lost. Also, serum potassium levels increase.

*Creatinine clearance.* An excellent indicator of renal function, this test requires a timed 12- or 24-hour urine collection and a blood sample. It determines how efficiently the kidneys are clearing creatinine (a by-product

## Endoscopic removal of bladder and ureteral calculi

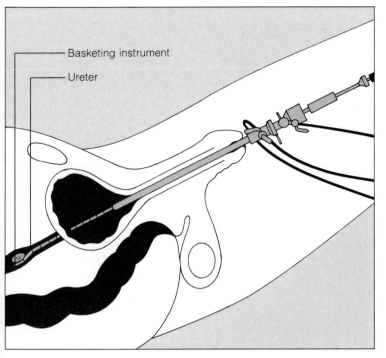

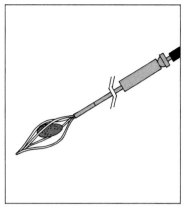

To perform stone basketing, a method of removing a ureteral calculus (shown top left), a basketing instrument is passed through a cystoscope into the ureter, beyond the calculus. Once in position, the basket is opened and twisted to catch the calculus. (See detail above.)

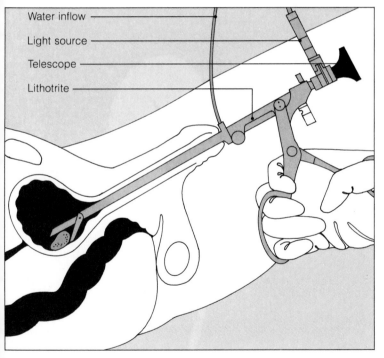

To perform litholapaxy (shown bottom left), the bladder is filled with saline solution, a lithotrite is inserted into the bladder to grab and crush the calculus, and the fragments are aspirated.

of creatine metabolism) from the blood. Decreased clearance rates indicate damage to the nephrons.

*Blood gas analysis.* In uncompensated metabolic acidosis from renal tubule malfunction, serum bicarbonate levels will be low, and so will pH. Compensated metabolic acidosis is reflected by normal pH and decreased $PCO_2$. Serum bicarbonate levels remain low, reflecting renal loss of bicarbonate.

**Treatment to save renal function**
Treatment aims to relieve obstruction and its symptoms as quickly as possible, to prevent or eradicate infection, and to preserve renal function. Such treatment includes catheterization, surgery, endoscopic removal of calculi (see *Endoscopic removal of bladder and ureteral calculi*), ureteral stents, and antibiotic therapy to prevent or eradicate infection. If the obstruction has an extrinsic cause, other

treatment, such as radiation to treat a pelvic tumor, may be needed. However, the patient with a ureteral or bladder calculus may require only conservative treatment—increased fluids and analgesics—since most calculi pass spontaneously.

It's hard to predict how much renal function will be regained with successful treatment. Often, relieving the obstruction causes prompt improvement and alleviates uremia. Renal function may continue to improve for up to a year after the relief of acute renal failure from obstruction. However, obstruction of significant duration may need additional treatment, such as short-term dialysis.

**Catheterization.** Initially, catheterization is done to relieve distention and to measure residual urine. This procedure also may relieve the obstruction if the obstruction results from prostatic enlargement or urethral stricture. The diameter of the catheter used depends on the degree of urethral obstruction. Sometimes lubrication aids catheter placement; but if the catheter can't be passed beyond the obstruction, it shouldn't be forced. This would cause edema and, possibly, other complications. Report inability to pass the catheter beyond the obstruction to the doctor.

If the obstruction resides above the bladder, anterograde or retrograde approaches may be tried, depending on diagnostic test results.

In ureteral obstruction, a retrograde approach is the treatment of choice. The doctor threads a catheter into each ureter with the aid of a cystoscope. Sometimes instrumentation and irrigation alone are enough to correct the obstruction.

**Basketing technique.** If a calculus is found in the distal ureter, it may be removed by the *stone basketing* technique. Again with the aid of a cystoscope, a special catheter con-

## Ureteral stents

Stents are used to support and maintain patency of tubelike structures such as the ureters. Stents can be placed in an anterograde fashion during cystoscopy, or they can be placed surgically in a retrograde fashion, using a percutaneous approach. Ureteral stents may be used temporarily, after removal of an obstruction or after repair of ureteral damage, to allow for healing and to maintain patency of an edematous ureter, or permanently, to maintain patency when the ureter is compressed by an inoperable extrinsic obstruction. Patients with permanent stents are usually terminally ill or poor surgical risks.

**Retrograde**

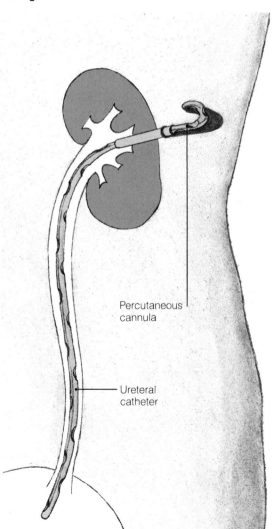

Percutaneous cannula

Ureteral catheter

**Anterograde**

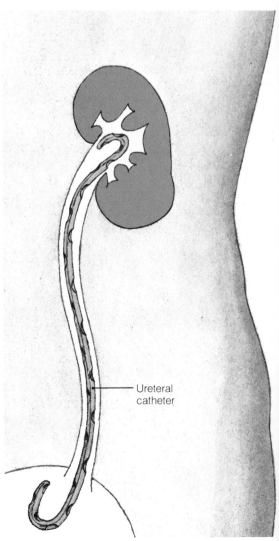

Ureteral catheter

taining a small wire basket folded into its tip is passed up the ureter past the obstruction. Once in position, the basket is opened and carefully drawn backwards, snaring the obstruction. The small wire basket and its capture are then withdrawn through the bladder and urethra.

Since the narrow ureteral lumen may show some edema, a urethral catheter is inserted and left in place for several days to ensure adequate drainage. Stone basketing must be performed carefully to avoid perforating the ureter.

If the ureteral obstruction cannot be removed cystoscopically, an anterograde approach—involving percutaneous, nephrostomy, pyelolithotomy, or ureterolithotomy—may be necessary.

**Surgical approaches.** In *nephrostomy,* a curved clamp is inserted through a fistula created in the renal pelvis and worked through the pelvis into a calyx and through the renal parenchyma to the other side of the organ. The clamp then grasps the tip of a Malecot catheter, which is then pulled back through the kidney and positioned in the pelvis, where it's secured by its expandable tip. Although this procedure provides immediate drainage relief, it should be used only as a temporary measure because of the risks—infection, stone formation, bleeding, and accidental tube displacement—that come with prolonged use.

*Percutaneous nephrostomy* involves insertion of a flexible catheter and guide wire through a puncture wound in the patient's flank under local anesthetic. The catheter is moved to the renal pelvis using fluoroscopy or ultrasound, and a contrast medium can be injected to visualize the collecting system and any obstruction. The drainage catheter is prone to clog because of its small diameter. However, the procedure is useful in septic-obstructed patients who are poor surgical risks.

When longer or permanent renal pelvic drainage is required, insertion of a permanent nephrostomy tube or other diversion, such as an ileal conduit, cutaneous ureterostomy, continent vesicostomy, or cystostomy, may be done, especially if the obstruction is extrinsic, such as a pelvic or abdominal mass.

*Pyelolithotomy* and *ureterolithotomy* involve surgical removal of renal calculi from the pelvis and ureter, respectively.

A *ureteral stent,* usually a thin catheter, is threaded via either the renal pelvis or the bladder into the ureter to maintain its patency in the presence of an obstruction, such as an

abdominal malignancy that constricts the ureter, or, postoperatively, during healing after removal of a ureteral or ureteropelvic junction obstruction. Stents can be left in place indefinitely but should always be considered a potential source of infection.

**Lithotripsy.** Bladder calculi are commonly removed by lithotripsy techniques. In *litholapaxy,* a stone is crushed by a lithotrite inserted via the urethra, and the fragments are removed by irrigation. It's indicated when a stone is soft enough to crush or shatter and when not contraindicated by associated disease. *Lithotripsy* also involves use of a lithotrite and an electrode. After the bladder is filled with a nonconducting fluid such as glycine, the electrode is advanced into the bladder until it contacts the stone, which disintegrates after a few bursts of high-voltage current.

The newer lithotripsy techniques, used in some centers, are *percutaneous ultrasonic lithotripsy* (PUL) and *extracorporeal shock wave lithotripsy* (ESWL).

In PUL, an ultrasonic probe is inserted into the renal pelvis through a nephrostomy tract and positioned against the stone. The doctor disintegrates the stone with pulses of ultrasound, and the fragments are suctioned out. Other instruments may be passed through the nephrostomy tract if necessary.

In ESWL, a noninvasive procedure, the patient is anesthetized and placed in a water bath. His affected kidney is positioned under water over an electric spark generator, which creates high-energy shock waves that shatter the stone without damaging surrounding tissue. The patient may receive 500 to 1,500 shocks in 30 to 60 minutes; the stone is broken down into fine gravel that is excreted normally. (See *Lithotripsy disintegrates renal calculi,* pages 130 and 131.)

**Antibiotic therapy.** To control UTI from urine stasis due to an obstruction, broad-spectrum antibiotics are given until urine culture and sensitivity test results are obtained. Then, treatment is specific to the infecting organism. Since some broad-spectrum antibiotics, such as the aminoglycosides (tobramycin, gentamicin), are potentially nephrotoxic, renal function parameters must be monitored before and during their administration.

Serum creatinine levels are measured before antibiotic treatment to check for renal insufficiency, and drug dosages are adjusted accordingly. Therapeutic drug levels must be carefully monitored and maintained to achieve serum levels adequate to sterilize the urinary tract without damaging kidney tissues with toxic drug levels.

## NURSING MANAGEMENT

Nursing care of obstructive uropathy begins with a thorough patient history, followed by a systematic physical examination. These two steps provide the subjective and objective data you'll need to formulate nursing diagnoses, to set care goals, and to plan and evaluate interventions. When taking the patient history, performing the physical examination, and carrying out your care plan, realize that the nearness of the urinary tract to the genitalia may cause the patient to be fearful and anxious. In many patients, this fear is often compounded by lack of knowledge of medical or biological terms to explain symptoms and concerns. So try to be sensitive to their feelings, and encourage them to express their concerns.

### Take patient history

To obtain a good patient history, it's essential to put the patient at ease. Your concern and acceptance are essential for good communication, not only in this instance, but also for your patient teaching and other care.

After you've made the patient comfortable, ask about his chief complaint. Does he have pain? Where? Has he seen blood in his urine or noticed changes in urination patterns? Pain generally localizes to one flank or radiates to the groin or vulvar region; it may appear suddenly or may have been present for a while. Flank pain may be a dull ache or, if it results from renal colic, an excruciating spasm that leaves the patient diaphoretic, breathless, and unable to sit still without writhing in agony. Renal colic is commonly described as the most severe pain one can experience; it usually causes a patient to seek immediate treatment.

Next, ask him if he experiences bladder fullness and retention. He may describe these symptoms as tightness, fullness, or a feeling of severe pressure on internal organs. If bladder distention is severe, he may also experience respiratory discomfort from pressure on the diaphragm.

Ask the patient to describe any changes in urination—the inability to void, voiding in small amounts, pain or burning with urination (dysuria), or excessive urination at night (nocturia). The male patient, especially, may have difficulty initiating urination, so the force of urination may be less than usual, or it may be interrupted. Changes in patterns of urination may be acute or may develop insidiously over weeks or months.

Also ask him if he's noticed any changes in urine color. Normally, urine color varies from light yellow to light amber. With hematuria, it's dark amber or smoky brown. Both occult and frank blood in the urine require immediate attention.

Gastrointestinal symptoms (such as diarrhea, constipation, or anorexia) or altered menstrual patterns may also indicate an extrinsic obstruction, such as uterine disease or an abdominal mass.

Does the patient have a history of renal calculi, neurogenic bladder, or other urinary tract abnormalities? Recurrent UTIs may result from obstruction. A history of previous urologic surgery may indicate the site and cause of subsequent obstruction. Ask him if he's been immobilized recently; prolonged immobilization, particularly if accompanied by dehydration, may cause renal calculi.

After pinpointing symptoms of obstruction, check for signs and symptoms of infection, uremia, or malignancy. If infection is present, the patient may report fever, chills, and sometimes vomiting. Uremia may cause nausea, vomiting, weight loss, weakness, pallor, pruritus, and altered behavior. General malaise, fatigue, and lethargy may be present with uremia, malignancy, or infection.

Get a medication history including antihistamines, antihypertensives, beta blockers, anticholinergics, antidepressants, and antiparkinsonian agents. Many different drugs can cause urinary retention.

Throughout your questioning, try to assess the patient's understanding of his disorder and his ability to participate in therapy. Keep your assessment current, because metabolic or electrolyte abnormalities may temporarily obscure the patient's understanding or may modify signs and symptoms. In making your psychological assessment, consider the patient's age and how his self-concept, self-worth, and body image may affect his feelings about his disorder. Realize that since the organs of urination are also part of his sexual organs, he may be anxious about past, present, or future sexual activity.

### Perform the physical examination

*Obtain baseline vital signs,* weight, and urinary output. Elevated body temperature, pulse, and respiration rate suggest infection. Elevated blood pressure may suggest renal failure or fluid overload. When urinary obstruction causes renal failure, respiratory changes, such as tachypnea (increased rate of respirations) or hyperpnea (increased rate or depth of respirations), may occur as the body tries to compensate for metabolic acidosis. Hyperpnea is also called Kussmaul's breathing.

When you weigh the patient, ask him about his usual weight and fluid intake. Compare his usual weight to his present weight. Fluid retention may increase body weight; when assessing fluid retention, remember that a pint of fluid (500 ml) equals a pound of weight.

Next, *assess the genitourinary tract.* To rule out prostate gland enlargement, perform a rectal exam. Males over age 50 or those with changes in urination should have annual rectal examinations. Prostate enlargement may result from benign hyperplasia or prostatic carcinoma. In the former, the prostate is symmetrically enlarged; in the latter, it's usually irregularly enlarged with hard, palpable nodules. Also, inspect the penis for urethral drainage. If drainage is present, send a specimen to the laboratory for culturing before the patient urinates.

When examining a female patient, *perform a pelvic examination* to rule out pelvic disease or pelvic masses such as ovarian tumors. She should have yearly pelvic examinations, especially if she's over age 35.

*Assess the abdomen* using inspection, percussion, and palpation. Normally, the bladder lies below the symphysis pubis and is not visible on inspection. A distended bladder is symmetrically enlarged, producing a rounded abdominal contour and displacement of the umbilicus toward the head. Percussion produces a tympanic resonance in a distended bladder.

Look for any distortion of abdominal or flank contours, which may suggest underlying abnormality. For example, you may detect enlarged polycystic kidneys as readily palpable abdominal masses; if so, palpate them gently because they frequently bleed. Rupture of the cysts, with bleeding, may cause clots that obstruct one or both ureters.

*Percuss the costovertebral angle or flank*—the area between the vertebral column and the lower rib cage border. The kidneys lie beneath this angle. To palpate this angle, help the patient sit, or turn him to the opposite side. Then percuss the flank area with the ulnar surface of your fist. In kidney or perinephric infection, the patient will feel tenderness and pain over the costovertebral angle.

*Look for an incision* on either side of the groin area, which may indicate a renal transplant. The transplanted kidney is easily palpable and subject to obstruction, just as any other kidney would be. Again, palpate gently. You may induce some involuntary urine loss during percussion or palpation.

## Formulate nursing diagnoses

After you've pinpointed the site and cause of obstruction, you're ready to formulate appropriate nursing diagnoses and to carry out a nursing plan to prevent complications. Consider the following possible diagnoses.

**Knowledge deficit related to diagnostic testing.** Your goals in this diagnosis are to reduce the patient's anxiety; to prepare him physically; to keep him well-hydrated before and after tests, especially those using contrast media; and to enable him to achieve normal voiding within 6 hours after testing (unless the obstruction has not been removed).

Prepare the patient for the test both mentally and physically. Describe the test so he knows what to expect and what to do. Your explanation helps ensure his cooperation and better test results. If ordered, cleanse the bowel thoroughly. Before and after procedures using a contrast medium, encourage fluid intake and monitor intake and output. Also, be alert for a hypersensitivity reaction to the contrast medium (pruritus, sneezing, wheezing, dyspnea, flushed skin).

For procedures that include urethral catheterization, explain to the patient that he may experience some voiding discomfort for a few hours after the procedure. Encourage increased fluid intake, unless contraindicated, and monitor the character and volume of urine output for 24 hours after the procedure. Report low urine output or hematuria. Watch for dehydration. Also watch for infection by monitoring the patient's temperature for 24 hours. If a calculus was the source of obstruction, strain all urine. Also, administer prophylactic antibiotics, as ordered.

Consider your interventions effective if the patient is relaxed and cooperative; if urinary output is normal within 6 hours after testing; and if no signs or symptoms of dehydration, hypersensitivity, infection, or severe bleeding or discomfort exist.

**Knowledge deficit related to surgery.** Your goals are to ensure that the patient understands the proposed surgery and knows what (continued on page 132)

# Lithotripsy disintegrates renal calculi

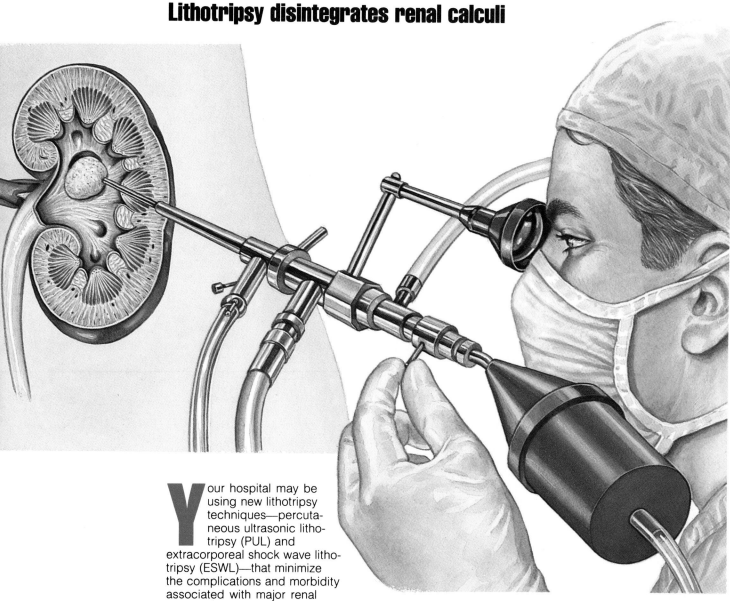

Your hospital may be using new lithotripsy techniques—percutaneous ultrasonic lithotripsy (PUL) and extracorporeal shock wave lithotripsy (ESWL)—that minimize the complications and morbidity associated with major renal surgery and reduce the required hospitalization time. For these techniques to be effective, a calculus should be accessibly located within the renal pelvis, calyx, or upper ureter. However, ESWL can't be used if the calculus is radiolucent (the procedure relies on X-rays for positioning) or sits low in the ureter, shielded by the pelvic bones.

### Percutaneous ultrasonic lithotripsy
In this procedure (see above), ultrasound is used to shatter renal calculi. The first step is establishing a nephrostomy tract. After injection of a local anesthetic, a doctor or radiologist inserts a nephrostomy tube under fluoroscopic guidance. After establishing the tract, he replaces the nephrostomy tube with angiographic wires. Then he progressively dilates the tract and inserts a universal nephroscope to visualize the calculus. He determines the size of the stone and confirms the extraction method. Possible methods, other than lithotripsy, include basket extraction or the use of forceps. The same or next day, after the tract is established (using general or local anesthesia), the doctor or radiologist inserts a tube resembling a small cystoscope into the kidney's collecting system and up against the calculus. Then he passes an ultrasonic probe through the tube, up against the stone, and shatters it into fragments that are continuously removed by suction. If fragments remain, irrigation can be performed; infrequently, if a large piece of calculus remains, further manipulation with forceps or basket extraction is necessary.

Twenty-four to forty-eight hours after this procedure, a nephrotomogram is taken to check for fragments. If no leakage or residual fragments exist, the doctor removes the nephrostomy tube. If there is no pain, fever, or extravasation (leakage of fluid into a body cavity) within 24 to 48 hours, the patient is discharged.

## Extracorporeal shock wave lithotripsy

This noninvasive procedure uses spark-induced shock waves propagated through water to break a calculus into fine particles (see diagram at right). Before undergoing ESWL, the patient receives epidural or general anesthesia and is put in a water bath. (See below.) In the water, enough shock waves are emitted to break the calculus into fine particles; usually, 500 to 1,500 shock waves are emitted in a 30- to 60-minute period. To avoid disrupting the patient's cardiac rhythm, the shock waves are synchronized to the patient's R waves and fired during diastole. Within a few days after this procedure, most fine calculus particles pass out in the patient's urine.

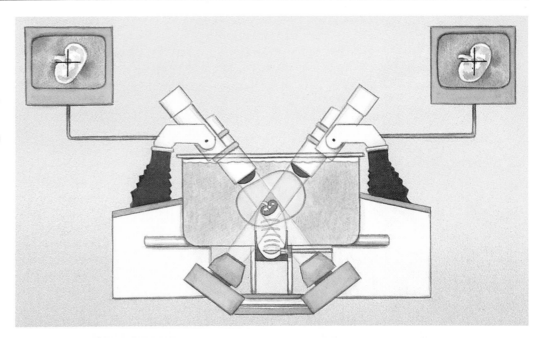

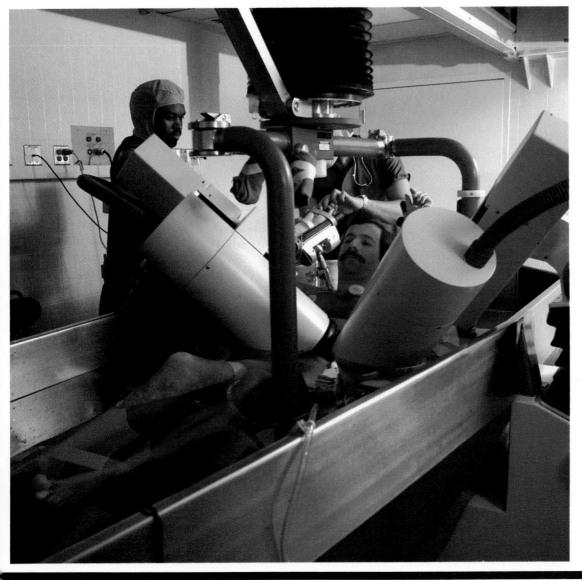

to expect before and after the procedure and to reduce his anxiety level.

Explain any perioperative procedures, especially those requiring the patient's cooperation, such as deep-breathing exercises. Explain the surgery in language he can understand, using diagrams if necessary. If he's about to undergo a urinary diversion, teach him about the type of stoma he'll have and about its care. If possible, have him wear a water-filled appliance on his abdomen to give him the "feel" of an ostomy. Arrange for an enterostomal therapist to visit the patient, or arrange contact with a support group.

If the patient is scheduled for PUL or ESWL, explain these procedures to him (see *Lithotripsy disintegrates renal calculi,* pages 130 and 131). Inform him that with PUL he may experience pain associated with nephrostomy tube insertion, but that PUL and ESWL should otherwise be pain-free. Also, make sure he realizes that the length of hospitalization will vary with the number of stone fragments and the amount of residual edema of the renal pelvis. If possible, arrange for him to examine the ESWL apparatus; point out its components and explain their use. The day before PUL, be sure the patient understands nephrostomy tube placement and the PUL procedure, including the possible use of I.V. medication, expected bloody urine, passage of stone fragments, and the need for frequent postprocedural nephrotomograms. Make sure he understands he may not eat or drink after midnight.

After the procedure, take his vital signs frequently; give him a clear, liquid diet, as tolerated; and change the dressing frequently. Also, irrigate the nephrostomy tube frequently to eliminate clots and to ensure patency. If the tube is obstructed, the patient will experience pressure-like pain within the flank area, leakage of urine at the nephrostomy tube insertion site, decreased urine output, and possible temperature elevation. Maintain an accurate intake/output record. Watch for hematuria; immediately after PUL, the urine may be frankly bloody or dark, with or without clots. Hematuria should decrease markedly within 24 hours. Notify the doctor if urine output decreases to less than 30 ml/hour after patency of the nephrostomy tube is assured. Also, strain all urine for fragments. Watch for other possible complications: fluid extravasation, residual calculi or fragments, and infection.

Before ESWL, tell the patient not to be alarmed by the sound of the shock generator. After the procedure, strain the patient's urine. Give analgesics and antiemetics, as ordered and as needed. Tell the patient to increase his fluid intake to 8 to 10 glasses a day and to walk about as much as he can to pass the stone particles more easily.

Consider your interventions effective if the patient understands the procedure, is reassured about it, and cooperates fully.

**Potential for anxiety related to exposure of the genital area and possible changes in body image or function.** Your goals are to establish rapport with the patient, to show respect for his privacy, and to help rid him of unrealistic fears and reduce realistic fears.

Before talking to the patient, try to ensure as much privacy as possible. Then gain his confidence by making him realize you've dealt with patients with similar conditions before. If necessary, provide him with basic information on genitourinary tract anatomy and physiology, using diagrams and terminology that he can understand. Inform him about the treatment regimen and its expected outcome. Maintain an accepting, nonjudgmental attitude toward a patient whose sexual behavior, preferences, or philosophy differs from yours. Encourage him to share his feelings and to ask questions.

Consider your interventions successful if the patient understands his condition, can express his feelings about it, and shows no verbal or nonverbal signs of anxiety or fear.

**Potential for discomfort or altered pattern of urinary elimination from insertion or removal of an indwelling (Foley) catheter.** In this diagnosis, your goals are to alleviate the patient's discomfort, pain, or anxiety resulting from Foley catheter placement; to prevent UTI; to prevent or detect early voiding complications following catheter removal; and to maintain adequate hydration.

Before catheter insertion, ensure the patient's privacy, and make sure he is comfortable and properly draped. Lubricate the catheter to ease its passage. If you can't pass the catheter beyond an obstruction, do not force it because you could aggravate local edema and complicate the obstruction. Instead, notify the doctor.

Assess a Foley catheter regularly. Prevent kinks and loops in tubing, and always keep the collecting container below bladder level. To avoid catheter displacement and discomfort, securely tape tubing to the patient's inner thigh.

Prevent infection by cleansing the catheter and meatus regularly, according to hospital policy, and by checking for redness or drainage. Encourage the patient to maintain a fluid intake of approximately 3,000 ml/day unless contraindicated. Be alert for signs of catheter obstruction—decreased urine output (< 30 ml/hour); severe, persistent bladder spasms; suprapubic distention on palpation or percussion; urine leakage around the catheter; and blood clots or mucus in catheter tubing. Don't open the drainage system unless absolutely necessary. If you must open the system (for example, for direct irrigation), prevent contamination of open tubing ends, and reconnect the system as soon as possible. Obtain urine specimens. without opening the system, via rubber ports.

Also, record urine color, odor, and amount every shift. Report cloudiness, mucus shreds, hematuria, or strong odor.

Your interventions are successful if the catheter is patent and draining freely; daily urine output is within normal limits and without unusual or foul odor; the patient shows no fever or chills; the skin around the catheter is clean, and discomfort from the catheter is minimal; and, after catheter removal, normal voiding resumes without hematuria or dysuria.

**Potential for discomfort related to passage of a renal calculus.** Your goals are to relieve symptomatic discomfort, to precisely monitor visible urine elements, and to maintain adequate hydration.

Document the location, quality, and duration of pain. Give antispasmodics or morphine, as ordered. Apply heat over the flank area to help relieve pain. If the patient is nauseated, get an order for antiemetics immediately— once the patient begins vomiting, antiemetics are less effective. Document the effects of all medications. Unless otherwise ordered, encourage ambulation to help move the calculus and to stop pain. Supervise the patient's ambulation after narcotic administration.

To keep the patient hydrated, administer intravenous infusions, as prescribed, especially if he is vomiting. The patient may be losing considerable amounts of fluid through perspiration or vomiting; notify the doctor if intake and output differ significantly or if you have difficulty assuring parenteral fluid administration as prescribed.

Monitor vital signs to check for infection resulting from urinary stasis related to obstruction. Give antibiotics as ordered. Since some antibiotics, particularly aminoglycosides, are nephrotoxic, monitor serum creatinine levels daily.

Strain all urine before disposal. Note color, amount, odor, and formed elements. Send all formed elements for analysis. Teach the patient to strain and evaluate his own urine.

Consider your interventions effective if the patient no longer experiences colic pain, is sufficiently hydrated, and is free of infection.

**Potential for alteration in skin integrity related to urinary diversion.** Your goals are to prevent skin excoriation and breakdown and to maintain patency of urinary drainage devices.

Care measures depend on the type of urinary diversion employed and on the type of stoma and collection device required (see *Urinary diversions define nursing care,* pages 134 and 135).

The patient with an *ileal conduit* or *cutaneous ureterostomy* will have a stoma on his abdomen that requires a wearable urine collection appliance. This must be placed correctly on the patient's skin to prevent leakage and excoriation. To change the appliance, place the patient in a supine position to eliminate skin folding, which may loosen the adhesive seal. Empty the urine pouch by turning the drain valve. To remove the appliance, apply soap and water or adhesive solvent while gently pushing the skin away from the pouch. Wash the skin around the stoma with water to remove any crystal deposits. Dry excoriated areas thoroughly, and cover them with a thin layer of skin barrier ostomy cement or karaya powder. To prevent skin irritation and to enhance appliance adhesion, apply the skin barrier as close to the edge of the stoma as possible. When the cement becomes tacky, place the appliance over the stoma. Change the entire appliance every 3 to 5 days or whenever leakage occurs.

Empty the urine pouch when it's one-third to one-half full to prevent the appliance from pulling away from the stoma.

The patient with a *continent vesicostomy* requires stoma catheterization to allow urine drainage. To do this, remove the gauze pad covering the stoma, and carefully cleanse the area around it. Slowly insert a clean, lubricated catheter into the stoma; when urine flow stops, remove the catheter and dry the skin around the stoma thoroughly to prevent irritation. Apply a sterile gauze sponge over the stoma to keep it clean.

*(continued on page 136)*

# Urinary diversions define nursing care

Urinary diversion provides an alternative for urine excretion. You need to understand and recognize the many types of urinary diversion as each needs different nursing care.

The most common reason for diversion is an invasive bladder tumor needing total cystectomy, but diversion can also relieve ureteral or urethral obstruction from stricture, trauma, neurogenic bladder, congenital defect, prostatic malignancy, or severe renal or ureteral damage from chronic infection.

Diversion may be permanent or temporary. Nephrostomy and cystostomy may be used to create permanent diversion to relieve obstruction from an inoperable tumor or to create temporary diversion to relieve obstruction from a calculus or ureteral edema. Permanent urinary diversions with stomas include ileal conduit, cutaneous ureterostomy, and continent vesicostomy. Common diversionary measures are reviewed here.

For *nephrostomy*, a catheter is inserted transcutaneously through the flank into the renal pelvis. The free end of the catheter is connected to a urine collection bag. Maintaining catheter patency is essential since obstruction results in urine

**Nephrostomy**

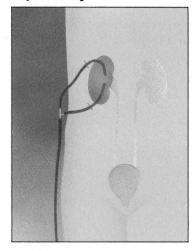

collection in the renal pelvis (which has a capacity of only 5 to 8 ml).

In *cystostomy*, a catheter is inserted transcutaneously through the suprapubic area into the bladder. Since the catheter is prone to obstruction by the bladder wall and is connected to a urine collection bag, irrigation with sterile saline solution is necessary to help maintain catheter patency.

For an *ileal conduit*, a 6" to 8" (15- to 20-cm) segment of the ileum is excised, and the resulting ileum ends are anastomosed. The ureters are implanted into the ileal segment. Then one end of the ileal segment is

closed with sutures, and the opposite end is brought through the abdominal wall to form a stoma. Although the ileal segment remains supported by the mesentery, it is isolated from, and does not impede, normal bowel function. Because the inner lining of the ileum can absorb water and electrolytes, the ileal segment should be as short as possible to avoid kinking and urinary stasis. However, excessive tension on the stoma must be avoided. This procedure requires use of an external collection device.

For *cutaneous ureterostomy*, ureters are diverted to the abdomen or flank to form a stoma or stomas. Ureterostomy requires use of an external collection device since urine flow is constant. Types of ureterostomies include:
• *Loop ureterostomy*. Ureters are brought to the skin surface in a loop to form a single stoma.
• *Double-barrel ureterostomy*. Both ureters are brought to the skin surface to form side-by-side stomas.
• *Transureteroureterostomy*. One ureter is anastomosed to the other and brought to the skin surface to form a stoma.
• *Bilateral ureterostomy*. Both ureters are brought to the skin surface to form widely separated stomas.

**Cystostomy**

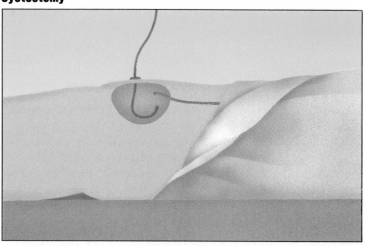

**Ileal conduit**

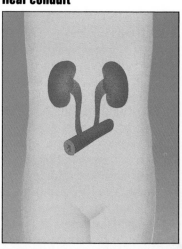

• *Unilateral ureterostomy.* One ureter is brought to the skin surface to form a stoma.

For *ureterosigmoidostomy,* both ureters are anastomosed to the sigmoid colon to allow urine to flow into the colon and out of the rectum. The linings of the sigmoid and rectum also serve as absorptive sites. One problem of this procedure is hyperchloremic metabolic acidosis from sodium chloride and hydrogen absorption. Meanwhile, bicarbonate and potassium levels decrease. Calcium levels may increase, causing renal and urinary calculi. Also, magnesium levels may decrease. No external collection

## Ureterosigmoidostomy

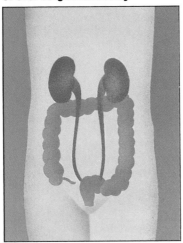

device is needed since urinary control is maintained via the rectum; but a rectal catheter may be inserted at night to allow for drainage while sleeping.

For *continent vesicostomy,* a tube is formed from part of the bladder wall. One end of the tube is brought to the skin to form a stoma. At the internal end of this tube, a nipple valve is created from the bladder wall, and the urethral neck is sutured closed so urine won't drain out unless a catheter is inserted through the stoma into the bladder pouch. An external collection device is not necessary since drainage is achieved with catheterization.

## Cutaneous ureterostomy

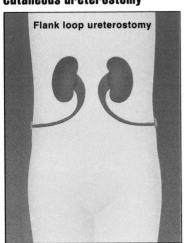

Flank loop ureterostomy

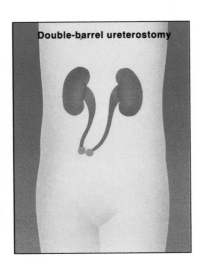

Double-barrel ureterostomy

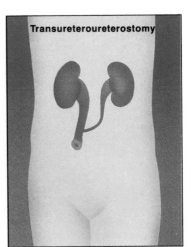

Transureteroureterostomy

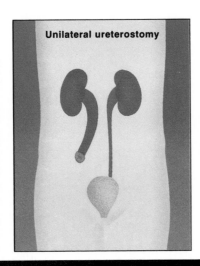

Bilateral ureterostomy

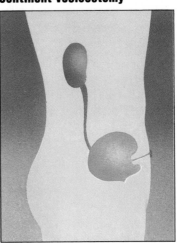

Unilateral ureterostomy

## Continent vesicostomy

## Urine pH identifies calculi

Renal calculi have different chemical compositions, depending partly on whether the patient's urine pH is acidic or alkaline. A patient with acidic urine tends to form uric acid, amorphous urate, or calcium oxalate crystals. A patient with alkaline urine tends to form triple phosphate, calcium carbonate, or calcium phosphate crystals. (See crystals below.) Often, a patient who voids a certain type of crystal tends to form the same type of calculus.

To test urine pH:
• Dip the test area of a reagent strip (such as Combistix) in a fresh urine specimen, and remove it immediately. (See top left photo.) Remove excess urine by tapping the strip against a clean surface or the side of the reagent strip container.
• Compare the color on the reagent strip to the chart on the container. (See top right photo.) The chart on the photograph above is only a representation and should not be used in place of the chart on the Combistix package.

**Testing for urine pH**

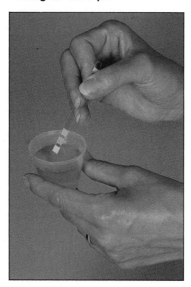

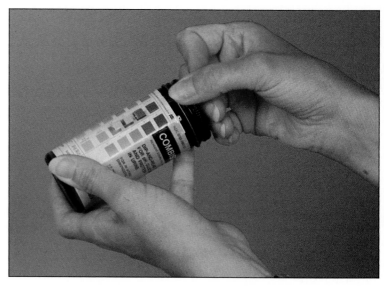

**Crystals found in acidic urine**

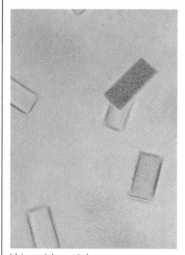

Uric acid crystals

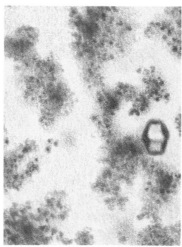

Amorphous urate crystals

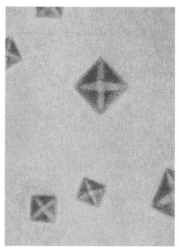

Calcium oxalate crystals

**Crystals found in alkaline urine**

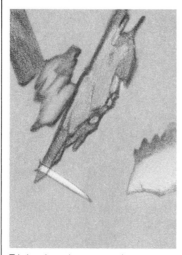

Triple phosphate crystals

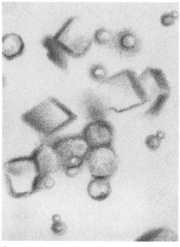

Calcium carbonate crystals

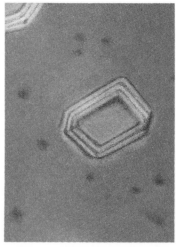

Calcium phosphate crystals

The patient with a *nephrostomy* or *cystostomy* must maintain tube patency to prevent urine backflow to the kidney and to avoid skin problems. To maintain adequate urine flow, irrigate a blocked nephrostomy tube, as ordered, and irrigate a cystostomy tube, as needed. When irrigating a nephrostomy tube, use no more than 5 ml of solution since the renal pelvis holds no more than 4 to 8 ml of fluid at one time. Use sterile irrigation technique to avoid introducing pathogens directly into the renal system.

Change wet nephrostomy and cystostomy tube dressings since wet dressings can cause excoriation or bacterial contamination of the renal pelvis or bladder. Use aseptic technique.

To provide maximum drainage absorption, pad the area around the tube with extra absorbent dressings. Treat erythematous areas with protective ointments (petrolatum, A and D ointment) to prevent further skin breakdown. Also, use nonallergenic adhesive tape to secure dressings.

After surgery for calculus removal, expect the patient to have a ureteral catheter and a retention catheter in place. If he's had a pyelolithotomy, a Penrose drain in the incision prevents local extravasation of urine into surrounding tissues. Change the dressing over the drain to keep skin dry and to prevent excoriation and infection.

Consider your interventions effective if the patient's urinary diversion remains patent and free of infection and if the stoma site is comfortable and free of excoriation.

**Knowledge deficit related to calculus prevention.** Teach the patient how to prevent calculus formation. Depending on the type of calculus he tends to form, teach him the appropriate diet. To maintain adequate hydration, instruct him to drink 12 to 16 glasses of water a day or more, if necessary, to compensate for excess perspiration. Explain the rationale, dosage, and potential side effects of prescribed medication. Make sure he understands the relationship between medication, diet, and urine pH, and teach him how to test urine pH, if necessary.

You know your care is effective if the patient's pain is reduced or absent, he does not experience nausea and vomiting, and he is adequately hydrated.

**Potential for complications from nephrostomy tube placement.** Your goals in this diagnosis are to prevent complications from nephrostomy tube placement, to make sure urine drains freely through the system, and to keep the patient free of infection and adequately hydrated.

Make sure that the drainage system is functioning properly. See that tubes that are usually taped, but sometimes sutured, to the patient's flank area have not dislodged. If they have, notify the doctor immediately. Also make sure the collecting container is below kidney level and tubing is not kinked.

To prevent infection (a major threat since the tube is placed directly within the renal pelvis), use sterile technique when changing the dressing, and check the dressing frequently for drainage or odor. Watch for other signs and symptoms of infection, such as fever or chills.

Maintain fluid intake of 3,000 to 4,000 ml/day, unless contraindicated. Accurately record the character and volume of tube drainage, which is usually pink to amber in the first 48 hours. Report bright red drainage or reduced drainage. Irrigate the nephrostomy tube, if ordered, using sterile technique. Also, don't instill more than 5 ml of irrigant at once unless otherwise directed.

Your interventions are effective if urine drains freely and the patient shows no signs or symptoms of infection.

**Potential for complications related to presence of a ureteral catheter.** Your goals are to maintain patency of the system and to keep the patient free of infection.

Make sure the catheter is taped securely to the patient's thigh, and be careful, when moving him, to avoid dislodging it. Teach the patient how to maneuver in bed to prevent accidental displacement. Carefully record fluid intake and tube output so you can assess hydration.

If ordered, irrigate the catheter; if you are not proficient in catheter technique, find someone else to irrigate the catheter. In any event, sterile technique must be maintained.

Your interventions are effective if urine is draining freely through the system and the patient shows no signs or symptoms of infection (fever, chills, or foul-smelling drainage).

## Keys to care: Monitoring and support

Your careful assessment techniques can often help to correctly diagnose an obstructive disorder early on. And your care plan (based on psychological support) to combat sexual and other fears, your monitoring of the treatment's progress, and your practice of scrupulous aseptic technique should ensure an uneventful recovery for your patient.

**Points to remember**

- Infection accompanying urinary tract obstruction can lead to renal deterioration if not rapidly treated and eradicated.
- Suspect urinary tract obstruction if urine flow stops suddenly, with or without an indwelling (Foley) catheter in place, or if high urine output alternates with little or no output.
- Obstruction can be asymptomatic and should be suspected in patients found to be azotemic—those with increased BUN and serum creatinine levels.
- Noninvasive tests, such as ultrasound and computerized tomography scan, carry minimal risk to the patient because they can detect and delineate obstruction without using contrast media.
- The urinalysis results of a patient with obstruction are usually normal. However, with infection, white cells or bacteria are present. If the patient has a calculus, he may excrete crystals of the same composition as the calculus.
- When you assess the patient, always consider the possibility that he may have only one functioning kidney.
- A physical examination for a patient with obstruction requires a rectal examination in the male and a pelvic examination in the female.
- Maintaining adequate hydration is essential, especially before and after diagnostic tests that use contrast media.

# 7 TREATING INFECTION

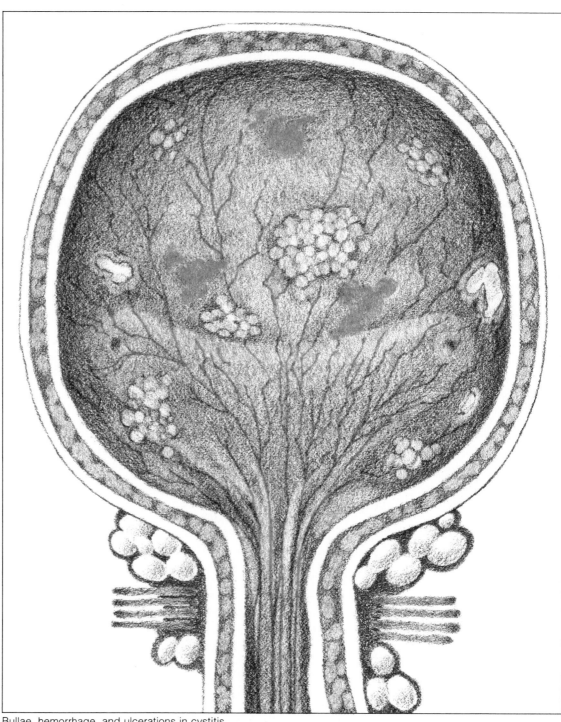

Bullae, hemorrhage, and ulcerations in cystitis

Urinary tract infections (UTIs) are often easily diagnosed and cured. Still, they present an important clinical challenge. And not just because they're so common. UTIs are typically difficult to localize as involving the urethra, bladder, or ureters; they may spread to involve the kidneys in life-threatening infection; and they show a discouraging tendency to recur after treatment.

Learning to identify the various signs and symptoms of UTIs is essential and can be lifesaving. It requires thorough understanding of inflammation and infection and of their specific effects in UTIs, as well as practiced assessment skills.

## UTI: Upper or lower
Urinary tract infection describes the presence of bacteria in any part of the urinary tract. It can occur as an infection of the urethra (urethritis) or of the urethra and bladder (cystitis); these two disorders are commonly lumped together as "lower" UTIs. When infection involves the kidneys (pyelonephritis), it is sometimes called an "upper" UTI. Lower UTIs usually respond well to treatment, but pyelonephritis is more refractory and can severely damage the kidneys. It causes approximately 15% of deaths from end-stage renal disease.

Although few patients with UTI become septic, instrumentation of the urinary tract, especially with an indwelling (Foley) catheter, is the most common cause of gram-negative bacteremia and death from such infection.

Viruses, yeasts, and fungi sometimes cause UTIs, but bacteria are the usual pathogens. Typically, a first infection recurs in about 25% of patients. Unresolved bacteriuria, associated with inadequate initial treatment, usually results from bacterial resistance to drug therapy. In almost all patients, recurrent lower UTI results from reinfection by the same or a new causative organism. In about 1% of patients, recurrence of UTI reflects persistent infection that results from renal calculi, chronic bacterial prostatitis, or an infected structural anomaly.

An uncomplicated UTI is not associated with underlying structural or neurologic lesions. Most commonly caused by *Escherichia coli,* such infection usually marks the first few episodes of UTI in females. An uncomplicated UTI usually responds well to drug treatment.

A complicated UTI occurs when repeated bacterial infections cause inflammatory changes or when urinary tract obstructions or neurologic lesions inhibit urine drainage. Complicated UTI may persist, despite drug therapy, until the underlying obstruction or voiding abnormality is corrected.

## Who gets UTI?
UTIs affect people of all ages. (See *Age and sex variations in incidence of urinary tract infection,* page 140.) They're especially common in women—an estimated 25% to 35% of all women between the ages of 20 and 40 have at least one episode of cystitis. UTIs are a leading contributory cause of death in elderly, debilitated patients and can be a life-threatening complication in patients with severe neurologic disorders (such as neurogenic bladder). Perhaps most importantly, UTIs cause roughly 40% of all nosocomial infection; about 80% of these nosocomial UTIs result from catheterization.

## Women at greater risk
More women than men develop UTIs because of their shorter urethra and its proximity to the anus. Some women may also be susceptible to colonization of the vaginal vestibule and urethra with *E. coli.* Such risk increases with age, sexual activity, and pregnancy (before and after delivery).

In males, incidence of UTI is about 1% up to age 50 but rises sharply, up to 15% thereafter, due primarily to anatomic abnormalities of the urinary tract, such as bladder neck obstruction secondary to prostatic enlargement. Any obstruction (strictures, calculi, tumors, prostatic hypertrophy, neurogenic bladder) increases the risk of UTI because it causes urinary stasis, which invites bacterial invasion. So does vesicoureteral reflux, which may result from congenital weakness at the junction of the ureter and the bladder. Aging, debilitation, diabetes, and other conditions that promote accumulation of residual urine in the bladder also magnify the risk of developing UTI.

## Catheterization and other risks
The risk of nosocomial UTIs from catheterization is significant in females, in the elderly, and in critically ill patients. However, the duration of catheterization, the quality of catheter care, and the potential for cross-contamination also influence the frequency of such infection.

Pyelonephritis can result from an infection *(continued on page 142)*

## Age and sex variations in incidence of urinary tract infection

Urinary tract infection (UTI) affects women more commonly than men, but its incidence increases with age in both sexes. In women, childbearing, sexual activity, and relaxation of the pelvic floor may cause age-related increases. Even in nulliparous women, aging significantly increases susceptibility to infection.

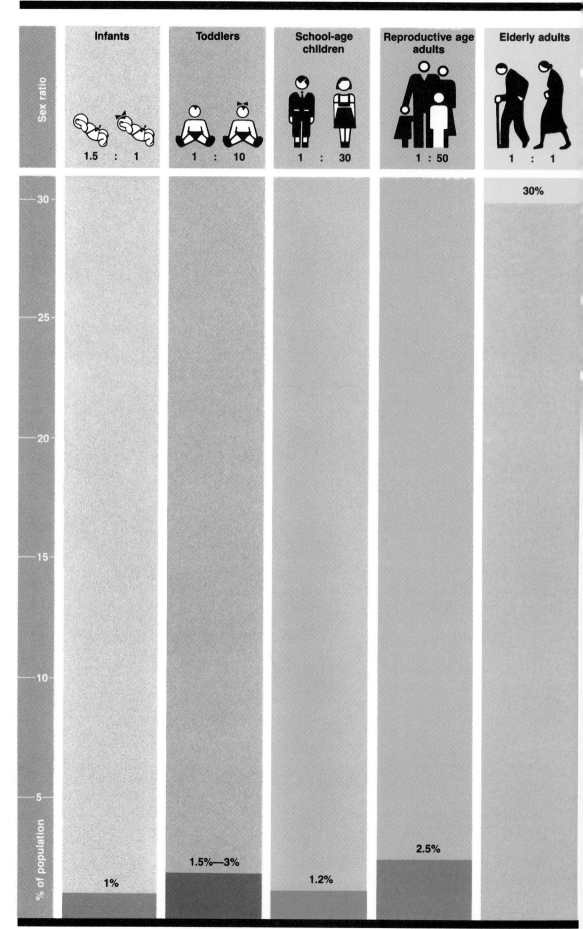

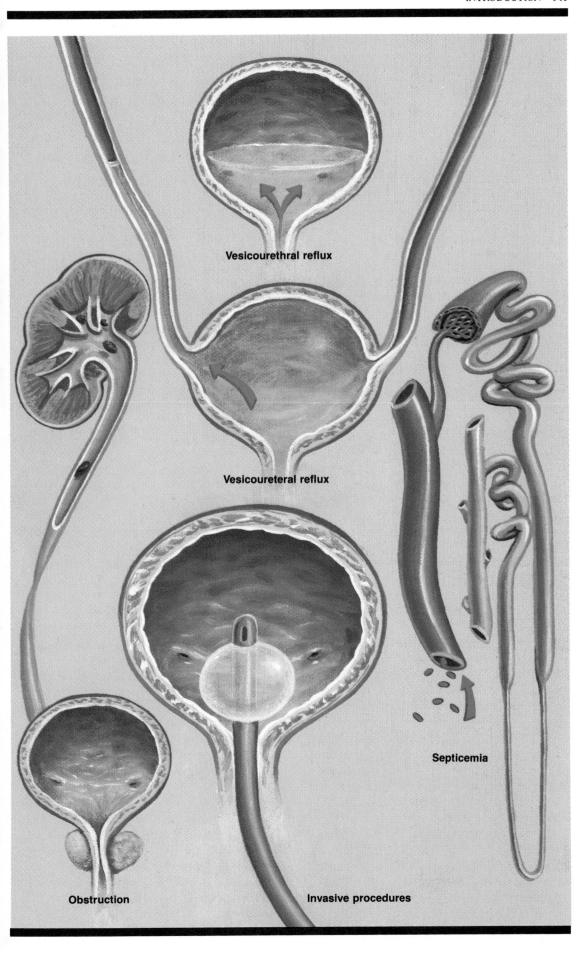

**Vesicourethral reflux**

**Vesicoureteral reflux**

**Septicemia**

**Obstruction**

**Invasive procedures**

# Major risk factors in urinary tract infection

Urinary tract infection (UTI) can result from obstruction, invasive procedures, vesicourethral or vesicoureteral reflux, or septicemia.

*Obstruction* (strictures, calculi, tumors, prostatic hypertrophy, neurogenic bladder) of urine flow anywhere along the urinary tract leads to urinary stasis, thus inviting bacterial infections.

*Invasive procedures* (catheterization, cystoscopy, and urologic surgery) allow bacteria to enter the urinary tract. In catheterization especially, bacteria ascend to the bladder through the urine in the catheter lumen or up the mucous sheath outside the catheter. Invasive procedures may result in UTI in both sexes.

*Vesicourethral* or *vesicoureteral reflux* refers to backflow of urine into the bladder or into one or both ureters and, in some cases, into the renal pelvis. Reflux can occur during voiding because of an incompetent vesicoureteral junction and is common in children.

*Septicemia*, usually the result of untreated bacteremia, spreads to the kidneys, causing cortical and perinephric abscesses.

## Pathologic bladder mucosa changes in cystitis

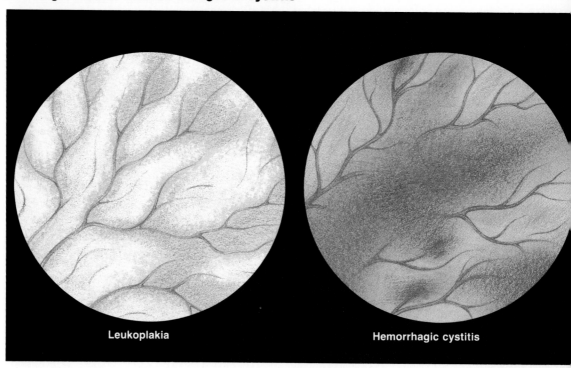

Leukoplakia

Hemorrhagic cystitis

of the lower urinary tract that ascends to the kidney and damages the renal parenchyma. In such cases, persistent bacteriuria increases the risk of damage to the renal cortex. (See *Major risk factors in urinary tract infection,* page 141.)

### PATHOPHYSIOLOGY
Bladder urine is normally sterile because of antibacterial defense mechanisms of the bladder and urine. These defense mechanisms include the flushing action of the urine and its normally low pH and high osmolality, which retard bacterial growth; the mucopolysaccharide factors in the bladder mucosa that discourage adherence and growth of organisms; and the antibacterial property of the urethral mucosa. (Although bacteria may be present in the lower urethra, their number diminishes toward the bladder.) The male's urethra is better protected than the female's, since the male urethra is longer, is bathed in antibacterial prostatic fluid, and is anatomically further removed from fecal contamination.

### Ascending and descending infections
When urologic defenses break down, bacteria enter the urinary tract through the urethra (the primary route of infection in older children and adults), the blood, or, possibly, the lymph. Most of the bacteria associated with

UTI occur in the intestinal flora. *E. coli,* the most common bacterium, is found in about 80% of patients with a first infection. Other infecting bacteria include *Proteus, Pseudomonas, Klebsiella, Aerobacter,* enterococci, and rarely, staphylococci, which may cause UTI following urinary tract instrumentation or drug therapy. However, in patients with neurogenic bladder, an indwelling catheter, or a fistula between the intestine and bladder, simultaneous infection with multiple bacteria may cause UTI.

In both men and women, infection usually ascends from the urethra to the bladder. Pathogenic bowel organisms migrate to the urinary tract through person-to-person contact (hands, bedpans, catheters), soiled bed linens, and bathing. In women, these infecting organisms can also reach the urinary tract through use of vaginal douches and sprays, which can force fluid into the bladder, and through wiping the perineum from back to front.

Although less common, descending or hematogenous infections result from blood-borne bacteria and can severely infect the kidney. For example, staphylococcal bacteremia commonly spreads to the kidney, causing cortical abscesses that may progress to perinephric abscess. Bacteria may also enter the urinary tract through the lymph, most commonly in infancy.

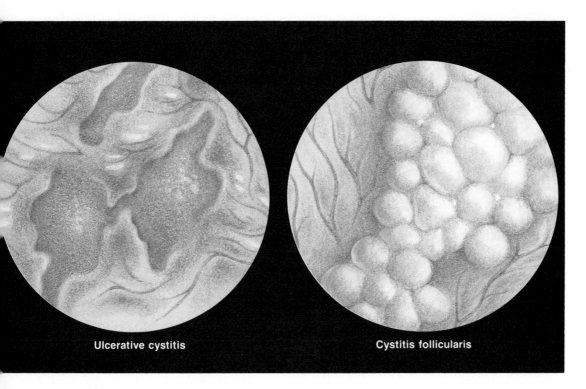

Ulcerative cystitis

Cystitis follicularis

## Inflammatory and immune responses

Bacterial infection causes injured tissues to release histamines and other substances. These stimulate increased blood flow to the affected area and increase capillary permeability. Macrophages in the tissue begin phagocytosing the invading bacteria; they're also joined by neutrophils from the bloodstream, as well as by additional macrophages and monocytes from adjacent tissues. In fact, the white blood cell (WBC) count may rise as high as 30,000/mm³.

Meanwhile, phagocytosis triggers the immune system, whose two major components—humoral and cell-mediated response—produce substances that destroy the pathogens by *lysis* or by enhancing phagocytosis. (See *The immune response to bacterial invasion,* page 144.)

## The aftermath of infection

Inflammatory and immune mechanisms produce pathologic changes in the affected tissues. Acute cystitis results in hyperemia of the bladder mucosa and edema plus infiltration with polymorphonuclear leukocytes. This process eventually replaces healthy mucosa with a friable, hemorrhagic surface with shallow, exudative ulcers. Persistent infection leads to chronic cystitis, with more edema and extreme piling up of the epithelium, eventually resulting in fibrous thickening of the tunica propria and loss of bladder wall elasticity. In cystitis follicularis, a special form of chronic cystitis, WBCs accumulate in lymph follicles within the bladder mucosa and underlying wall, thereby causing bacteriuric bumps or nodules. (See *Pathologic bladder mucosa changes in cystitis.*)

## Signs and symptoms of UTI

Lower UTI (cystitis and urethritis) and upper UTI (acute or chronic pyelonephritis) usually produce characteristic signs and symptoms. Acute cystitis, for example, produces urinary frequency and urgency, dysuria, nocturia, suprapubic discomfort, low back pain, and, occasionally, hematuria. Usually, though, it doesn't produce chills, fever, or flank pain. However, if these symptoms are present, underlying acute bacterial prostatitis must be ruled out.

Acute pyelonephritis causes abscesses and pus-filled channels to develop in the renal parenchyma, whereas chronic pyelonephritis causes parenchymal scarring.

Clinical features of acute pyelonephritis include chills and fever, unilateral or bilateral flank pain, urinary frequency and urgency, dysuria, nocturia, malaise, nausea and vomiting, and, occasionally, hematuria. Bacteremia is possible and may lead to signs and symptoms of septic shock. (See *Septic shock,* pages 152 and 153.)

144    TREATING INFECTION

## The immune response to bacterial invasion

When foreign substances, such as bacteria, invade the body, two types of immune response reinforce the defense by white blood cells: antibody-mediated (humoral) immunity and cell-mediated immunity. Both types involve lymphocytes that share a common origin in stem cells of the bone marrow. B cells evolve directly in humoral immunity, whereas T cells, in order to mature, rely on the thymus.

In *humoral* immunity, antigen-stimulated B cells differentiate into plasma cells and produce immunoglobulins (antibodies) that disable bacteria and viruses before they can enter host cells. These antibodies circulate in the blood.

In *cell-mediated* immunity, T cells move directly to attack invaders, particularly within cell walls. Three T-cell subgroups trigger the response to infection. *Helper T cells* spur B cells to manufacture antibodies. *Effector T cells* carry out the direct antigen-killing mission of T cells. In addition, effector cells produce lymphokines—proteins that induce inflammatory response by attracting lymphocytes, macrophages, and other blood cells to the battleground and that mediate the delayed hypersensitivity reaction. *Suppressor T cells* regulate both T and B types of immune response.

Macrophages, scavenger cells of the reticuloendothelial system, also affect both types of immune response by presenting antigens in the proper orientation to B cells for recognition and to T cells for destruction. And macrophages themselves are activated by lymphokines to destroy foreign agents.

Each time foreign substances, such as bacteria, invade the body, both T and B cells preserve a "memory" of this encounter, which provides long-term immunity to many significant diseases.

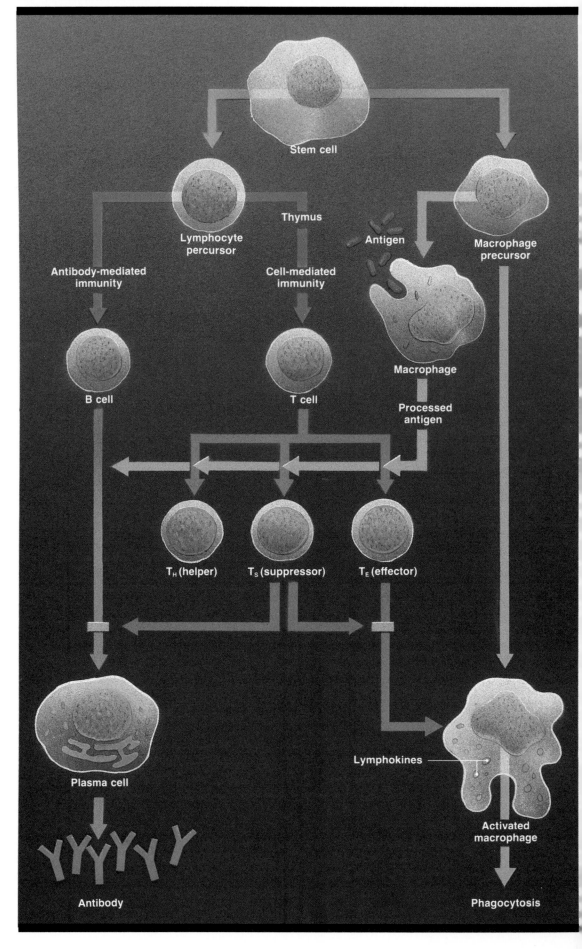

# MEDICAL MANAGEMENT

UTIs can be difficult to identify. They typically cause pain in the flank or lower abdomen with or without fever, but these symptoms are nonspecific. In some patients with UTI, bacteriuria is present without symptoms; or, typical UTI symptoms may be associated with low or sterile bacteria counts (abacteriuria), as in urethral syndrome. (See *Urethral syndrome.*)

Even with overt bacteriuria, clinical signs and symptoms don't reliably distinguish renal infection from bladder infection. For example, a patient with symptoms of pyelonephritis clearly exhibits renal involvement, but absence of symptoms does not rule out infection. Studies show that many women with symptoms restricted to the lower urinary tract also have silent renal infection.

## Diagnostic testing

Urinalysis and culture-and-sensitivity tests help detect lower and upper UTI, confirm diagnosis, identify the causative organism, and help direct drug treatment. Further testing includes localization studies to help distinguish between lower and upper UTI. Diagnostic testing may also include imaging and cystoscopic tests to visualize structural abnormalities or obstructions that contribute to infection.

**Urinalysis.** A clean-catch midstream urine specimen (preferably the first-voided morning specimen), revealing a bacterial count over 100,000/ml, confirms lower UTI. (See *The clean-catch specimen: Avoiding contamination,* page 149.) However, since bacteria require 30 to 45 minutes to reproduce in urine, lower counts do not necessarily rule out infection, especially if the patient is voiding frequently. Suprapubic needle aspiration reliably detects bacteriuria in such borderline patients, since bacteria found in urine collected under aseptic technique from the renal pelvis, ureters, or bladder indicates infection. Catheterization, which can infect or reinfect the bladder with urethral bacteria, should be avoided. Two consecutive clean-catch specimens are required for reliable test results if the patient is receiving drug treatment.

Before collection, meticulous technique is required to clean the perineal area thoroughly to avoid contamination, especially in women susceptible to recurrent infections. In such women, large numbers of *E. coli* may colonize the vaginal vestibule and urethra. However, antibacterial agents, such as hexachlorophene, should be avoided during clean-catch preparation since they may inhibit bacterial growth and result in spurious urine culture results.

**Urine cultures and sensitivity tests.** Diagnosis requires urine cultures to identify the infecting organism. However, isolation of known pathogens doesn't necessarily confirm UTI since specimens are commonly contaminated by organisms from the urethra and external genitalia. To distinguish between true bacteriuria and contamination, it's necessary to know the number of organisms in a milliliter of urine, estimated by colony-counting, which reliably differentiates between infection and contamination.

Pus in the urine indicates inflammation, which is reflected as an elevated WBC count. However, a normal WBC count does not exclude a UTI and cannot replace culturing in the diagnosis of UTI. WBC casts in the urine indicate renal involvement.

Drug sensitivity testing determines the infecting pathogen's sensitivity to specific drugs and permits individualized drug therapy.

**Localization tests.** These tests distinguish between renal and bladder infections by localizing the site of infection. Invasive procedures for localizing infection include cystoscopy, ureteral catheterization, and serial cultures from each kidney. These procedures are considered accurate if collection technique is meticulous, but they involve risks associated with instrumentation and the possible need for anesthesia. Therefore intensive efforts are under way to develop accurate noninvasive tests for localizing the site of infection. Localization tests currently under development are described below; despite advances, test results are not consistently reliable.

*The Fairley bladder washout technique* requires bladder catheterization. Too time-consuming and complex to be adapted for clinical use, this test is used to evaluate the accuracy of other localization tests, such as the antibody-coating and the lactic dehydrogenase (LDH) isoenzyme procedures. The Fairley bladder washout test involves a series of urine cultures and instillation of a solution of neomycin and Elase and washout with sterile water.

The neomycin sterilizes the bladder; thus, in lower UTI, subsequent cultures should be negative. In upper UTI, one or more cultures taken after washout should be positive, or they should show significantly increased bacterial count over the bladder washout specimen.

# Managing prostatitis

Prostatitis, inflammation of the prostate gland, may be acute or chronic. Prostatic infection, especially chronic prostatitis, is the most common cause of recurring urinary tract infection in men. Prostatitis most often results from the presence of gram-negative bacteria. The infection probably spreads to the prostate by the hematogenous route or from ascending urethral infection, invasion of rectal bacteria by way of the lymph system, or reflux of infected bladder urine into prostate ducts. Less commonly, prostatitis results from infrequent or excessive sexual intercourse or from urethral instrumentation, such as cystoscopy or catheterization. Chronic prostatitis usually develops as a result of bacterial invasion through the urethra.

Acute prostatitis begins with sudden moderate-to-high fever, chills, low back and perineal pain, urinary frequency and urgency, nocturia, dysuria, general malaise with arthralgia and myalgia, and varying degrees of outlet obstruction. Clinical features of chronic bacterial prostatitis vary but may include sensations of chronic perineal fullness, low back pain, and dysuria, sometimes associated with a slight urethral discharge. Unlike the acute form, chronic prostatitis is rarely accompanied by fever or major illness.

Rectal examination usually reveals a highly tender, enlarged prostate. Diagnosis depends on comparison of urine cultures before and after prostatic massage. In general, bacterial prostatitis is confirmed by the presence of at least 10 times more bacteria in the post-prostatic massage specimen than in either the urethral or bladder specimen.

Treatment for acute prostatitis includes sulfonamides and co-trimoxazole (sulfamethoxazole-trimethoprim), depending on drug sensitivities and patient allergies. Treatment continues for 30 days to prevent the de-velopment of chronic prostatitis. In severe cases, drug therapy includes an aminoglycoside, such as gentamicin or tobramycin. Patients receiving these drugs require hospitalization and should be observed for side effects, such as ototoxicity and nephrotoxicity.

In chronic prostatitis, drug therapy frequently includes co-trimoxazole. Minocycline, doxycycline, and carbenicillin may also be used. Drug therapy continues for a minimum of 6 weeks; if necessary, the course may be repeated. If the infection persists, treatment may include low doses of co-trimox-azole, methenamine mandelate, methenamine hippurate, or nitrofurantoin to suppress a related urinary infection. If drug therapy fails in chronic prostatitis, treatment may include transurethral resection of the prostate, which requires removal of all infected tissue to be successful. Total prostatectomy is curative but may cause impotence and incontinence. In both acute and chronic prostatitis, supportive therapy includes bed rest, analgesics, stool softeners, adequate hydration, sitz baths, and, possibly, antipyretics. Suprapubic needle aspiration of the bladder may relieve urinary retention. If prolonged bladder drainage is required, a suprapubic cystotomy may be performed to avoid the risk of infection from urethral instrumentation.

Nursing management involves administration of drugs and patient teaching, especially about the prescribed drug. If the patient is taking co-trimoxazole, he should take the drug exactly as prescribed for the entire time period. Because this drug contains a sulfonamide (sulfamethoxazole), the patient should drink several glasses of water or other liquid every day. He should also be alert for signs of gastrointestinal upset and should take the drug with meals or extra fluids if this occurs.

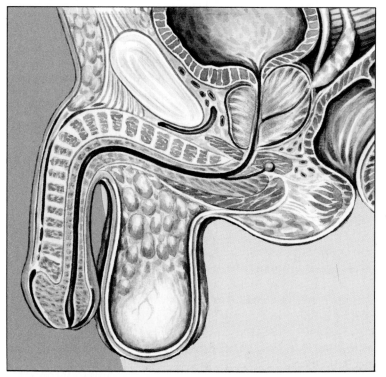

Enlarged prostate causing bladder outlet obstruction

*Antibody-coating,* a noninvasive localization test, is an immunofluorescence technique involving incubation of bacteria in urinary sediment with fluorescein-conjugated antihuman globulin. The test includes a microscopic search for antibody-coated (fluorescent) bacteria to differentiate bacteria in the renal parenchyma from those in the bladder. Bacteria from the renal parenchyma demonstrate fluorescence resulting from exposure to circulating immunoglobulins; bladder bacteria do not since they are relatively protected from these immunoglobulins.

*LDH isoenzyme studies* take advantage of the fact that isoenzyme patterns differ in serum, in normal urine, and in lower and upper UTIs. In pyelonephritis, elevated levels of $LDH_5$ result from damaged renal cortical tissue.

Definitive noninvasive localization techniques would permit earlier and more intensive drug therapy in patients who are at risk for renal damage from an upper UTI; however, both the antibody-coating localization test and the LDH isoenzyme pattern technique require further evaluation.

**Antibody studies.** These tests detect the presence or absence of a vaginal antibody that acts specifically against colonization of the vaginal vestibule by *E. coli.* Women resistant to urinary infections rarely have fecal enterobacteria in the vaginal vestibule; they possess a specific vaginal antibody against their own fecal *E. coli.* However, susceptible women have no vaginal antibody to combat such colonization. This suggests that susceptibility to recurrent lower UTI may result from an immunologic defect. Such a defect involves a lack of a specific vaginal antibody, which may inhibit bacterial adhesion to epithelial surfaces.

**Imaging tests.** Radiographic tests are usually not part of the diagnostic workup for initial UTI; but, if necessary, they may be done to evaluate first infections in males and children. These tests visualize conditions, such as obstructions, congenital malformation, and reflux, that may cause urine stasis and predispose the kidney to infection.

*Excretory urography* visualizes the renal parenchyma, calyxes, and pelvis, as well as the ureters, bladder, and, in some cases, the urethra. Obstruction anywhere along the urinary tract causes delayed excretion of the injected contrast medium, revealing dilation of the urinary drainage system proximal to the obstruction. The degree of dilation depends on the severity and duration of the obstruction. In addition, excretory urography may demonstrate calculi and renal ischemia and, in children, may show ureteropelvic junction obstruction and congenital abnormalities.

*Voiding cystourethrography* reveals bladder contour, adequacy of voiding, and the presence or absence of vesicoureteral reflux. This test can also reveal prostatic enlargement, urethral strictures, and diverticula. *Ultrasonography* and *computerized tomography (CT) scanning* are used to help evaluate the kidney for suspected infection and abscess.

**Cystoscopy.** This test allows visual examination of the interior of the bladder for signs of inflammation (redness, edema), cysts, leukoplakia, trabeculations, and foreign bodies or calculi. It is also used to rule out carcinoma in patients with chronic UTI, bladder irritability, and gross hematuria. In addition, this test may detect various congenital anomalies, such as ureteroceles, duplicate ureteral orifices, or urethral valves in children.

## Treatment: Drugs preferred
Treatment of UTI centers on drug therapy to eradicate the pathogen from the urinary system and to prevent or treat recurrence. Preventing progressive renal disease is especially important.

Drug therapy, of course, depends on the cause, symptoms, patient's age and sex, whether this is the initial infection or a recurrence, level of renal function, and infection site. For example, high concentrations of drugs can effectively treat superficial infection of the bladder mucosa. In contrast, more intensive and prolonged therapy is required for pyelonephritis and prostatitis. (See *Managing prostatitis.*)

Initially, medical treatment is usually identical for all patients with suspected UTI, since distinguishing between upper and lower UTI is often difficult. Currently, the *response* to antimicrobial therapy is considered the best available guide to patient management.

**Conventional 10- to 14-day therapy.** This is typically used to treat recurrent infections. Recurrent UTI may indicate renal or deep bladder tissue infection, or it may indicate noncompliance. Prolonged therapy, for 6 to 12 weeks, is generally required for male patients with recurrent infection. Drugs of choice include tetracycline; ampicillin or amoxicillin; an oral cephalosporin, such as cephalexin; nalidixic acid; cinoxacin; sulfamethoxazole-trimethoprim; and nitrofurantoin. Methenamine mandelate or methenamine hippurate with ascorbic acid may be administered to acidify the urine (resulting in release of formaldehyde when urine pH is maintained at or below 5.5). Therapy continues for 6 months or longer in persistent or continuing recurrence of UTI. In susceptible patients, conscientious follow-up and prophylactic treatment are essential.

**Single-dose drug therapy.** This form of treatment is considered a major advance in the management of the most common form of UTI—acute, uncomplicated UTI of the adult female. Single-dose therapy consists of amoxicillin, sulfamethoxazole-trimethoprim, or sulfisoxazole, given orally, or kanamycin, administered I.M. Side effects are less common in single-dose therapy than in conventional therapy. Also, the patient's response, as indicated by sequelae and follow-up culture results, helps direct further treatment.

Single-dose regimens are not recommended for uncooperative patients who may not be available for follow-up, for patients with symptomatic pyelonephritis, or for those with indwelling catheters or anatomic abnormalities of the urinary tract. Similarly, single-dose therapy is not usually recommended for male patients with UTI with presumed prostatic tissue invasion. These patients require a full course of drug therapy.

**Other drug regimens.** A sulfonamide, such as sulfamethoxazole, or ampicillin, amoxicillin, or cephalexin, administered for 7 to 14 days, is used to treat asymptomatic bacteriuria in pregnant women. If untreated, asymptomatic bacteriuria is associated with a 40% incidence of acute pyelonephritis later in pregnancy. Tetracycline is avoided throughout pregnancy, as are sulfonamides in the last month, because of the risk of hyperbilirubinemia and kernicterus to the newborn. Treatment of asymptomatic bacteriuria in women who are not pregnant is controversial.

Acute pyelonephritis requires aminoglycosides (tobramycin) and third-generation cephalosporins (cefotaxime), since the usual causative organisms may resist ampicillin, cephalothin, and sulfonamides. Phenazopyridine (Pyridium) may be used temporarily as a local urinary analgesic, but its prolonged use is contraindicated because of the significant risk of adverse reactions.

Some patients with UTI may require surgery to correct structural anomalies, urinary tract obstruction, vesicoureteral reflux, or other causes of urinary stasis.

## NURSING MANAGEMENT

Nursing management of UTI involves explaining diagnostic tests and teaching the patient how to deal with his current infection and how to prevent a recurrence. Your care extends to psychological support and counsel for the depressed patient who fears infection and recurrence that may require time off from work and possible withdrawal from sexual activity. Your care also includes helping to prevent nosocomial infections. Begin planning your care with an accurate assessment based on a thorough nursing history and physical examination.

### Getting a history

Focus your questions on the patient's chief complaint. Explore its severity, duration, frequency, and the degree of resulting disability. When a UTI is present, the chief complaint usually centers on difficult urination.

**Assess urinary patterns.** Question the patient about changes in urination, and relate them to his fluid intake. *Polyuria,* abnormally high urine output in relation to fluid intake, may occur in a UTI as well as in diabetes mellitus, in diabetes insipidus, and in some stages of renal failure. *Urgency,* a sudden, severe need to void, may indicate cystitis, bladder hypertrophy from early obstructive disease, uninhibited neurogenic bladder, or a foreign body or calculi in the lower urinary tract.

Urination normally occurs every 4 to 5 hours (normal capacity 500 ml), depending on fluid intake. *Frequency,* a common symptom of reduced bladder capacity, usually results from acute inflammation, neurogenic overstimulation or lack of inhibition, carcinoma, calculi, bladder hypertrophy, extravesical compression from fibroids, or pregnancy.

Ask the patient how often he normally wakes in the night to void and if this pattern has changed. *Nocturia,* the passing of large volumes of urine at night, usually results in a need to void two or more times during the night. Typically, nocturia may result from late evening use of diuretics or from increased fluid intake. In an elderly patient, fluid may accumulate in the lower extremities during the day, but when he reclines in bed at night, fluid reenters the circulatory system and is excreted, resulting in increased urine output.

*Dysuria,* painful urination, commonly results from lower UTI. However, it may also result from nonbacterial inflammation due to calculi, a foreign body, or a tumor. The patient

# he clean-catch specimen: Avoiding contamination

Correctly done, the clean-catch midstream urine specimen provides a virtually uncontaminated specimen. Explain the procedure to the patient carefully. Provide illustrations to emphasize correct collection technique, if necessary.

### efore the procedure
Instruct the patient to cleanse the periurethral area (tip of the penis, or labial folds, vulva, and urinary meatus) with soap and water, and then wipe the area three times, each time with a fresh 2″ x 2″ gauze pad soaked in povidone-iodine solution or, if you're using a commercial kit, with the wipes provided.

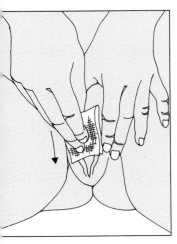

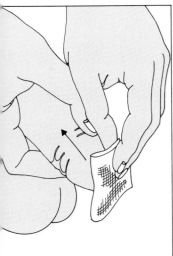

Instruct the female patient to separate her labial folds with the thumb and forefinger; to wipe down one side with the first pad and discard it; to wipe the other side with the second pad and discard it; and finally, to wipe down the center over the urinary meatus with the third pad and discard it. Stress the importance of cleansing from front to back to avoid contaminating the genital area with fecal matter. Instruct the uncircumcised male patient to retract his foreskin to effectively cleanse the meatus and to keep it retracted during voiding.

### The procedure
• Tell the female patient to straddle the bedpan or toilet to allow labial spreading. She should continue to keep her labia separated with her fingers while voiding.
• Instruct the patient to begin voiding into the bedpan, urinal, or toilet, because the urinary stream washes bacteria from the urethra and urinary meatus. Then tell the patient to void directly into the sterile container, collecting about 30 to 50 ml at the midstream portion of the voiding. The patient can then finish voiding into the bedpan, urinal, or toilet. The first and last portions of the voiding are discarded. (If the patient's urinary output must be measured, pour the remaining urine into a graduated container. Remember to include the amount in the specimen container when recording the total amount voided.)

### After the procedure
• Take the sterile container from the patient, and cap it securely. Avoid touching the inside of the container or the lid. If the container is soiled, clean it and wipe it dry.
• Wash your hands thoroughly to prevent cross-contamination, and tell the patient to do the same.
• Label the container with the

patient's name and room number, type of specimen, collection time, and suspected diagnosis, if known. If a urine culture is to be performed, note any current antibiotic therapy on the laboratory request slip. Send the container to the laboratory immediately, or place it on ice to prevent specimen deterioration and altered test results.

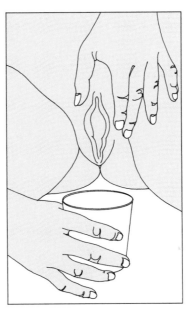

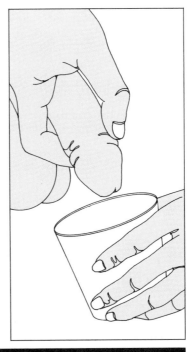

# Prevent contamination in catheterization

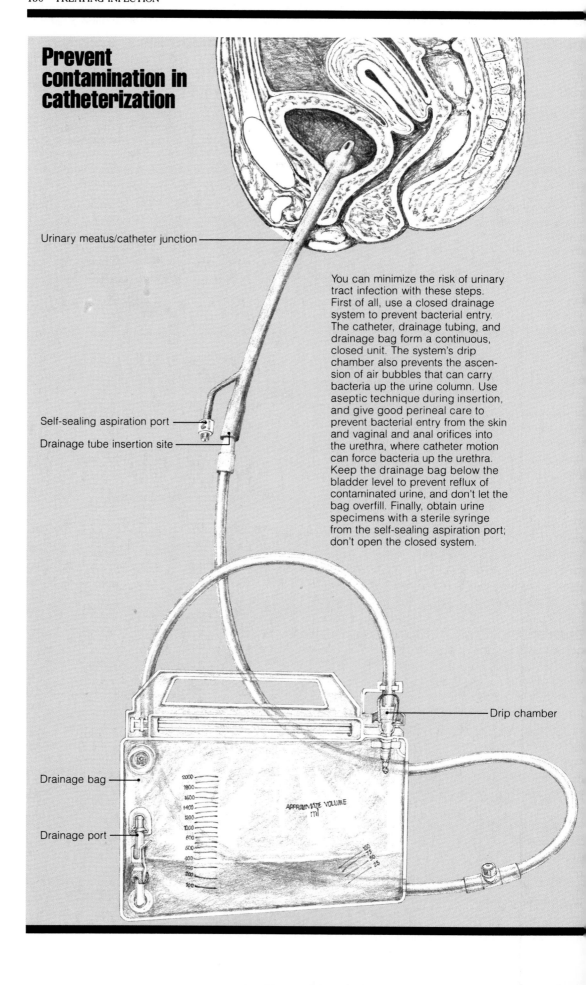

Urinary meatus/catheter junction

Self-sealing aspiration port

Drainage tube insertion site

Drainage bag

Drainage port

Drip chamber

You can minimize the risk of urinary tract infection with these steps. First of all, use a closed drainage system to prevent bacterial entry. The catheter, drainage tubing, and drainage bag form a continuous, closed unit. The system's drip chamber also prevents the ascension of air bubbles that can carry bacteria up the urine column. Use aseptic technique during insertion, and give good perineal care to prevent bacterial entry from the skin and vaginal and anal orifices into the urethra, where catheter motion can force bacteria up the urethra. Keep the drainage bag below the bladder level to prevent reflux of contaminated urine, and don't let the bag overfill. Finally, obtain urine specimens with a sterile syringe from the self-sealing aspiration port; don't open the closed system.

ay complain of pain in the bladder area, perineum, and/or urethra before, during, or after voiding. In acute inflammation of the urethra, prostate, and bladder, pain frequently results from mechanical irritation of inflamed tissue.

*Enuresis,* the involuntary loss of urine, usually occurs at night. It is most commonly caused by obstruction, infection, or neurogenic bladder dysfunction and may be psychogenic in some patients. In children, enuresis may be related to anatomic abnormalities that interfere with normal urine flow. (By age 5, about 85% of children are dry.) Ask the patient about hesitancy (delay in initiating the stream), intermittency (interruption of urinary stream), decreased amount and force of stream, and postvoid dribbling. Common causes of these symptoms include prostatic enlargement, obstructive urethral lesions (urethral stricture, carcinoma), and neurogenic bladder.

**Ask about pain.** Pain may or may not accompany changes in voiding pattern. Bladder pain may be described as a continuous, dull discomfort if due to infection, or the pain may be characterized as an intermittent, sharp spasm in the suprapubic area if due to overdistention.

Sudden obstruction associated with passage of a calculus can cause exquisite pain accompanied by diaphoresis, fainting, nausea, and vomiting, whereas the pain of chronic, progressive obstruction may be less severe. In renal or ureteral colic, severe pain results from distention of the ureter and renal pelvis due to passage of calculi. When the natural peristaltic flow of urine is interrupted, resulting distention above the obstructive calculus or blood clot causes hyperperistalsis and paroxysmal spasms of the ureter.

Urethral pain, accompanied by dysuria and burning, most often results from inflammation or a foreign body in the urethra. Characteristically, prostatic pain may be described as a vague discomfort or fullness in the perineal and rectal areas, or as low back pain, which results from acute inflammation of the prostate.

**Investigate hematuria immediately.** The cardinal sign of urologic disease, hematuria always mandates a complete urologic workup to rule out malignancy, calculi, or inflammation. If the patient notices hematuria at the beginning of urination (initial hematuria), urethral disease is the most common cause. If hematuria occurs at the end of urination (ter-

minal hematuria), the disease is near the bladder neck or posterior urethra. If it occurs throughout the urinary flow (total hematuria), suspect disease in the bladder neck or higher. In about 60% of patients, hematuria originates from the lower and midurinary tract; commonly, it results from bladder neoplasms. Hematuria may also result from cystitis, calculi, varices of the bladder, diverticula with tumor, and postradiation changes. Prostatic bleeding from benign prostatic hypertrophy is the most common cause of hematuria in males over age 60.

**Review the medical and family history.** A history of diabetes mellitus, hypertension, blood dyscrasias, or neoplasm may affect diagnosis and treatment of UTI. Has the patient had surgery or medical treatment for renal or urinary calculi, or urologic reconstructive surgery? Does he have a history of recurrent UTI? As a child, did he have frequent UTIs, or surgery for urologic problems? This may indicate a history of flow abnormalities with urinary stasis. Determine if the patient has been hospitalized recently for UTI and if catheterization was performed. This may offer clues to nosocomial infection. Ask appropriate questions about the patient's family history to obtain clues to familial or genetically related urinary tract disease. If the patient's history reveals previous infection or inflammation, inquire about perineal hygiene, sexual activity, gynecologic problems in females, and obstructive symptoms and prostatitis in males.

## The physical examination: Establishing a baseline
Weigh the patient and take his blood pressure, pulse, respirations, and temperature. Hypertension may alert you to possible renal dysfunction. Focus your examination on the following key areas.

**Examine the abdomen.** The normal empty bladder cannot be palpated. Palpate the kidney; this may elicit pain in pyelonephritis. In urinary retention, palpating the patient's bladder area may reveal an oval-shaped mass and produce lower abdominal pain. Inspect the lower pelvis; a rounded swelling, dull to percussion, may indicate a distended bladder. Next, palpate the patient's groin; enlarged lymph nodes may be related to an inflammatory process.

**Examine the genitalia.** Look for signs of inflammation (redness, swelling, irritation, ex-
*(continued on page 154)*

**Emergency management**

# Septic shock

Septic shock causes inadequate blood perfusion and circulatory collapse. It occurs in up to 30% of patients with bacteremia, a complication most commonly resulting from instrumentation or surgery of the genitourinary tract. Although women may develop septic shock, the risk is highest in elderly males after prostatic surgery. The average mortality is about 50%. The onset of septic shock is subtle and, if undetected, progresses rapidly to cardiovascular failure. Early detection and prompt, aggressive treatment provide the best chance for recovery.

**Clinical and laboratory findings**
Clinical and laboratory findings vary with the stage of septic shock. *In early shock,* signs and symptoms include chills and fever, warm, dry skin, mental confusion, moderate tachycardia, and increased respiration. Hemodynamic findings indicate diminished urine output and increased urine concentration, mildly decreased blood pressure, and normal central venous pressure. Characteristic metabolic findings reveal mildly decreased $PO_2$ and $PCO_2$, normal or slightly elevated blood lactate, low serum potassium, normal serum sodium, and usually an increased white blood cell count with a shift of differential to the left.

*In late shock,* symptoms include possible chills and fever, pale, moist skin, marked disorientation and tachycardia, and increased respiration. Hemodynamic findings indicate oliguria and sharply decreased blood pressure and central venous pressure. Metabolic findings include sharply decreased $PO_2$, sharply increased $PCO_2$, elevated blood lactate, elevated serum potassium, low serum sodium, and a decreased white blood cell count with a shift of differential to the left.

## Pathogenesis of septic shock

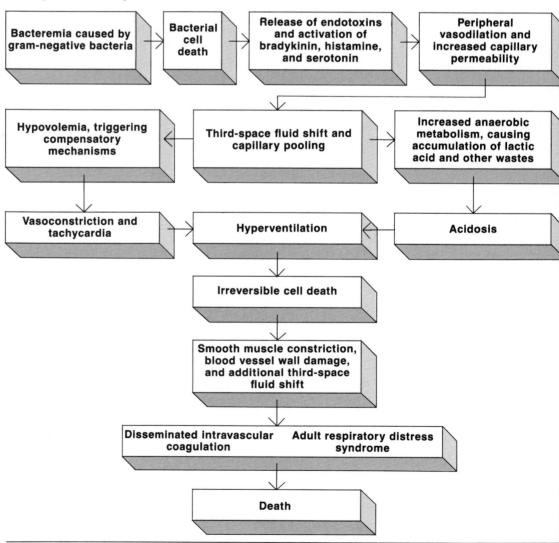

## Nursing interventions

Prompt nursing action may save the patient's life.

**Control infection.** Give antibiotics as soon as they're ordered. *Minutes count!* Look for phlebitis, since antibiotics (such as cephalosporins and gentamicin) initially given while cultures are being made can cause nephrotoxicity and other severe effects.

**Watch vital signs and ABGs.** Take vital signs at least hourly. When septic shock threatens, watch for hypotension and rising heart and respiratory rates. Report these at once.

Report all lab work and arterial blood gas (ABG) levels right away so the patient's treatment can keep up with the changing clinical status. Watch for decreasing pH and $PO_2$. If the pH falls below 7.35 and $PO_2$ below 80 mm Hg, report it.

**Restore fluid balance.** The patient in shock needs replacement fluids because increased capillary permeability causes fluid leakage into surrounding tissues. To monitor the amount of fluid you can safely give, check blood pressure, pulse, temperature, and urine output often, and, if possible, central venous or pulmonary artery pressure. To prevent fluid overload, use this rule: *replacement rate equals urine output plus 30 ml/hr.* Ensure adequate fluid early; this avoids risking an overload later, when it may cause cardiac or respiratory failure.

**Improve cardiovascular function.** Effective perfusion depends on sufficient fluid to restore normal blood volume, on sufficient cardiac output and oxygenation, and on careful drug therapy.
• In septic shock, tachycardia reflects the body's attempt to maintain cardiac output against vasodilation and leakage. Administer dopamine, as ordered, to increase cardiac output, to improve perfusion, and to correct hypotension and hemodynamic imbalance.

• Observe the patient for side effects, including a marked decrease in pulse pressure or, if dopamine is stopped, marked hypotension. To restore blood pressure, administer norepinephrine, if ordered. Report decreased urine output (less than 30 ml/hour) at once.
• Give cardiotonic glycosides (digoxin), as ordered, to improve myocardial contractility and to regulate heart rate.
• In advanced septic shock, give oxygen to combat breathing problems and to keep $PO_2$ between 80 and 100 mm Hg.
• In late septic shock, give corticosteroids to stabilize the process of cell membrane rupture, to strengthen cardiac contractions; to inhibit release of myocardial depressant factor from an ischemic pancreas, and possibly to aid cell glucose metabolism.

**Reduce fever.** Control fever with aspirin, acetaminophen suppositories, or a cooling blanket, if necessary. Monitor the patient's temperature and check the automatic probe against a standard glass thermometer. If you use a cooling blanket, give good skin care, and apply mineral oil to help prevent skin breakdown.

**Watch for complications.** Respiratory failure is the most likely complication in septic shock.
• *Shock lung.* Watch for dyspnea, tachypnea, cyanosis, grunting respirations, and intercostal retractions. Report these signs at once. They indicate shock lung, or adult respiratory distress syndrome, which results in edematous, stiff lung tissue and reduced compliance. The shock-lung patient requires intubation and ventilatory support.

After the patient stabilizes, continue to observe him for respiratory distress, which can recur long after other abnormalities have disappeared.
• *Dysrhythmias.* These can occur if the patient remains in shock despite adequate fluid administration. Dopamine strengthens contractile force

and increases renal and other visceral blood flow. Isoproterenol reduces venous pooling and acts as a strong myocardial stimulant. In early septic shock, increased beta-adrenergic stimulation probably increases pulse rate and myocardial contraction. Excessive beta-adrenergic stimulation can also cause dysrhythmias, signaling septic shock long before other evidence.
• *Oliguria.* Monitor urine output closely and report any downward trend. Output below 30 ml/hour indicates a serious decrease in renal perfusion, either because the patient isn't getting enough fluid or because his kidneys are about to fail.

The patient may be given mannitol or furosemide to combat oliguria. Monitor blood urea nitrogen (BUN) and creatinine levels, vital signs, electrolytes, and acid-base balance.

In severe shock, after the patient's stabilized, he may have kidney damage. Continue to check urine output hourly. If BUN and creatinine levels continue to rise, report them. Weigh the patient daily and check him for dependent edema.
• *Vascular complications.* Be alert for petechiae, ecchymoses, epistaxis, hemoptysis, hematuria, upper and lower GI tract bleeding, or oozing of blood from I.V. sites—signs of disseminated intravascular coagulation. If sepsis is severe, order a complete blood count and coagulation studies every 12 hours, noting their trends.

Keep the patient clean and dry, and turn him often to prevent skin breakdown and respiratory complications.

**Give psychological support.** To weather septic shock, the patient requires all the support he can get. By relieving his anxiety and reducing sympathetic stimulation, you'll lower his needs for oxygen and cell nutrients.

**After shock.** Continue to monitor for infection. Also, observe for any sign of septic shock's return or for late complications.

coriation) or for discharge from the urethral meatus or vagina. Note the character and color of the discharge. Send foul-smelling, profuse, purulent, or yellow discharge to the laboratory for culturing. A profuse, yellow discharge may be related to gonorrhea or other infection. Note the position of the urinary meatus: in the female, a posterior meatus (close to the vagina) may increase susceptibility to UTI. In the male, inspect the penis for discharge or swelling of the urethral area. In an uncircumcised male, retract the foreskin to inspect the urethral area. Also, look for urine stains on the patient's clothing; if present, they may indicate urinary frequency or urgency.

### Formulate nursing diagnoses

Once you've completed a thorough initial assessment, you're ready to formulate nursing diagnoses, subject to revision as the patient's condition changes.

Use the following sample nursing diagnoses to help develop appropriate nursing interventions for a patient with UTI. Focus your nursing care on the patient's immediate needs and well-being and on preventing recurrent infections.

**Alteration in patterns of urinary elimination related to an inflammatory process within the urinary tract.** Your goals include maintaining fluid and electrolyte balance and preventing urinary retention. To meet these goals, measure and document fluid intake and output, and encourage oral fluid intake of 2,000 to 3,000 ml/day, unless contraindicated. Provide comfort measures to reduce painful urination. Provide easy access to a bathroom, bedpan, or urinal, and, if needed, help the patient assume a comfortable position for urination. Periodically inspect his bladder area for distention.

Your interventions are effective if electrolyte levels are maintained within normal limits, the patient's daily fluid output equals his intake, and his voiding pattern has returned to normal.

**Alteration in comfort related to UTI.** Your goals are to minimize pain and to make the patient comfortable by maintaining fluid and electrolyte balance and by achieving good hygiene. To meet these goals, administer drugs, as ordered. Since these drugs may be started before results of drug sensitivity tests are received, you may have to change the initial drug therapy. Administer phenazopyridine, a urinary analgesic, as ordered, and

warn the patient that this drug causes reddish orange urine. Also, if ordered, administer antispasmodics to relieve acute discomfort associated with UTI.

Monitor and document pain relief. Stress the importance of maintaining a fluid intake of approximately 2,000 to 3,000 ml/day, unless contraindicated, to help flush bacteria from the urinary tract. Suggest warm sitz baths for relief of perineal discomfort, if ordered, or sparing application of heat to the lower abdomen. Instruct the patient to avoid using vaginal sprays, douches, or bubble bath preparations since these may irritate the urethral meatus.

Your interventions are effective if the patient complies with the prescribed regimen and reports feeling comfortable.

**Potential for infection or injury related to catheterization.** Your goals are to maintain adequate urinary drainage, to prevent nosocomial infections that may lead to septic shock, and to prevent tissue trauma. To meet these goals, wash your hands before the procedure, and use aseptic technique during catheter insertion. Studies show that the use of aseptic technique by nurses who are specially trained in catheter care can significantly reduce the incidence of catheter-associated UTI.

Thoroughly cleanse the meatus with soap and water followed by povidone-iodine to remove surface bacteria that may contaminate the catheter. Also, use a closed drainage system. (See *Prevent contamination in catheterization,* page 150.) To help minimize tissue trauma and to allow secretions to drain out alongside the catheter, use a catheter with a smaller diameter than the urinary meatus. Be sure to lubricate the catheter tip with water-soluble lubricant. This permits easier insertion and also helps to minimize tissue trauma.

In females, tape the catheter to the inner thigh on the side where the drainage bag is to hang to avoid undue traction on the bladder. In males who require an indwelling catheter for a prolonged period, tape the catheter to the abdomen to avoid urethral trauma at the penoscrotal junction and to prevent fistula formation.

Always keep the drainage bag below the level of the patient's bladder to prevent reflux of contaminated urine into the bladder. Don't allow kinking or twisting of the drainage tube, which can inhibit urine flow and cause urine stasis and bacterial growth. To lessen this risk, empty the drainage bag at least every 8 hours. Cleanse the bag's outflow spout with povidone-iodine after emptying. If drainage appears cloudy or foul-smelling, obtain a specimen and send it to the laboratory for culturing. Obtain the urine specimen from the self-sealing aspiration port with a 25G needle and syringe. Remove the needle, and empty the syringe contents into the specimen container. This avoids pushing urine through the needle's small lumen, which would result in a breakdown of urine components and a false reading.

Be alert for other characteristic signs and symptoms of UTI, such as fever and chills, which require immediate treatment to avoid the risk of septic shock. (See *Septic shock,* pages 152 and 153.) Frequently cleanse the urinary meatus of encrusted material with an antimicrobial, such as povidone-iodine, and inspect the area for redness, blisters, or suppurative drainage.

Your interventions are successful if urine flow is unobstructed and if the patient is free of residual trauma and UTI after catheterization.

**Knowledge deficit related to recurrent UTI.** Your goal is to prevent the recurrence of UTI by teaching the patient about the importance of fluid intake, compliance, and perineal hygiene. To meet this goal, encourage the patient to drink several glasses of water and other liquids daily, even after he completes the prescribed course of drug therapy. Tell him not to postpone urination, even though he may experience the urge to void more frequently because of the increased fluid intake. Tell the female patient with a history of recurrent UTI to urinate and to drink two glasses of water after intercourse. Following this suggestion may make her more comfortable. Instruct the patient with an inflamed trigone to change position during intercourse to avoid irritation. Tell the patient to seek prompt medical advice for unusual vaginal discharge, itching, or dysuria.

Emphasize the importance of following the prescribed drug regimen exactly, and give the patient information about possible adverse effects. Teach female patients to wipe the perineum from front to back to avoid spreading fecal bacteria from the rectum to the urethra. Also, instruct them to wear loose, nonrestrictive clothing and to avoid nylon undergarments which retain moisture. Cotton is preferable.

Your teaching is effective if the patient un-derstands and complies with your instructions and if he demonstrates no evidence of recurrent UTI.

**Potential for anxiety related to exposure of the genital area and discussion of personal habits.** Your goals are to achieve effective verbal communication and to convey your respect for the patient's privacy. To meet these goals, explore your own feelings about discussing problems associated with the genitalia. Provide as much privacy as possible for examinations and discussions with the patient. Maintain a professional, objective approach and an accepting, nonjudgmental attitude regarding the patient's sexual preferences and habits. Convey your experience in dealing with patients with similar conditions. In addition, provide the patient with basic knowledge of genitourinary tract function. Use simple terms and illustrations, if appropriate, and answer the patient's questions as completely as possible.

Your teaching is effective if it significantly reduces the patient's anxiety and helps him to willingly express feelings about information related to genitalia.

**Sleep pattern disturbance related to nocturia.** Your goal is to help the patient achieve adequate sleep. To meet this goal, instruct the patient to void before bedtime. Also tell him to avoid drinking fluids for 2 to 3 hours before bedtime. Encourage him to communicate his anxious feeling about his inability to sleep. To help the patient relax or sleep, administer a sedative, as ordered. Provide appropriate comfort measures before bedtime. These may include a sitz bath, back rub, clean clothes and linen, or other soothing measures.

Your interventions are effective if the patient can sleep comfortably without undue interruption.

## Reducing the UTI threat

Clearly, management of infectious disorders of the urinary tract has improved in recent years. No longer are all UTIs treated alike; upper UTI generally requires more intensive therapy than lower UTI. (However, the search continues for definitive, noninvasive localization tests that reliably distinguish between renal and lower tract involvement.) Also, single-dose drug therapy is an improvement over traditional 7- to 14-day therapy. Your role, involving skilled assessment, patient care, and teaching, as well as scrupulous attention to aseptic technique, is critical for control of UTI.

 **Points to remember**

- Urinary tract infection (UTI) accounts for more than 40% of nosocomial infections. About 80% of these UTIs result from urethral catheterization.
- Prevention of nosocomial UTI requires good hand-washing technique, thorough patient education, and avoidance of urethral catheterization when possible.
- The clean-catch midstream procedure of collecting urine samples minimizes contamination.
- Even when bacteriuria is present, the ability to differentiate between renal and bladder infection is currently limited by a lack of reliable infection-localizing tests.
- Single-dose drug therapy is a major advance in the management of the most common form of UTI—acute, uncomplicated UTI in the adult female.

# 8 MANAGING INCONTINENCE AND RETENTION

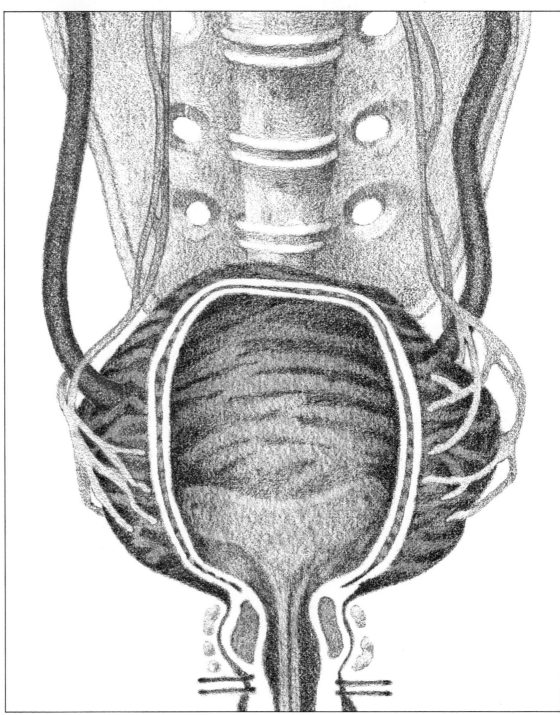

Atonic bladder

Urinary incontinence is not in itself life-threatening. But it's always a serious matter because of its potential impact on the patient's life. However minor, incontinence is always potentially embarrassing. When severe or total, it's socially disabling and causes severe psychological distress, as well as urinary tract infection and skin maceration.

Incontinence is an intensely private matter; you'll be challenged by the need to maintain the patient's dignity and feelings of self-worth and to control the urinary disorder as quickly and effectively as possible.

A thorough understanding of urinary tract pathophysiology and assessment, combined with your skill, concern, and dedication, will enable you to help your patient understand his disorder and the limitations imposed by it and achieve a renewed sense of independence, reduced stress levels, and a good attitude toward rehabilitation. In this chapter, you'll learn about urinary incontinence and retention, their medical and nursing management, and how to arrive at useful nursing diagnoses that will help you alleviate your patient's symptoms and deal successfully with his emotional problems.

## Causes: Organic and functional

Urinary incontinence may result from anything that interferes with bladder or urethral sphincter control. Organic causes may include congenital disorders, acquired disorders, and neurogenic bladder. *Congenital disorders* produce lifelong and complex urinary dysfunction. Such disorders include bladder exstrophy, epispadias, spina bifida with myelomeningocele, and ectopic ureteral orifice. *Acquired disorders* include stress incontinence, urge incontinence, incontinence associated with surgery or trauma, and paradoxical (overflow) incontinence. *Neurogenic bladder* is a complex condition involving any bladder disturbance provoked by a nervous system lesion.

Urinary retention may follow surgery or delivery and may result from uterine myomas or urethral strictures; from spinal anesthetics or other drugs; or from anorectal problems, such as fecal impaction or hemorrhoids. It may also stem from psychological causes.

Functional incontinence, associated with psychological causes, may result from various maladaptive behaviors, such as manipulation, regression, depression, dependence, or insecurity. For example, older patients who are susceptible to organic incontinence may also neglect bladder control if they are depressed or otherwise poorly motivated.

## PATHOPHYSIOLOGY OF INCONTINENCE

Because urinary tract dysfunction may result from the interplay of so many different congenital, acquired, physical, or systemic disabilities, urinary incontinence can rarely be attributed to a single cause.

### Congenital malformations

Urinary incontinence results from various structural anomalies, chief of which are bladder exstrophy, epispadias, spina bifida with myelomeningocele, or ectopic ureteral orifice distal to the external sphincter. (See *Congenital anomalies affecting the urinary system,* page 158.)

**Bladder exstrophy.** A complicated, serious genitourinary anomaly, bladder exstrophy is marked by the absence of part of the lower abdominal wall and the anterior bladder wall, with the posterior bladder wall everted through the defect. The exposed ureteral orifices discharge urine externally. Bladder exstrophy is usually associated with skeletal and intestinal malfunctions and is invariably associated with genital defects. In males, the scrotum is unusually small and cleft. In females, the clitoris is cleft, and the labia majora widely separated. In both sexes, the pubic arch is open, the ischia are widely separated, and the urethral sphincters are incomplete.

If exstrophy is not corrected, the persistent urine flow excoriates and ulcerates the bladder and surrounding skin; infection constantly threatens; and malignant changes are possible if the patient survives to adulthood. Fortunately, bladder exstrophy is rare.

**Epispadias.** Absence of the upper wall of the urethra can be a complete or a partial and minor deformity. Complete epispadias occurs in both sexes. In females with epispadias, the clitoris and prepuce are cleft, and the labia and pubic bones are widely separated. In males with complete epispadias, the entire urethra is exposed, appearing as a large groove on the dorsum of the penis. The pubic bones are usually separated and may be rudimentary. Usually, the external sphincter is incompletely developed, causing incontinence.

**Spina bifida with myelomeningocele.** This severe genetic defect results from incomplete closure of the embryonic neural tube during the first trimester of pregnancy. Occurring generally in the lumbosacral area, it's charac-

# Congenital anomalies affecting the urinary system

## Spina bifida

Myelomeningocele —

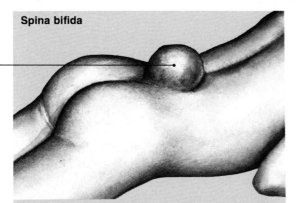

In *spina bifida*, defective development of vertebrae allows a portion of the spinal cord and meninges to protrude through the defect, causing outpouching. Urinary tract dysfunction may result from neurologic dysfunction caused by this anomaly.

## Exstrophy of bladder in male

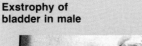
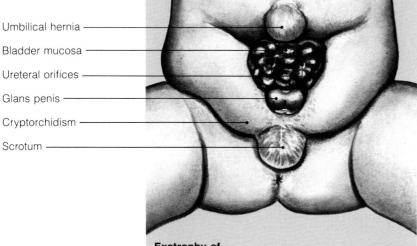

Umbilical hernia —
Bladder mucosa —
Ureteral orifices —
Glans penis —
Cryptorchidism —
Scrotum —

## Exstrophy of bladder in female

Umbilical hernia —
Bladder mucosa —
Ureteral orifices —
Divided clitoris —
Vagina —

In *bladder exstrophy*, the lower anterior abdominal wall and the anterior bladder wall are absent. The bladder mucosa is turned inside out, exposing the ureteral orifices.

## Ectopic ureteral orifices

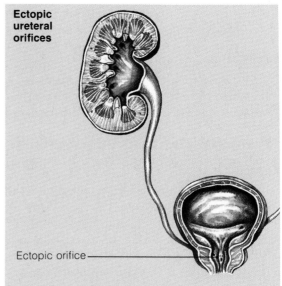

Ectopic orifice —

## Complete duplication of the ureter

Opening of ureter from right inferior renal pelvis —

Opening of left ureter —

Opening of ureter from right superior renal pelvis —

*Ectopic ureteral orifices* (top) may occur in many urinary system sites, such as the urethra, bladder neck, and trigone in females and the trigone, bladder neck, and prostatic urethra in males. Complete duplication of the ureter (above) may also create ectopic openings, as here in the bladder neck.

## Complete epispadias

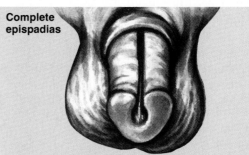

In *epispadias*, the upper wall of the urethra is absent and may be exposed as a large groove on the dorsum of the penis. In addition, the external sphincter may be incompletely developed.

terized by protrusion of spinal contents into an external sac containing meninges, cerebrospinal fluid, and a portion of the spinal cord or nerve roots distal to the conus medullaris. This disabling condition causes permanent neurologic dysfunction, such as flaccid or spastic paralysis.

**Ectopic ureteral orifice.** A unilateral malplaced ectopic ureter may contribute to incontinence, but, more commonly, two ureters arise on one side of the bladder. An ectopic ureteral orifice causes incontinence when the orifice opens distal to the external urethral sphincter (in most cases, the ectopic ureter comes from the kidney's upper pole). This condition is more frequent in the female than the male, because in the male the ectopic ureter almost always terminates proximal to the external sphincter. Occasionally, the ectopic ureteral orifice opens into the vas deferens, seminal vesicle, ejaculatory duct, or prostate in the male, or into the urethra, vagina, uterus, or fallopian tubes in the female.

## Disorders caused by trauma or surgery

Incontinence may result from certain traumatic or surgical procedures, such as pregnancy, labor, and vaginal delivery in females and transurethral resection and other prostatectomies in males.

**In females.** Incontinence may result from vesicovaginal fistula, an anomalous connection between the bladder and vagina that may occur during pregnancy or vaginal delivery, when genitourinary structures undergo extensive anatomic changes, or as a result of hysterectomy or therapy for cervical cancer.

Even normal labor and delivery traumatizes the bladder; and prolonged labor greatly increases the risks of significant bladder injury. During pregnancy, continuous pressure against the bladder from the gravid uterus can cause ischemia, bladder tissue necrosis, and subsequent fistula formation. Such necrosis can be extensive, involving the trigone, ureters or urethra. Fortunately, vesicovaginal fistulas resulting from obstetric problems are rare in the western world; however, they're still a serious problem in other countries.

Because surgical trauma associated with hysterectomy also causes fistulas, their incidence has increased with the rising number of hysterectomies. The rate of fistula formation is higher after abdominal hysterectomy—1 in 1,000, compared to 1 in 2,500 after vaginal hysterectomy. This may be related to the fact that indications for the abdominal approach

include some diseases that distort the bladder, such as myomas and endometriosis.

Invasive cancer of the cervix and radiation therapy also cause vesicovaginal fistulas. They occur in 0.5% to 2% of women receiving radiation for carcinoma of the cervix.

**In males.** Continence control in males focuses on the proximal urethral sphincter (bladder neck and prostatic urethra) and on the distal urethral sphincter (external striated muscle sphincter at the level of the seminal crest). Other factors, such as transmission of intraabdominal pressure to the urethra and the anatomic position of the bladder neck and urethra, are probably unimportant.

Total incontinence may result if at least two of the three mechanisms involved in male continence—bladder neck smooth muscle fibers, prostatic urethral smooth muscle fibers, and striated muscle fibers of the external sphincter—have sustained damage. Continence after transurethral resection of the prostate (TURP) is maintained mainly by the external sphincter.

Total incontinence following a TURP almost always results from injury to the external sphincter and either the bladder neck or the prostatic urethral muscle fibers, or both. Other surgical procedures associated with a high incidence of postsurgical male incontinence include perineal or retropubic prostatectomy (about 30% of patients) and suprapubic prostatectomy (about 15% of patients). Also, after radical prostatectomy for carcinoma, about 10% to 15% of patients may be incontinent.

## Stress incontinence: Generally a female problem

In this type of incontinence, urine leakage occurs when bladder pressure equals or exceeds urethral resistance. It occurs almost exclusively in females, especially after vaginal delivery and menopause. It may also occur in healthy, nulliparous women upon sudden exertion, such as coughing, sneezing, or laughing with a full bladder. Normally, the proximal 3 cm of the urethra prevents urine leakage from the bladder by maintaining continuous autonomous tension in the urethral wall. But with stress incontinence, a lax vesical neck closes sluggishly and opens promptly with increased abdominal pressure.

Pathologically, stress incontinence represents a paraurethral structural weakness rather than bladder dysfunction. The causes most frequently implicated in this disturbing symptom are anomalous urethral length, an abnormal urethrovesical angle (see *The ureth-rovesical angle: Critical to continence),* and defective transmission of increased intraabdominal pressure. A short urethra tends to "telescope" on itself when the patient is vertical, which decreases urethral tube resistance and causes leakage.

Paraurethral structural weakness results from vaginal delivery, gynecologic surgery, congenital defect, prolonged increased intraabdominal pressure from tumors or heavy lifting, or normal loss of elastic tissue associated with aging. The weakened support structures may also allow pelvic structures to sag into the vaginal vault, resulting in cystocele, which may be accompanied by a prolapsed uterus.

Stress incontinence may also occur in men in association with neurogenic bladder or iatrogenic urethral injury involving the external sphincter.

### Urge incontinence: An irritable bladder
Incontinence following a sudden, strong urge to void is thought to be due to uncontrolled contraction of the detrusor muscle. Normally, the detrusor muscle does not contract between voiding. Unlike stress incontinence, which is generally associated with straining activity, urge incontinence occurs randomly. It may be caused by abnormal stimulation of the detrusor muscle related to an "irritable" bladder resulting from infection; inflammation; an upper motor neuron lesion; or other bladder irritants such as calculi, foreign bodies, diverticula, or tumors.

Urge incontinence may also signal a psychological disorder. It may appear with varying severity during psychosocial and environmental stress.

### Overflow incontinence
When the bladder cannot empty and becomes overdistended, intravesical pressure eventually overcomes urinary sphincter resistance, resulting in a dripping-type overflow, or paradoxical, incontinence. When enough urine is released, intravesical pressure drops sufficiently to allow the sphincter to regain competence. The patient with this condition may complain that the bladder does not feel empty and that he frequently voids small amounts of urine.

In patients with bladder obstruction, such as occurs with benign prostatic hypertrophy, overflow commonly results from retention. As the prostate enlarges, it constricts the ure-

thra. The bladder compensates by hypertrophying. If the obstruction is not relieved, bladder diverticula can form.

Men with benign hypertrophy are particularly susceptible to overflow incontinence when treated with such drugs as atropine and scopolamine, which can interfere with the normal micturition reflex. Patients who receive these drugs before prostatectomy often experience distressing paradoxical incontinence on attempting to void for the first time after surgery.

Overflow incontinence may also follow spinal cord injury related to diabetic neuropathy, tabes dorsalis of syphilis, poliomyelitis, tumors, trauma, and local infections.

The patient with sensory paralytic bladder, caused by injury to the lateral spinal thalamic tracts, no longer perceives bladder filling and experiences chronic retention with overflow incontinence. On the other hand, the patient with a motor paralytic bladder, caused by injury to the motor outflow tracts at the S2, S3, or S4 level, perceives filling but cannot initiate micturition.

### Neurogenic bladder: Three major types
The term neurogenic bladder describes any bladder dysfunction that results from a central nervous system (CNS) lesion. The bladder is innervated by the S2, S3, and S4 spinal nerves and is also under the control of higher centers in the cerebrum's frontal lobe. The type of bladder dysfunction depends on the site of the lesion within the CNS. (See *Types of neurogenic bladder,* page 162.)

Neurogenic bladder disorders are broadly classified as upper motor neuron bladder, lower motor neuron bladder, and mixed motor neuron bladder.

**Upper motor neuron bladder.** This results from nerve damage above S2, S3, and S4. In this condition the reflex arc remains intact because the injury occurred above the sacral area, but cerebral control is interrupted. If a spinal cord injury or a tumor affects both motor and sensory fibers, the cord below the injury becomes hyperirritable, resulting in uninhibited contractions as the bladder fills. This, in turn, diminishes bladder capacity. Voiding becomes involuntary because the bladder lacks cortical inhibition and is incomplete because the bladder is spastic. The detrusor muscle may hypertrophy, which leads to vesicoureteral reflux, hydronephrosis, and permanent renal damage. The external sphincter and perineal muscles also become

# The urethrovesical angle: Critical to continence

**Normal angle**

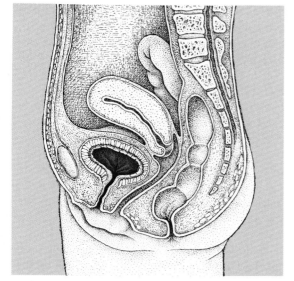

**Displaced urethra**

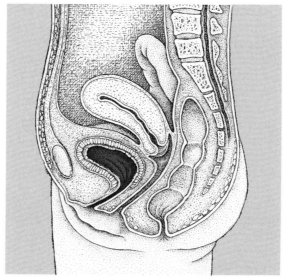

Stress incontinence, an almost exclusively female urinary problem, causes urine leakage due to paraurethral structural weakness, which is commonly caused by an abnormally short urethra or loss of tissue tone, which alters the *urethrovesical angle* to a straight line.

Normally, a urethrovesical angle of 90° to 100° (at the junction of the bladder and urethra) allows intraabdominal pressure to be transmitted equally to the bladder and urethra, thereby maintaining continence. If the upper urethra is displaced caudally to the pelvic dia-

phragm through loss of tissue tone, increased intraabdominal pressure is transmitted more to the bladder than to the urethra, so that intravesical pressure exceeds intraurethral pressure, causing incontinence.

Although urethrovesical angle displacement appears to be important in developing incontinence, the pelvic wall's integrity and the urogenital diaphragm can maintain continence in spite of an abnormal urethrovesical angle. Treatment includes Kegel exercises or surgery to restore the angle to normal.

---

spastic, resulting in increased urine flow resistance and retention of residual urine.

The clinical findings after a patient has incomplete cord injury, and in patients with a prolapsed lumbar disk, multiple sclerosis, or a cerebral lesion (such as a tumor or a cerebrovascular accident), are not so dramatic as they are in a patient with a complete upper motor neuron lesion. He retains bladder sensation, but cortical inhibition of the vesical stretch reflex is diminished or lost, resulting in frequent and involuntary voiding (urge incontinence). The voiding stream is unimpaired and no residual urine remains, but bladder capacity is diminished.

**Lower motor neuron bladder.** This bladder dysfunction results from nerve damage at the S2, S3, or S4 level. After such damage, the patient loses control of micturition because of interrupted nerve impulse transmission. Loss of bladder tone follows, preventing the patient from voiding by reflex bladder evacuation. As the bladder retains residual urine, the wall becomes stretched and flabby and prevents a sensation of fullness. Finally, overdistention causes bladder musculature damage, bladder infection from urinary stasis, and kidney infection from urine reflux. The bladder can

hold 1,000 ml or more of urine, but spontaneous voiding of small amounts does occur. This overflow incontinence commonly happens when the patient is moved from his bed to a chair. Since the patient lacks a sensation of fullness, he cannot stimulate bladder muscle contraction or inhibit urine dribbling. Other clinical findings associated with lower motor neuron bladder include absent or hypoactive peripheral reflexes, flaccid paralysis, absence of the bulbocavernous reflex, and loss of anal sphincter tone.

**Mixed motor neuron bladder.** This bladder disorder results from cortical damage from such causes as trauma, cerebrovascular aneurysm, brain tumor, and multiple sclerosis. It causes diminished perception of bladder fullness and a diminished ability to empty the bladder. Because this condition diminishes sensation and control, the patient with mixed motor neuron bladder usually feels urgency to void but cannot control the urgency.

## PATHOPHYSIOLOGY OF RETENTION

In urinary retention, the kidneys produce urine normally, but the urine is retained in the bladder for various reasons, including obstruction, pregnancy and childbirth, neoplasms, surgical trauma or preoperative and intraoperative drugs and fluid imbalance associated with surgery, and psychological problems.

### Causes of obstruction

Urethral obstruction may result from congenital urethral stenosis, benign prostatic hypertrophy, urethral calculi, fecal impaction, hemorrhoids, or tumor involving the bladder neck or urethra. Such obstruction may also result from perineal tissue edema following childbirth or local manipulation during surgical procedures, such as total hip replacement or lower-leg vascular surgery.

In females, urethral obstruction may follow estrogen deficiency associated with tissue changes caused by normal aging or trauma. This results in increased collagen deposition, which reduces elasticity of the distal urethra and meatus. In normal urination, bladder pressure and urinary flow increase, causing a normally elastic urethra and meatus to dilate so that urine flows easily. But an inelastic meatus may cause back pressure, turbulent flow, and incomplete emptying, all of which increase the risk of infection.

Other gynecologic conditions may lead to retention by causing urethral compression. Such conditions include uterine myomas that protrude through the uterus, distending the vagina and displacing the uterus, and a gravid uterus that impinges on the urethra.

### Retention after surgery

Postoperative retention is probably related to the type of anesthetic used, the timing of preoperative medication, and the patient's activity level after surgery. After certain types of surgery, especially intraabdominal procedures, such as a colectomy and total hip replacement, postoperative retention stems from the effects of surgical manipulation on sensory nerve activity to and from the bladder.

Postoperative urinary retention may also be related to low fluid intake, because the bladder takes longer to fill and its stretch receptors lose their sensitivity to fullness.

Drug-induced urinary retention is common and may result from the use of psychotropics, antihistamines, narcotics, antispasmodics, and sedatives, which interfere with normal

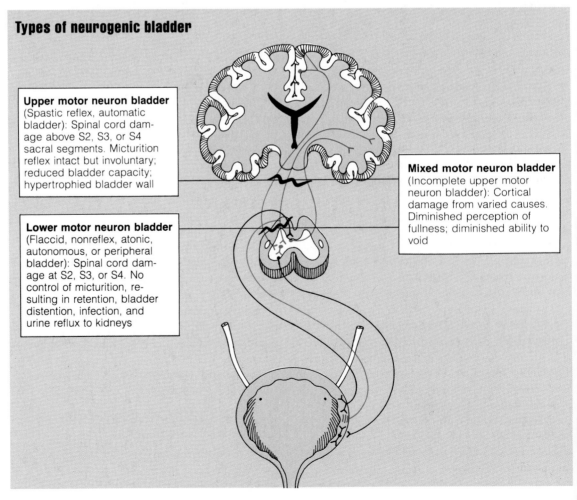

## Types of neurogenic bladder

**Upper motor neuron bladder** (Spastic reflex, automatic bladder): Spinal cord damage above S2, S3, or S4 sacral segments. Micturition reflex intact but involuntary; reduced bladder capacity; hypertrophied bladder wall

**Lower motor neuron bladder** (Flaccid, nonreflex, atonic, autonomous, or peripheral bladder): Spinal cord damage at S2, S3, or S4. No control of micturition, resulting in retention, bladder distention, infection, and urine reflux to kidneys

**Mixed motor neuron bladder** (Incomplete upper motor neuron bladder): Cortical damage from varied causes. Diminished perception of fullness; diminished ability to void

# Recognize drug-induced urinary retention

You should get a thorough medication history from your patient, including over-the-counter and prescription drugs that may cause urinary retention. Hospitalized patients are predisposed to retention caused by the preoperative drugs or anesthetics listed below.

*Antispasmodics and anticholinergics,* such as atropine, belladonna, Donnatal, and Librax, inhibit the muscarinic action of acetylcholine at postganglionic neuroeffector sites. Small doses may inhibit salivary and bronchial secretions; larger doses reduce ureter and bladder tone and motility, causing urinary retention.

Trihexyphenidyl hydrochloride, an anticholinergic, is used with levodopa (see *antiparkinsonian drugs* at right) and with phenothiazines. Because of its parasympatholytic effects, this drug should be used cautiously in obstructive bladder disease and benign prostatic hypertrophy. Benztropine mesylate, similar to atropine, has antihistaminic and anticholinergic effects and could cause retention.

*Antihistamines* antagonize histamine at the $H_1$ histamine receptor but do not block histamine release. They have anticholinergic effects and may cause frequent or difficult urination or urinary retention.

*Antipsychotics* include members of several distinct classes: phenothiazines, thioxanthenes, butyrophenone, molindone (a dihydroindolone derivative), and loxapine (a dibenzoxazepine). Their effects are similar; these drugs are thought to act as postsynaptic dopamine receptor antagonists. In addition, they exert anticholinergic effects, including urinary hesitancy or retention.

*Antiparkinsonian drugs,* such as levodopa, occasionally cause urinary retention. Levodopa is a dopamine precursor that crosses the blood-brain barrier and is converted to dopamine in the basal ganglia.

*Antihypertensives,* such as methyldopa, may cause urinary retention. Hydralazine hydrochloride lowers blood pressure by a peripheral vasodilating effect through direct relaxation of vascular smooth muscle. This drug also maintains or increases renal and cerebral blood flow.

---

micturition. (See *Recognize drug-induced urinary retention.*)

Psychogenic urinary retention occurs in postpubertal girls and women but occurs infrequently in men. It may accompany psychological or social trauma, such as divorce, surgery, or self-punishment or punishment of others for some perceived wrongdoing. This kind of chronic retention can be severe enough to cause anatomic changes in the urinary tract.

## MEDICAL MANAGEMENT

Because male and female mechanisms of continence differ, medical management of urinary incontinence varies with the patient's sex. No single diagnostic test can reliably identify the cause of the incontinence. A combination of tests must be selected after evaluating the patient's history, physical examination, and radiographic studies. The history should focus on the patient's past and current voiding patterns and on his overall physical and emotional health as the underlying reason for the incontinence may not be readily apparent. A comprehensive physical examination should be performed with special attention to the genitourinary tract.

In females, a thorough pelvic examination is mandatory. The doctor visualizes the anterior vaginal wall, using a Sims' speculum placed on the posterior vaginal wall. He examines the urethral meatus for swelling, tenderness, and discharge and evaluates the incontinent patient with a full bladder. The patient is asked to bear down while the meatus is observed. A spurt of urine from the meatus confirms stress incontinence; however, the absence of a spurt does not necessarily rule it out. Further vaginal exploration determines the presence or absence of vaginal and pelvic relaxation. The patient is asked to bear down while the vaginal wall is observed for bulging. Any bulging is considered abnormal, possibly indicating a cystocele.

*The Bonney-Read-Marshall* test (vesical neck elevation test) is done to identify incontinence related to loss of the posterior urethrovesical angle. The patient's bladder is filled with sterile water (approximately 150 to 200 ml) through a catheter until she feels the desire to void. The catheter is removed, and the patient is asked to strain downward or cough and to perform Valsalva's maneuver. If urine leaks out at the peak of Valsalva's maneuver, the doctor elevates the vagina with two fingers, making sure not to compress and obstruct the urethra, and has the patient repeat the ma-

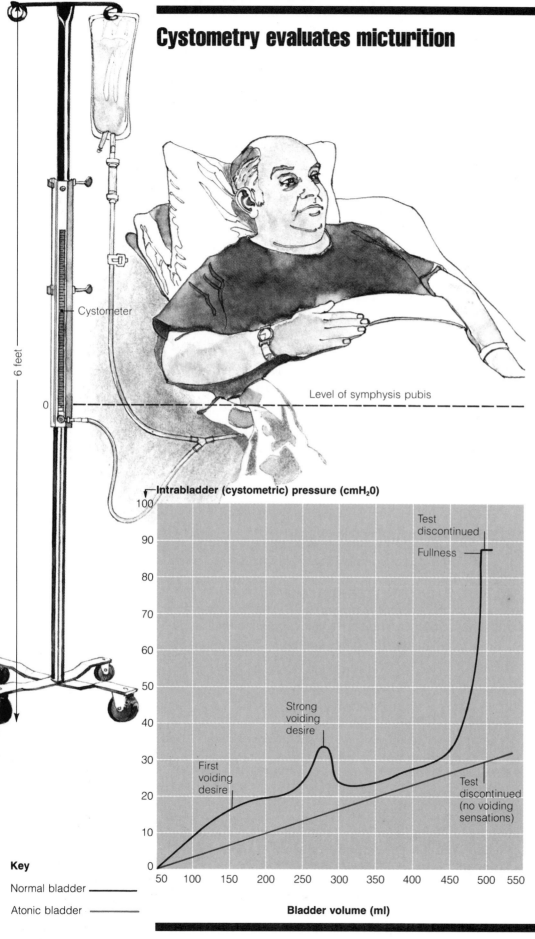

# Cystometry evaluates micturition

**C**ystometry assesses the bladder's neuromuscular function by measuring the efficiency of the detrusor muscle reflex, intravesical pressure and capacity, and the bladder's reaction to thermal stimulation. Qualities of the urinary stream and the bladder's reaction to thermal stimulation may give pathophysiologic information.

First, the patient voids into a device that gauges amount, flow, and time of voiding. Time and effort required to initiate the stream, its strength and continuity, and terminal dribbling are also noted.

Next, as the patient lies supine on an examination table, a catheter is passed into his bladder to measure residual urine, if any. Difficult catheter insertion may indicate an obstructed meatus or urethra.

The patient's response to thermal sensation is then tested by instilling sterile water or saline solution into the bladder, followed by an equal volume of warm fluid. He's asked to describe what he feels (discomfort, the need to void, nausea, or flushing).

After the fluid is drained from the bladder, the catheter is attached to the cystometer, and fluid is dripped into the bladder; the patient is asked to tell when he feels the first urge to void, then when he feels he must void. The related pressure and volume is automatically plotted. When his bladder is full, he's asked to void, and maximal intravesical pressure is noted. If no more tests are needed, the catheter is removed.

The first voiding desire normally occurs at about 150 ml of infused fluid; strong voiding desire, at 250 to 300 ml; and maximum capacity, at 300 to 500 ml. If uninhibited contractions occur (normally they shouldn't), they may indicate stroke, multiple sclerosis, or spinal cord pathology. The simplified diagram here illustrates the cystometric principle.

**Key**

Normal bladder ————

Atonic bladder ————

neuver. If urine doesn't leak, the test is positive. With the patient standing upright, the doctor repeats the test. A spurt of urine at the peak of Valsalva's maneuver indicates stress incontinence. Leakage that occurs several seconds after the maneuver, or a stream or dribble of urine, indicates other incontinence mechanisms.

External anal sphincter tone is assessed to evaluate the perineal musculature. The sphincter muscle tone and the patient's ability to contract the muscle are assessed digitally; voluntary contractions indicate that the pelvic floor's innervation is intact. Preserved muscle tone in the absence of voluntary contraction indicates a suprasacral lesion, whereas diminished tone implies a sacral lesion or a peripheral nerve problem.

Further neurologic examination should include evaluation of the motor system, reflexes, and sensation. Patients with quadriplegia and paraplegia may suffer any number of neurogenic bladder dysfunctions.

## Diagnostic tests

Accurate diagnosis of urologic dysfunction is based on radiologic, cystoscopic, uroscopic, and urodynamic procedures that enable the doctor to visualize urethral and bladder conditions and to evaluate urinary system performance. Because these tests are themselves commonly associated with significant risk of infection and because infection may cause misleading test results, these tests should be done *after* urinary tract infection is ruled out.

**Excretory urography.** This test, also known as intravenous pyelography, involves I.V. administration of a radiopaque dye that is filtered by the kidneys and excreted through the urinary tract. Excretory urography enables the doctor to identify the size, location, and configuration of the kidneys, ureters, and bladder. In an incontinent patient, postvoiding films may demonstrate abnormal dye retention, which may indicate a bladder neck obstruction. The test is most important when studying possible ureteral ectopia since it may reveal the presence of the redundant collecting system.

**Retrograde cystography.** These X-ray studies of the bladder are made after retrograde instillation of a radiopaque dye through a urethral catheter. Cystography helps diagnose conditions that may be causing neurogenic bladder or stress incontinence. This test clearly outlines the bladder, demonstrating bladder diverticula, vesicovaginal fistula, and

contrast media extravasation that may occur behind the bladder through a structural defect.

**Urethrography.** This radiographic X-ray examination of the urethra is performed to outline the inner size and shape of the urethra and to check for possible extravasation through a defect. In males, films are taken after a thick radiopaque substance is injected into the urinary meatus. In females, the procedure requires a less viscous material and a special catheter. The examination may show stenotic or dilated urethral areas. Urethrography can also be done in an antegrade fashion (voiding cystourethrography.)

**Cystourethroscopy.** Used as a diagnostic tool and as a treatment, this procedure combines the use of a cystoscope and a urethroscope. As a diagnostic tool, cystoscopic examination may identify bladder tumors and calculi. It also allows evaluation of bladder capacity and urinary reflux, permits collection of urine from each kidney and collection of biopsies, and can be used as an adjunct to retrograde ureteropyelography. In treatment, cystoscopy is invaluable for retrieving foreign bodies from the bladder, resecting tumors, fulgurating bleeding points, dilating constricted ureters, implanting radium, and resecting large obstructing prostate glands.

**Cystometry.** This test measures intravesical pressure during bladder filling. It provides information about detrusor muscle stability (see *Cystometry evaluates micturition*), the bladder's reaction to thermal stimulation, and intravesical pressure and capacity.

**Uroflometry.** This screening test evaluates the micturition phase of the lower urinary tract. The urinary flow rate represents the urine volume expelled through the urethra per unit of time; it's the result of detrusor or abdominal contractions, or both, acting through or against the resistance presented by the urethra's size. In men under age 50, the normal flow rate is about 20 to 25 ml/second; in men over age 50, the normal rate decreases. Females have slightly lower flow rates than men. An abnormal urinary flow rate may indicate an obstruction or detrusor muscle abnormalities.

**Catheterization for residual urine.** The urine volume retained in the bladder after voluntary micturition is determined by catheterizing a patient immediately after voiding. Normally, no residual urine is present, but authorities disagree over what constitutes a "significant" amount of residual urine. Residual urine may result from detrusor muscle dysfunction, obstructive uropathy, diverticula, or psychogenic inhibition. Absence of residual urine confirms effective micturition.

**Electromyography (EMG).** Usually done in conjunction with cystometry, electromyography is sometimes used to evaluate the relationship of perineal muscle activity to detrusor muscle contraction. Perineal muscle activity can be recorded with special anal or urethral electrodes. Although this test is useful for assessing neurogenic bladder dysfunction, it provides information only about striated or voluntary muscle activity, not about smooth muscle activity.

**Urethral pressure profile (UPP).** Methods of measuring urethral pressures have been developed to help evaluate urethral smooth muscle function. A UPP is a record of pressure generated throughout the urethra. It's obtained by inserting and then withdrawing a recording catheter through the urethra at a predetermined rate. Low pressure readings that reveal ineffective smooth muscle tone along the urethra may suggest incontinence; high readings may demonstrate excessive muscle tone and indicate a cause of urinary retention. A high pressure reading may also indicate strictures or urethral narrowing. The UPP should be evaluated together with an EMG to differentiate between spasms of striated and smooth muscles. Also, because detrusor muscle contraction may cause falsely high pressure readings, simultaneous bladder pressure measurement during cystometry may help further differentiation.

### Treatment: Conservative modalities

Managing incontinence begins by ruling out or treating urinary tract infections as these increase bladder irritability. Many conservative approaches can be used to treat urination disorders. For example, treating chronic cough and allergies may help ease incontinence by preventing sporadic increases in intraabdominal pressure. Similarly, a regular bowel elimination schedule will prevent excessive pressure arising from the lower gastrointestinal tract. Weight loss programs and pelvic exercises to strengthen the perineal muscles and increase sphincter control also help treat incontinence and prevent its recurrence.

**Perineal muscle training.** In the female, Kegel exercises specifically help stress incontinence. The patient is positioned in a chair with her legs slightly apart and her feet flat on the floor. This position ensures that the exercises will use perineal, rather than the glu-

teal, muscles. She is told to contract the pelvic muscles as though she were stopping a stream of urine, repeating the maneuver ten or more times at least four times a day. She's instructed to try to start and stop the urine stream several times while voiding to learn how the exercise should be done and to see if she is doing it correctly. Once she has learned the correct technique, she should be warned not to continue it during urination, to avoid possible urinary retention. She must continue to use these exercises as long as she has the problem; persistence is essential if the exercises are to achieve success.

**Bladder training.** A bladder training program has been used successfully in patients with neurogenic bladder dysfunction. Such training is commonly combined with intermittent or continuous catheterization to prevent overdistention; it requires close cooperation between the patient and nurses. (See *Training the neurogenic bladder.*)

**Biofeedback training.** Biofeedback, a reinforcement technique to gain control over involuntary (autonomic) nervous system responses, has been applied to bladder control. It is used primarily in pediatric and adolescent patients to try to "retrain" their neurologic pathways to achieve a normal voiding reflex.

**Catheterization.** Simple urethral catheterization is commonly used to relieve urinary retention: suprapubic catheterization, which is a surgical procedure, is used much less often. In *urethral catheterization* using aseptic technique, a straight or retention catheter is inserted into the urethral meatus, through the urethra, beyond the internal sphincter, and into the bladder. A straight catheter is preferred if it is to be removed as soon as the bladder is drained. An indwelling (Foley) catheter is used when it must remain inside the bladder for an undetermined amount of time. It is kept in place with an inflated balloon near the catheter tip and is attached to a drainage bag.

A *suprapubic catheter* may be inserted by a doctor, usually under local anesthesia. The patient's bladder must be distended. Using sterile technique, the doctor inserts a catheter or a trocar and cannula through a small incision in the abdominal wall into the bladder. Once the trocar and cannula are in place, he removes the trocar and threads the catheter through the cannula. He then sutures or seals the catheter into place. When the suprapubic catheter is removed, the muscle layers of the

# Training the neurogenic bladder

Bladder training in patients with spinal cord injuries aims to provide a method of emptying the bladder regularly in an acceptable manner with as little residual urine as possible, to preserve the urinary tract, and to protect it from infection and calculi formation. Eventually, the patient may be weaned off his catheter, or he may be instructed in how to give himself intermittent catheterization at home.

An *upper motor neuron* bladder does not receive a voiding signal from the brain, so it behaves reflexively, without a controlling impulse. The patient must learn to recognize some other common signs of a full bladder, such as sweating, restlessness, and abdominal discomfort, and to induce spontaneous (reflex) voiding.

He can try to induce voiding by stimulating trigger areas: by stroking his inner thigh, abdomen, or genitalia; by pulling the pubic hair or digitally stimulating the anal sphincter; or by lifting his buttocks up and down off the commode.

These techniques can be used in a bladder training program such as this one:
• The patient's catheter is removed in the morning and in the evening.
• He is given a glass of fluid hourly; after 3 hours he tries to void by stimulating a trigger area, as described above.
• If he voids, the residual urine is checked immediately. If it is less than 100 ml, the training can continue; if it's more, the catheter is reinserted and another training session is scheduled later.

A *lower motor neuron* bladder has no spontaneous voiding reflex since the sacral reflex arc is not intact. To compensate for this, the patient must apply pressure to the bladder by performing Credé's maneuver, by straining downward against a closed epiglottis (Valsalva's maneuver), or by contracting the abdominal muscles to bring pressure to bear on the bladder.

This patient's training program is similar to that for an upper motor neuron patient, except that his program continues with residual urine of less than 50 ml, and the catheter is reinserted if residual urine exceeds that amount.

bladder quickly close over the incision, so sutures are usually not needed.

The most common problem with suprapubic catheterization is poor drainage caused by mechanical obstruction, clogging with sediment and clots, or obstruction of the catheter tip by the bladder wall. However, with good insertion technique, the procedure carries less risk of urinary tract infection than the more commonly used Foley catheters.

The use of *clean intermittent catheterization (CIC)* has become the treatment of choice for vesicourethral dysfunction and has saved many neurogenic bladder patients from major reconstructive surgery. In patients with neurogenic bladder disorders associated with a hyperactive external sphincter, CIC makes continence possible.

## Pharmacologic treatment increasing
Drugs are now being used more frequently to treat urinary incontinence or retention.

**Anticholinergics.** Indicated for detrusor hyperactivity, these drugs act at the parasympathetic ganglia and at the smooth muscle receptors by competing with acetylcholine for receptor sites of smooth muscles, thus decreasing bladder contractility. Atropine, the prototype of this group, is now seldom prescribed because of its lack of selectivity and numerous side effects. Synthetic analogues have been developed that are more specific than atropine. These anticholinergics lower intravesical pressure, ease bladder spasm, and increase bladder capacity. Methantheline (Banthine) is used most widely; propantheline (Pro-Banthine), also used with some success, can be administered in smaller doses to achieve the desired effects. Oxybutynin (Ditropan) suppresses bladder contraction and spasm. Valethamate, a new anticholinergic, is used in some centers. Its side effects are generally limited to larger doses.

**Cholinergics (cholinesterase inhibitors).** Neostigmine (Prostigmin) can help prevent and treat detrusor muscle atony in the absence of obstruction.

Bethanechol (Urecholine) is particularly useful in urologic disorders because of its affinity for smooth muscles. It acts by stimulating detrusor muscle postganglionic cells and gastrointestinal tract smooth muscles, which results in a desire to void. Bethanechol can be used in primary urinary retention associated with acute or chronic neurogenic atony of detrusor muscles. It also helps reduce residual urine and counteracts urinary retention associated with treatment of hypertension with ganglionic blocking agents. Given orally, it has no significant effects on heart rate, blood pressure, bronchial tone, or salivation. However, given subcutaneously, bethanechol loses its selectivity and causes symptoms of cholinergic stimulation. These symptoms are most pronounced if the drug is given I.V. or I.M.; therefore I.V. or I.M. bethanechol is contraindicated. When bethanechol is given subcutaneously, atropine should be available to antagonize the drug's effects.

Bethanechol should not be given to asthmatic patients and should be used cautiously during pregnancy and in patients with hyperthyroidism and coronary artery disease. Side effects of cholinergics include increased salivation, bronchial secretions, intestinal motility, skin temperature elevation, pupil contraction, and bradycardia. Absorption from the gastrointestinal tract is erratic, so the dosages and schedule for each patient often must be determined by trial and error.

Such drugs as ephedrine and phenylephrine (adrenergics) and imipramine (an antidepressant) are sometimes given to promote continence by increasing resting urethral pressure. Propranolol, an adrenergic blocker, may be used in patients with angina or hypertension, for whom ephedrine and related agents are contraindicated. However, the use of any drug in a patient with cardiovascular disease must be evaluated by a cardiologist.

### Surgical treatment
Surgical intervention is needed when conservative management doesn't correct incontinence.

**In females.** Occasionally, incontinence can be surgically corrected by increasing urethral length if the urethra has been damaged in gynecologic or obstetric procedures. In *anterior urethropexy*, the anterior urethral wall or roof is sutured to the periosteum of the overlying symphysis while the urethra is in an elongated position. This serves to increase urethral resistance; often, this procedure alone restores continence.

Other types of surgery for incontinence aim to elevate and displace the vesical neck forward in such a way as to restore the proper urethrovesical angle. The surgical procedure and approach (vaginal or suprapubic) are determined by the presenting symptoms and the degree of pelvic relaxation. Generally, the suprapubic approach produces the best results and minimizes the risk of recurrence.

The most common operation for stress incontinence is the *Marshall-Marchetti-Krantz procedure.* This suprapubic approach involves suspending the urethra and vesical neck by suturing the anterior vaginal wall on each side to the periosteum of the pubic bones and to the lower rectal fascia. When the periosteum is in poor condition, as in older patients, Cooper's ligament in the vesical neck region is used instead with satisfactory results.

The *Pereyra procedure* substitutes the rectal fascia for the periosteum to anchor the suspended structures from above. This method was developed to prevent recurrent urethrovesical angle prolapse and the painful periostitis that sometimes develops postoperatively. An endoscopic vesical neck suspension is being used increasingly to treat stress incontinence. Again, the objective is to restore the normal urethrovesical angle.

Urethral obstruction and its attendant infection and urination problems occur frequently. Two accepted ways to deal with urethral or meatal stenosis are urethral dilation with sounds and urethrotomy with a urethrotome.

**In males.** TURP is the generally accepted method of removing prostatic lesions and most enlarged prostate glands. This procedure, which does not require an incision, carries minimal morbidity and mortality. The surgeon inserts a resectoscope into the urethra and removes excess tissue with a cutting device inserted through the resectoscope. The resectoscope has an insulated sheath that prevents urethral damage and a movable tungsten wire loop that cuts the prostatic tissue with high-frequency current controlled by a foot pedal. The surgeon operates by looking through a telescope onto the illuminated field. The area is irrigated through the resectoscope, and tissue debris falls into the bladder and is washed out. Hospitalization for this procedure is brief, and recovery is rapid.

The only other reason for surgery is dribbling-type incontinence. Most therapeutic efforts are directed at increasing urethral resistance by plications of tendons, fasciae, and muscle slings or by prosthetic devices that press on the bulbomembranous urethra. One such device uses a silicone gel prosthesis placed against the proximal urethra and tied by Marlex strips around the body of the ischiocavernous muscle. With normal detrusor and abdominal muscle function, passive urethral compression can provide continence when the bladder neck and proximal urethral sphincter activity have been affected.

An artificial urinary sphincter is increasingly common in treating persistent urinary incontinence. (See *The artificial urinary sphincter,* page 170.) This device has produced good results in many different types of incontinence, including stress incontinence, postprostatectomy incontinence, and epispadias with incontinence. An artificial sphincter can also successfully treat other congenital anomalies, such as myelomeningocele and bladder exstrophy.

**Correcting congenital anomalies.** Surgery for epispadias is undertaken after the child passes age 30 months, when bladder control would normally be established. The procedure involves releasing constricting tissue, repairing the urethral deficit, and constructing a functioning, cosmetically acceptable penis. To control incontinence, an attempt is made to construct a functional sphincter. Epispadias repair may be done in one step or in several. After repair is complete, the child will experience some difficulty in learning to void and to control his bladder since this is a new function.

When sphincter control cannot be established but rectal control is normal, the option of urinary diversion is considered. These procedures are not done frequently and should be the last resort after several attempts to facilitate normal control of urination.

Surgical correction of bladder exstrophy is difficult. Attempts at repair by closing over the bladder; constructing a vesical sphincter; repairing the epispadias; and bringing together the ventral fascia, muscle, and skin have mostly failed. Reconstruction begins in stages, starting in the first 48 hours of life with bladder closure in the neonate. This converts the exstrophic bladder to a severe form of epispadias. This is followed by vesicourethral reflux correction and then bladder neck reconstruction for continence. Because this anomaly is complex, and because urinary control may not be achieved, reconstructive efforts may be disappointing. The treatment of choice is cystectomy and urinary diversion.

The treatment of myelomeningocele is also difficult. Presently, most patients with myelomeningocele are treated with drugs, intermittent catheterization, or both; use of corrective surgery is declining. In many patients, surgical treatment of incontinence has led to further impairment of bladder emptying and acceleration of upper tract damage. Sling operations, urethral plications, and implantable devices that exert pressure on the urethra have been proposed for incontinence. Bladder neck repair, transurethral resection, and pudendal nerve sections have been tried for retention. Most of the surgical treatments have proved disappointing. However, the artificial sphincter may bring greater success as this device is perfected.

## NURSING MANAGEMENT
Nursing management of the patient with urinary incontinence or retention begins with the taking of a thorough patient history followed by a systematic physical examination. These two steps provide the subjective and objective data you'll need to formulate nursing diagnoses, set care goals, and plan and evaluate interventions.

### Take patient history
History-taking elicits details about the causes and symptoms of neurovascular disorders affecting the patient's urinary tract, about his home and work environments, and about any drugs he's taking.

**Get a medication history.** Find out what over-the-counter and prescription drugs the patient is taking because many drugs promote incontinence or retention by interfering with the neurologic reflex that controls micturition. Drugs that exert parasympathetic and sympathetic effects may induce stress incontinence or urinary retention and may be responsible for urgency, frequency, and nocturia. Specific offenders include antihistamines, antispasmodics, sedatives, diuretics, and psychotropic drugs. (See *Recognize drug-induced urinary retention,* page 163.)

**Assess voiding and urine quality.** Focus the urologic history by asking the patient about any voiding pattern changes, such as significant changes in urinary output and increased or decreased voiding frequency. Ask the patient if hesitation precedes the onset of the urinary stream or if the stream's force has decreased. Ask if his urine has been bloody or turbid; hematuria may occur with renal colic attacks. Remember, however, that red blood cells and epithelial cells can be present even though they're not grossly visible. Ask about urine leakage or dribbling because this information can often define a specific cause for the incontinence, such as stress incontinence or urinary retention with overflow.

A history of allergies or recent respiratory infection and the accompanying symptoms, such as coughing and sneezing, may help diagnose stress incontinence.

**Evaluate pain.** Pain may signal a urinary tract infection that must be ruled out as a

## The artificial urinary sphincter

Surgically implanted, the inflatable sphincter permits the patient to apply intermittent urethral compression, allowing him to voluntarily reduce urethral resistance during voiding. The cuff is placed around the bladder neck, the deflating mechanism is placed in the scrotum, and the fluid reservoir is placed under the rectus muscle in the abdomen. The reservoir holds the fluid used to inflate the cuff.

The pumping mechanism is activated by squeezing the scrotal bulb. When the cuff is completely inflated, it seals the urethra. When the patient wishes to void, he squeezes the scrotal bulb, which deflates the cuff and opens the urethra by returning fluid to the abdominal reservoir. After a time, the urethral cuff reinflates automatically to maintain occlusive pressure against the urethra until the patient is ready to void again.

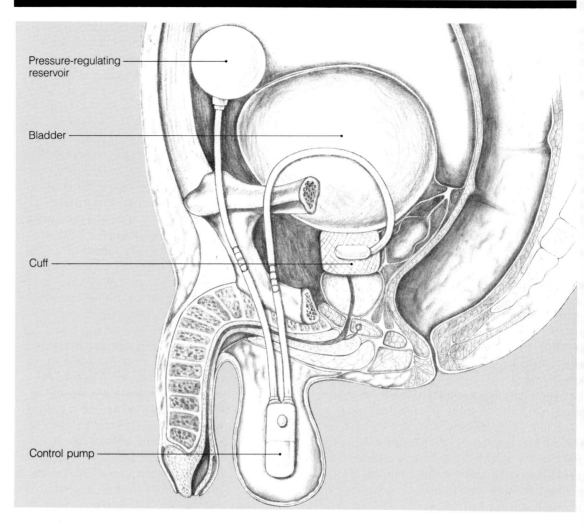

cause of symptoms before any other urologic diagnosis is made. Infections can be a primary problem or can occur secondary to other conditions, such as urine stasis. The patient's description of pain-related symptoms may help pinpoint the disorder. Question him about the onset, location, quality (somatic or focal pain versus visceral or diffuse pain), duration, and radiation. Eliciting ameliorating or exacerbating factors and associated symptoms, such as nausea, lightheadedness, and diaphoresis, may help identify the cause.

*Renal capsule distention* causes kidney pain that is felt as a constant, dull ache in the costovertebral angle, occasionally radiating to the periumbilical area. It could indicate hydronephrosis or pyelonephritis secondary to chronic urinary tract obstruction.

*Renal calculi* cause pain that's colicky and severe, but sporadic; the patient may not have sought medical advice after the initial attack.

*Ureteral pain* is colicky and severe and is produced by spasms of the renal pelvis and ureteral musculature. Ureteral pain radiates from the upper ureter and is associated with

pain in the ipsilateral testicle. Lower ureteral pain occurs in the scrotal wall in the male or in the ipsilateral labium in the female. Ureteral pain may indicate some inflammatory or obstructive process.

*Bladder discomfort* may be due to overdistention or inflammation. Pain from overdistention is generally located in the suprapubic area. Sometimes women describe this as a heaviness in the abdomen or as being "aware" of their pelvic area. Burning on urination is typical of these infections and is noted in the distal urethra in females and the prostatic urethra in males.

Does the patient have a history of urinary tract infections? Urethral pain occurs along the course of the urethra or at the meatus. By asking when the patient feels the pain, you may discover whether it originates in the bladder or in the urethra. Burning at the beginning of urination indicates urethritis; burning during and after urination indicates bladder infection.

**Get an ob/gyn history.** It's important to get a complete obstetric history, including the umber of pregnancies, deliveries, and abortions. Ask the patient about the duration of labor and the type of deliveries she has experienced. Surgical intervention in a delivery may predispose to continence problems.

The gynecologic history should include any preexisting or present gynecologic conditions, such as cystocele or uterine fibroids, and any gynecologic procedures or perineal surgery that has been done. If the patient has had a pelvic malignancy, find out where it was, how it was treated, and whether it recurred. Radiation injury contributes greatly to vesicovaginal fistulas, especially when radiation is teamed with surgery.

**Assess for prostate enlargement.** Ask the male patient about symptoms of prostatic hypertrophy. A man with significant prostatic enlargement may mention hesitation in starting a urine stream and a decrease in stream force. He may also complain that he does not feel he is emptying his bladder completely. Ask him if he has undergone prostatic surgery; transient incontinence may follow all types of prostatectomy procedures.

**Evaluate neurogenic status.** Ask the patient about congenital disorders, back problems, previous trauma, orthopedic or neurologic procedures, and any physical problems he may be aware of, such as paresthesias or arm or leg weakness.

A history of trauma, orthopedic or neurologic surgery, or paresthesias may help identify upper motor or lower motor neuron injury or disease.

If the patient has a congenital defect, you may gain more information about the disorder and its sequelae by letting the patient describe the condition in his own words. Intravertebral disk diseases may cause chronic inflammation of the spinal cord or may impinge on spinal nerves, which commonly results in urinary symptoms when the sacral part of the cord is involved.

**Ask about general health.** Include questions about recent weight gain, particularly in women; additional weight may further compromise a weakened pelvic floor. Get a psychosocial history (the patient's views of his illness and of himself; his coping mechanisms) to rule out the possibility of psychosomatic urologic symptoms. Women with psychological problems may manifest urinary symptoms; men, however, rarely do. Often, psychosomatic symptoms disappear with therapy, but surgical intervention is sometimes required.

## Perform the physical examination

In the physical examination, you'll be following through on the pertinent information you've gathered in the health history. Incorporate all body systems—including the genitourinary tract—in your direct examination.

The incontinent patient feels embarrassed and anxious and may be reluctant to talk about his condition. Try to put him at ease. See that the examination room is private, comfortably warm, and well-lit. As you discuss the examination procedure with him, note his appearance, posture, dress, and grooming, along with any idiosyncracies. Obtain vital signs, and inspect the patient's skin for scars, lesions, pigmentation, excoriation, and eruptions. Look for a bladder mass, asymmetry, or bladder contour; examine the abdominal wall for tension, tenderness, and hernia.

**Assess the kidneys and bladder.** Assess the kidneys for tenderness and masses by paraspinal palpation and percussion to evaluate costovertebral angle tenderness. Instruct the patient not to void before you examine the bladder. A distended bladder rises out of the pelvis and may be palpable above the symphysis. Percussing a full bladder produces a "kettledrum" sound. After the initial assessment, tell the patient to void, and percuss the bladder again to evaluate emptying.

**Assess the genitalia.** Establishing a good rapport with the patient before examining the genitalia is essential for a successful examination. An accepting attitude on your part can foster that rapport. Genital examination may cause anxiety for both the male and the female patient, because both sexes are susceptible to feelings of embarrassment and modesty. Sexual fears may be very real and wrapped up in cultural taboos. If a male patient experiences an erection during the genital examination, deal with it in a matter-of-fact, professional manner. Explain that this reaction is not uncommon and that it is nothing more than a physiologic response. Do not stop the examination or leave the room; merely proceed to examine another body area until the erection subsides. A firm, rather than soft, touch on the genitalia and a matter-of-fact, accepting attitude help reduce the chance of sexual stimulation.

Place a female patient in the lithotomy position, and drape her to avoid embarrassment. Before beginning, teach her to relax her abdominal muscles by deep breathing and by placing her hands on her abdomen. Explain (continued on page 174)

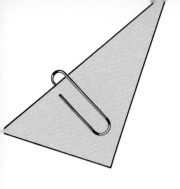

**PATIENT-TEACHING AID**

# How to catheterize yourself using clean technique

*Dear* _____

When you return home from the hospital, you won't have to use sterile technique to catheterize yourself. Just remember to take the few simple precautions outlined here.

In home self-catheterization, it's very important to strictly follow your catheterization schedule. Otherwise, you'll retain urine, which can lead to infection, a stretched bladder, or urine leakage. Never postpone catheterization for any reason, such as not having soap and water handy. Cleanliness is very important, but on the rare occasions when you can't wash, you must perform the procedure anyway to avoid the greater medical risks.

Remember that intermittent catheterization is only one component of controlling incontinence. By carefully regulating your fluid intake, you can help prevent incontinence and still maintain a good level of hydration. Also, you must remember to take your prescribed bladder medications regularly.

To catheterize yourself using clean technique, you'll need a rubber catheter, a clean washcloth, soap and water, a small package of water-soluble lubricant, and a plastic bag for used catheters. Also, obtain a container for draining urine if a toilet isn't available or if you need to measure your urine. Make sure you have good lighting. Before catheterization, try to urinate, then wash your hands.

**If you're a female**
Position yourself on a bed or toilet. Arrange your clothing so it's out of your way.

Separate your vaginal folds with one hand. Use downward strokes with the washcloth to wash the area thoroughly.

Lubricate the first 3″ (7.6 cm) of the catheter with water-soluble jelly.

Now you're ready for insertion. Hold the catheter as if it were a pencil, about ½″ (1.3 cm) from its tip. Keeping the vaginal folds separated, slowly insert the lubricated catheter about 3″ into your urethra. Press down with your abdominal muscles to empty your bladder. Allow all urine to drain through the catheter. When the urine stops draining, remove the catheter slowly.

Wash the catheter in warm, soapy water. Then rinse it inside and out, and dry it with a clean towel. Place it in the plastic storage bag for used catheters.

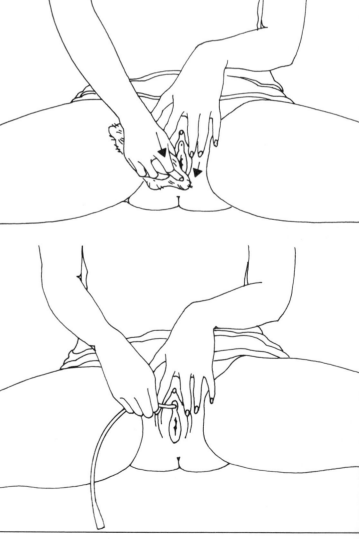

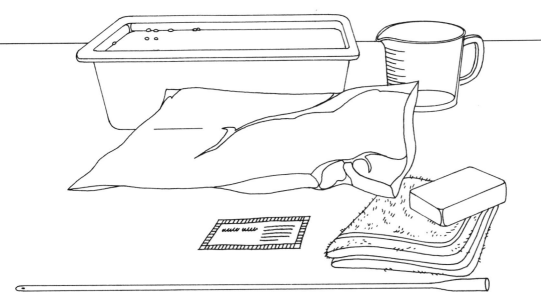

### If you're a male
Position yourself on a bed or toilet. If you're uncircumcised, pull back the foreskin of your penis and hold it back throughout the catheterization. Then wash the end of your penis thoroughly with soap and water.

Lubricate the first 7″ to 10″ (17.8 to 25.4 cm) of the catheter with water-soluble jelly.

Then hold your penis at a right angle to your body. Grasp the catheter as you would a pencil, and slowly insert it 7″ to 10″, until urine begins to flow. Then gently push the catheter 1″ farther. Allow all urine to drain.

When urine stops draining, slowly remove the catheter. Pull your foreskin forward again. Wash the catheter in warm, soapy water. Then rinse it inside and out, and dry it with a clean towel. Place the catheter in the used-catheter storage bag.

### Remember
Buy a new catheter supply each month or when catheters are brittle. Use each catheter only once. When you've used all but the last one, boil the catheters for 20 minutes. Drain the water and store the catheters in a clean towel. Each time you use a catheter, be sure to put it in the plastic storage bag for used catheters, not back with the clean catheters.

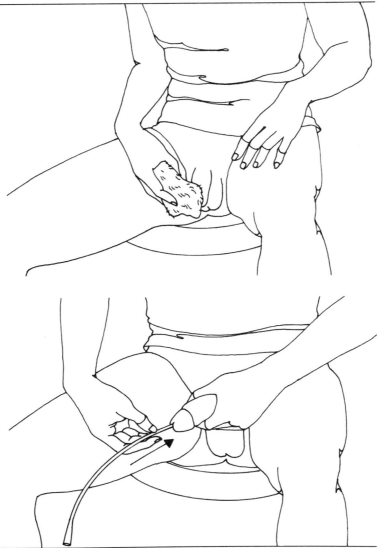

## Autonomic hyperreflexia

Characterized by paroxysms of hypertension, autonomic hyperreflexia occurs in patients with spinal cord injuries above the T6 level. It's a serious emergency, resulting from excessive autonomic response to normal stimuli. Systolic pressure may rise as high as 240 to 300 mm Hg. If untreated, hypertension may lead to seizures or stroke.

Symptoms of hyperreflexia include pounding headache, diaphoresis, gooseflesh above the lesion's level, nausea, chest pain, and nasal congestion. The disorder may be triggered by many stimuli, including bladder distention due to a plugged catheter or spastic sphincter. Other possible stimuli include constipation, fecal impaction, urinary calculi, severe bladder infection, or pain receptor stimulation from pressure sores or skin rashes.

Autonomic hyperreflexia can be treated by removing the trigger stimulus, if possible. If not, such drugs as diazoxide, hydralazine, or phentolamine may be given to control the hypertension. The patient and his family can be taught to avoid noxious stimuli and to recognize the symptoms of the disorder so that they may get immediate medical attention.

what you are going to do, and repeat the explanation as you do it.

The external genitalia may show evidence of dribbling from the urethra or excoriation of the labia and thighs; examine the urethral and vaginal openings for swelling, redness, exudates, and lesions.

Instruct the male patient to stand with genitalia exposed. Palpate and inspect the genitalia. Inspection may reveal dribbling from the meatus and excoriation of the scrotum or thighs from urine.

Many congenital defects of the urologic system involve associated defects in the penis and scrotum. Inspect the penis for any irregularities. The meatus should appear in the center at the top of the penis. In hypospadias, the meatus is on the inferior side of the penis. In epispadias, the meatus is displaced to the ventral side of the penis. Note any discharge from the urethral meatus, and obtain culture specimens, if necessary.

**Assess neurologic status.** Evaluating the patient's deep tendon reflexes provides information about segmental spinal cord function. Upper motor neuron abnormalities cause hyperactive reflexes; lower motor neuron damage causes diminished or absent reflexes.

The bulbocavernous reflex includes all the perineal striated muscle reflexes. Normally, the bulbocavernous muscle contracts upon being percussed. In males, elicit this reflex by squeezing the glans penis and monitoring external and sphincter contraction. For females, this test is not common.

Loss of pain, touch, and vibration reception in the skin suggests metabolic or toxic neuropathies, such as diabetes mellitus. Absence of deep sensation and pain suggests posterior column diseases such as tabes dorsalis. Localized sensory loss on the lateral leg suggests herniation of the intravertebral disk at the L4-to-L5 level or a nerve root problem at this level. Sensory loss on the lateral aspect of the foot may imply a problem involving the first or second sacral nerve roots.

### Formulate nursing diagnoses

After collecting information from the patient history and physical examination and after evaluating the patient's physical and emotional needs, you're ready to formulate nursing diagnoses that clearly explain the patient's problem and allow you to plan appropriate goals and interventions.

**Alterations in urinary elimination patterns related to stress incontinence.** Your goal is

to develop a regimen of daily care to establish a normal elimination pattern. Teach the female patient the importance of weight control because excess weight may decrease pelvic muscle tone. If the patient has a weight problem, involve the dietitian and family in creating an acceptable diet for her. Help her set realistic goals, and chart her progress. Instruct her in Kegel exercises to increase pelvic floor strength, and schedule them during activities of daily living (such as sitting, watching TV, or standing in lines).

Determine whether the patient smokes or has allergies or upper respiratory infections, all of which promote coughing or sneezing and precipitate stress incontinence. If the patient agrees to stop smoking, monitor her progress in a nonthreatening, supportive manner, explaining why this may help her attain continence. She may need to join a support group to stop smoking. If coughing still causes her to leak urine, suggest measures to relieve the cough or control her symptoms.

Identify activities that require straining or heavy lifting, and explain that these may precipitate stress incontinence. Teach the patient to modify them by using good body mechanics. Later, determine if she's noticed fewer symptoms after the recommended changes in activities. Your interventions are successful if the patient is losing weight safely and doing Kegel exercises properly, enabling her to hold her urine stream for increasing periods of time and strengthening her pelvic floor. Her vaginal vault and anal sphincter should have increased tension; if not, she may require surgery. She should be relieved of cough, allergic symptoms, and respiratory infections, and she should avoid or modify activities that precipitate stress incontinence.

**Knowledge deficit related to using CIC.** Your goals are to make sure the patient understands the principles of catheterization; to verify his correct self-catheterization technique; and to ensure that he protects himself from catheter-related urinary tract infections.

CIC carries less risk of infection than a Foley catheter, which may cause infection from continuous irritation of the urethra and bladder. Use of CIC also promotes greater patient independence and self-control.

Teach the patient how to perform the procedure (see *How to catheterize yourself using clean technique,* pages 172 to 173). To prevent nosocomial infection, you should teach the patient sterile technique while he's in the hospital. You should also teach him clean technique, which will be used at home.

Be sure to teach the female patient the location of the labia and the vaginal and urinary orifices, so she will be able to insert the catheter correctly.

Explain that the patient may still experience incontinence at times and that he may need to wear incontinent briefs or an external collection device between catheterizations. Plastic or rubber sheeting can be used to protect bedding. Emphasize the need to perform adequate skin care to prevent skin breakdown from contact with urine. Provide information on sources of needed supplies.

Your interventions are successful if the patient understands the procedure; if he demonstrates the ability to perform self-catheterization; and if he remains free from catheter-related urinary tract infections.

**Potential for disruption of skin integrity related to prolonged contact with urine.** Your goals in this diagnosis are to ensure that the patient has sensation in the perineum and to prevent skin breakdown.

If the patient has lost sensation in the perineum, teach him to do a self-examination with a mirror, or get a family member to do it. Explain why this is necessary to prevent infection and decubiti and to promote comfort. Cleanse and dry wet skin immediately.

Drying the area by exposure to a 40-watt light placed no closer than 12" (30 cm) to the skin may alleviate excoriation. The patient should be well draped for this procedure. Leave the light on for 10 minutes three times a day. Apply protective ointment, as ordered. Your interventions are successful if the patient properly assesses his perineal area for excoriation and if his skin is intact, with no redness, swelling, or excoriation.

**Disturbance in self-concept related to loss of body functions.** Your goal is to promote positive expression of productive interpersonal relationships. Provide an accepting and supportive atmosphere for the patient. Determine how a changed voiding pattern has affected his outside activities and sex life, and assess his emotions regarding incontinence.

Encourage him to express his feelings of anxiety, fear, anger, or helplessness. Give nonjudgmental care when cleaning the patient after an episode of incontinence. Explain to his family that it is merely a physiologic response to the patient's underlying condition. Promote feelings of self-worth by stressing the positive features in the patient's life (such as his abilities, sense of humor, accomplishments, and appearance).

Your interventions are successful when the patient has a good self-image and expresses—verbally and nonverbally—productive interpersonal relationships.

**Alteration in comfort related to frequency of, and burning of, urination.** Your goal is to make the patient as comfortable as possible and to prevent urinary tract infections. Administer drugs, as ordered. Explain the importance of taking them at the appropriate time and of taking the entire amount required, even after symptoms have abated. Encourage the patient to drink up to 2,000 ml of fluid daily, unless contraindicated, and explain that increased amounts of fluid dilute toxins in the urinary tract and flush medications from his kidneys. Encourage the patient to drink acid fluids (such as cranberry juice) to reestablish the bladder's acid pH and to discourage bacterial growth. Your interventions are successful if the patient experiences no discomfort related to urination and if infection is prevented or resolved.

**Alterations in urinary elimination patterns related to urinary retention or autonomic hyperreflexia related to urinary bladder distention.** Your goal is to enable the patient to prevent urinary retention and bladder distention. Be sure the patient has maximum privacy and is not rushed when trying to void. Elevate the head of his bed as much as possible to increase intraabdominal pressure. Advise him about techniques to stimulate voiding (such as running water in the sink, placing his hand in warm water, or pouring warm water over his perineum). Learn what drugs (prescription and over-the-counter) the patient is taking. Explain that some drugs encourage urinary retention, and discuss drug action and side effects. The doctor should be aware of all drugs, especially psychotropics, antihistamines, and antispasmodics, that the patient is taking. Your interventions are successful when the patient voids successfully.

## A satisfactory outcome

Your incontinent patient needs a lot of understanding, acceptance, and support. He and his family need to be educated and helped to deal with and make the most of his residual organic function. A good rehabilitation plan—including bladder training; use of prostheses, if necessary; diet; and drugs—will help your patient to reach his maximum potential and to return to a satisfying and secure life-style.

**Points to remember**

- Urinary incontinence may be caused by anything that interferes with bladder or sphincter control.
- Total incontinence after a transurethral prostatic resection almost always results from injury to the external sphincter and either the bladder neck or prostatic urethral muscle fibers, or both.
- Stress incontinence occurs almost exclusively in females.
- Clean intermittent catheterization has become the treatment of choice in vesicourethral dysfunction.
- Drug treatment of incontinence is becoming more prevalent, while surgical treatment is diminishing.

# APPENDICES

# Renal and urologic drugs

## Anticholinergics and antispasmodics

| Drug, dose, and route | Interactions | Side effects | Special considerations |
|---|---|---|---|
| **methantheline**<br>50 to 100 mg P.O. q.i.d.<br><br>**propantheline**<br>15 to 30 mg P.O. q.i.d. | *Digoxin:* elevated digoxin blood levels due to increased GI absorption. Monitor digoxin blood levels. | Drowsiness, dizziness, blurred vision, urticaria, mouth dryness, constipation, paralytic ileus, urinary hesitancy and retention, palpitations, confusion in elderly patients | Use cautiously in hot or humid environments to prevent drug-induced heat stroke. Give drug 30 to 60 minutes before meals and at bedtime. Bedtime dose can be larger and should be given at least 2 hours after the last meal of the day. Give smaller doses to the elderly.<br>  Instruct patient to avoid driving and other hazardous activities if he is drowsy, dizzy, or has blurred vision; to drink plenty of fluids to help prevent constipation; and to report any skin rash. Suggest sugarless gum or hard candy to relieve mouth dryness. |
| **oxybutynin**<br>5 mg P.O. b.i.d. or t.i.d. | *Digoxin:* elevated digoxin blood levels due to increased GI absorption. Monitor digoxin blood levels. | Drowsiness, mouth dryness, palpitations, transient blurred vision, urinary hesitancy or retention | Because oxybutynin suppresses sweating, its use during very hot weather may precipitate fever or heatstroke. Before giving drug, confirm neurogenic bladder by cystometry, and rule out partial intestinal obstruction in patients with diarrhea, especially those with colostomy or ileostomy. Periodically evaluate patient response to therapy by cystometry.<br>  Warn patient that drug may impair alertness or vision. |

## Antihypertensives

| Drug, dose, and route | Interactions | Side effects | Special considerations |
|---|---|---|---|
| **atenolol**<br>50 to 100 mg P.O. daily as a single dose | *Indomethacin:* decreased antihypertensive effect. Monitor blood pressure and adjust dosage.<br>*Lidocaine:* increased blood levels of lidocaine<br>*Prazosin:* increased hypotension<br>*Theophyllines:* decreased therapeutic effect of theophyllines | Bradycardia, hypotension, congestive heart failure | Always check patient's apical pulse before giving this drug; if slower than 60 beats/minute, withhold drug and call doctor. Monitor blood pressure frequently.<br>  Explain importance of taking drug, even when patient feels well. Tell him not to discontinue drug suddenly but to call doctor if unpleasant side effects develop. Counsel patient to take drug at regular time each day. |
| **captopril**<br>25 to 50 mg P.O. t.i.d. | *Indomethacin:* decreased antihypertensive effect | Leukopenia, hypotension, loss of taste, proteinuria, renal failure, skin rash | Question patient about impaired taste sensation. Should be taken 1 hour before meals. Monitor blood pressure and pulse rate frequently. |
| **clonidine**<br>0.2 to 0.8 mg P.O. daily in divided doses | *Tricyclic antidepressants:* decreased antihypertensive effect | Drowsiness, mouth dryness, constipation, orthostatic hypotension | Monitor blood pressure and pulse rate frequently. Dosage is usually adjusted to patient's blood pressure and tolerance. May be given to rapidly lower blood pressure in some hypertensive emergencies. Advise patient to avoid sudden position changes. Tell him to take last dose just before retiring. |
| **guanabenz**<br>4 to 8 mg P.O. b.i.d. | *CNS depressants:* increased sedation | Drowsiness, sedation, dizziness, weakness, mouth dryness | Advise patient to drive a car or operate machinery cautiously until CNS effects are known. Warn that drug may decrease tolerance to alcohol or CNS depressants. |
| **guanadrel**<br>20 to 75 mg P.O. daily in divided doses | *MAO inhibitors, sympathomimetics, methylphenidate, phenothiazines, tricyclic antidepressants:* decreased antihypertensive effect | Fatigue, dizziness, orthostatic hypotension | Monitor supine and standing blood pressure, especially during dosage adjustment. Warn that hot showers may cause hypertension. Inform patient that orthostatic hypotension can be minimized by rising slowly and avoiding sudden position changes. |
| **guanethidine**<br>25 to 50 mg P.O. daily | *MAO inhibitors, sympathomimetics, methylphenidate, phenothiazines, tricyclic antidepressants:* decreased antihypertensive action | Dizziness, weakness, orthostatic hypotension, nasal stuffiness, diarrhea, edema, weight gain, inhibition of ejaculation | Tell outpatient to avoid strenuous exercise, and warn that hot showers may cause hypotensive reaction. Inform patient that orthostatic hypotension can be minimized by rising slowly and avoiding sudden position changes. Give this drug with meals to increase absorption. |
| **hydralazine**<br>10 to 50 mg P.O. q.i.d. or 10 to 20 mg I.M. or I.V. q 4 hours. Switch to oral administration as soon as possible. | None significant | Sodium retention and weight gain, headache, lupus erythematosus-like syndrome, headache, tachycardia, angina | Monitor patient's blood pressure and pulse rate frequently. Watch closely for signs of lupus erythematosus-like syndrome (sore throat, fever, muscle and joint aches, skin rash). Call doctor immediately if any of these develop. Give this drug with meals to increase absorption. |
| **methyldopa**<br>500 mg to 2 g P.O. daily in divided doses; 500 mg to 1 g q 6 hours, diluted in D₅W, given I.V. over 30 to 60 minutes | *Lithium:* increased toxicity; lithium dose may have to be decreased | Sedation, decreased mental acuity, hemolytic anemia, edema and weight gain, orthostatic hypotension, mouth dryness | Weigh patient daily. Notify doctor of any weight increase. Inform patient that orthostatic hypotension can be minimized by rising slowly and avoiding sudden position changes. |

## Antihypertensives (continued)

| Drug, dose, and route | Interactions | Side effects | Special considerations |
|---|---|---|---|
| **metoprolol**<br>50 to 100 mg P.O. daily in two or three divided doses | *Barbiturates, indomethacin, rifampin, thyroid hormones:* decreased pharmacologic effect of metoprolol<br>*Chlorpromazine, cimetidine, oral contraceptives:* increased pharmacologic effect of metoprolol<br>*Lidocaine:* increased lidocaine blood levels<br>*Prazosin:* increased hypotension<br>*Theophyllines:* decreased therapeutic effect of theophyllines. | Bradycardia, hypotension, congestive heart failure | Monitor blood pressure frequently. If patient develops severe hypotension, notify doctor. Tell outpatient not to discontinue this drug suddenly; abrupt discontinuation can exacerbate angina and MI. Instruct patient to call doctor if unpleasant side effects develop. Food may increase absorption. Give consistently with meals. |
| **minoxidil**<br>10 to 40 mg P.O. daily | None significant | Edema, weight gain, hypertrichosis (elongation, thickening, and enhanced pigmentation of fine body hair), tachycardia | About 80% of patients experience hypertrichosis within 6 weeks of beginning treatment. Suggest a depilatory or shaving, and assure patient that extra hair will disappear within 1 to 6 months of stopping minoxidil. Advise patient not to discontinue drug without doctor's consent. |
| **nadolol**<br>80 to 240 mg P.O. once daily | *Indomethacin:* decreased therapeutic effect of nadolol<br>*Lidocaine:* increased blood levels of lidocaine<br>*Prazosin:* increased hypotension<br>*Theophyllines:* decreased therapeutic effect of theophyllines. | Bradycardia, hypotension, congestive heart failure, increased airway resistance | Always check patient's apical pulse before giving this drug. If slower than 60 beats/minute, withhold drug and call doctor. Tell outpatient not to discontinue drug suddenly but to call doctor if unpleasant side effects develop. This drug masks signs of shock and hypoglycemia. May be given without regard to meals. |
| **pindolol**<br>10 to 20 mg P.O. b.i.d. | *Indomethacin:* decreased therapeutic effect of pindolol<br>*Prazosin:* increased hypotension<br>*Theophyllines:* decreased therapeutic effect of theophyllines. | Fatigue, lethargy, congestive heart failure, hypotension, increased airway resistance, muscle and joint pain | Always check apical pulse rate before giving drug. If you detect extremes in pulse rates, withhold drug and call doctor. Tell outpatient not to discontinue drug suddenly to prevent exacerbation of angina and MI. This drug masks signs of shock and hypoglycemia. |
| **prazosin**<br>3 to 20 mg P.O. daily in divided doses | *Beta-adrenergic blockers:* increased hypotension | Dizziness, "first-dose syncope," palpitations, nausea, orthostatic hypotension, mouth dryness | If first dose exceeds 1 mg, patient may develop severe syncope with loss of consciousness. Increase dose slowly. Instruct patient to sit or to lie down if he feels dizzy. Inform him to avoid sudden position changes. |
| **propranolol**<br>80 to 160 mg P.O. daily in single dose (sustained-release capsule) or divided doses | *Barbiturates, indomethacin, rifampin, thyroid hormones:* decreased pharmacologic effect of propranolol<br>*Chlorpromazine, cimetidine, oral contraceptives:* increased pharmacologic effect of propranolol<br>*Lidocaine:* increased lidocaine blood levels<br>*Prazosin:* increased hypotension<br>*Theophyllines:* decreased therapeutic effect of theophyllines. | Fatigue, bradycardia, hypotension, congestive heart failure, increased airway resistance | Always check patient's apical pulse rate before giving this drug. If you detect extremes in pulse rates, withhold medication and call the doctor immediately. If patient develops hypotension, monitor blood pressure frequently.<br>    Don't discontinue abruptly; this can exacerbate angina and MI. This drug masks common signs of shock and hypoglycemia. Food may increase the absorption of propranolol. Give consistently with meals. |
| **timolol**<br>10 to 20 mg P.O. b.i.d. | *Indomethacin:* decreased therapeutic effect of timolol<br>*Lidocaine:* increased lidocaine blood levels<br>*Prazosin:* increased hypotension<br>*Theophyllines:* decreased therapeutic effect of theophyllines. | Fatigue, lethargy, hypotension, congestive heart failure, bradycardia, increased airway resistance | Always check apical pulse rate before giving drug. If you detect extremes in pulse rates, withhold drug and call doctor. Tell patient not to discontinue drug suddenly; abrupt discontinuation can exacerbate angina and MI. This drug masks common signs of shock and hypoglycemia. |

## Anti-infectives

| Drug, dose, and route | Interactions | Side effects | Special considerations |
|---|---|---|---|
| **amoxicillin**<br>750 mg to 1.5 g P.O. daily in divided doses q 8 hours | *Chloramphenicol, erythromycin, tetracyclines:* antibiotic antagonism. Give amoxicillin at least 1 hour before bacteriostatic antibiotics. | Nausea, diarrhea, maculopapular rash, urticaria | Before giving drug, ask patient if he's had any allergic reactions to penicillin. Give with food to prevent GI distress. Tell patient to take entire quantity, exactly as prescribed, even after he feels well. Amoxicillin and ampicillin have similar clinical applications. |
| **ampicillin**<br>250 mg to 1 g P.O., I.M., or I.V. q 6 hours | *Chloramphenicol, erythromycin, tetracyclines:* antibiotic antagonism. Give ampicillin at least 1 hour before bacteriostatic antibiotics. | Nausea, diarrhea, maculopapular rash, urticaria | If giving drug I.V., mix with dextrose 5% in water or a saline solution. Don't mix with other drugs or solutions. Give oral doses 1 to 2 hours before or 2 to 3 hours after meals to prevent impaired absorption. |
| **cefazolin**<br>500 mg to 1 g I.M. or I.V. q 6 to 8 hours | *Probenecid:* may increase cefazolin blood levels. Use together cautiously. | Thrombophlebitis at I.V. injection site, maculopapular skin rash, diarrhea | Avoid doses greater than 4 g daily in severe renal impairment. Before giving cefazolin, ask the patient if he's had any allergic reactions to cephalosporins or penicillin. Alternate injection sites if I.V. therapy lasts longer than 3 days. Use small I.V. needles in larger veins. |

## Anti-infectives (continued)

| Drug, dose, and route | Interactions | Side effects | Special considerations |
|---|---|---|---|
| **cinoxacin**<br>1 g P.O. daily in two to four divided doses for 7 to 14 days | *Probenecid:* may decrease urine levels of cinoxacin. Monitor for increased toxicity and reduced antibacterial effectiveness. | Dizziness, headache, nausea, photophobia, vomiting, abdominal pain | Obtain clean-catch urine specimen for culture and sensitivity tests before starting therapy, and repeat p.r.n. High urine levels permit twice-daily dosing. Report CNS side effects (dizziness, headache) immediately; they indicate serious toxicity and usually mean stopping the drug. Tell patient to take cinoxacin with meals to help decrease GI side effects. Warn him about photophobic effects of drug, and advise him to avoid bright sunlight. |
| **co-trimoxazole**<br>(sulfamethoxazole-trimethoprim)<br>160 mg trimethoprim/<br>800 mg sulfamethoxazole P.O. q 12 hours for 10 to 14 days | *Oral anticoagulants:* increased risk of bleeding. Monitor prothrombin time.<br>*Oral antidiabetics:* increased pharmacologic effect. Monitor for hypoglycemia.<br>*Phenytoin:* increased blood levels. Monitor for phenytoin toxicity. | Nausea, vomiting, diarrhea, erythema multiforme (Stevens-Johnson syndrome), generalized skin eruptions, epidermal necrolysis, exfoliative dermatitis, blood dyscrasias | Oral suspension is available for patients who cannot swallow large tablets. Note that "DS" product means "double strength."<br>Promptly report skin rash, sore throat, fever, or mouth sores—early signs of blood dyscrasias. Encourage fluid intake. |
| **doxycycline**<br>100 to 200 mg P.O. or I.V. daily | *Antacids (including NaHCO₃) and laxatives containing aluminum, magnesium, or calcium:* decreased antibiotic absorption. Give antibiotic 1 hour before or 2 hours after any of the above.<br>*Ferrous sulfate and other iron products, zinc:* decreased antibiotic absorption. Give doxycycline 3 hours after or 2 hours before iron administration.<br>*Phenobarbital, carbamazepine, alcohol:* decreased antibiotic effect. Avoid concomitant use if possible. | Epigastric distress, nausea, vomiting, diarrhea, skin rash, photosensitivity | Don't expose drug to light or heat. Protect from sunlight during infusion. Drug may be used in patients with renal impairment; it does not accumulate or cause a significant rise in BUN.<br>Watch for overgrowth of nonsusceptible organisms. Check patient's tongue for signs of monilia infection. Observe for diarrhea, which may result from local irritation or superinfection. Stress good oral hygiene. Superinfection requires stopping drug. Give with milk or food if GI side effects develop. |
| **gentamicin**<br>1.5 mg/kg I.M. or I.V. q 8 hours | *Bumetanide, ethacrynic acid, furosemide:* increased ototoxicity. Use together cautiously.<br>*I.V. penicillins:* separate gentamicin dose by at least 1 hour. Also, don't mix together in same I.V. container.<br>*Nondepolarizing muscle relaxants:* increased neuromuscular blocking effects. Use together cautiously. | Nephrotoxicity, ototoxicity, skin rash | Before start of therapy, weigh patient and obtain baseline renal function studies (urine output, specific gravity, urinalysis, BUN, creatinine levels, and creatinine clearance). Monitor renal function studies during therapy, and report signs of renal impairment. Ensure that the patient is well hydrated while taking this drug to minimize chemical irritation of the renal tubules. Evaluate the patient's hearing before and during therapy. Notify doctor if patient complains of tinnitus, vertigo, or hearing loss.<br>After completing I.V. infusion, flush line with normal saline solution. |
| **methenamine salts**<br>**(hippurate and mandelate)**<br>1 g P.O. one to four times daily | *Acetazolamide:* antagonizes methenamine effect. Use together cautiously.<br>*Alkalinizing agents:* inhibited methenamine action. Don't use together. | Nausea, vomiting, diarrhea, urinary tract irritation, skin rash | Obtain a clean-catch urine specimen for culture and sensitivity tests before starting therapy, and repeat p.r.n. Maintain urine pH at 5.5 or less. Use Nitrazine paper to check pH. Because *Proteus* and *Pseudomonas* tend to raise urine pH, urinary acidifiers are usually necessary when treating these infections.<br>Oral suspension contains vegetable oil. Administer cautiously to elderly or debilitated patients because aspiration can cause lipid pneumonia. If rash appears, withhold dose and contact doctor. |
| **nalidixic acid**<br>500 mg to 1 g P.O. q.i.d. for 7 to 14 days | *Oral anticoagulants:* increased risk of bleeding. Monitor prothrombin time. | Abdominal pain, nausea, vomiting, visual disturbances, photosensitivity | Obtain clean-catch urine specimen for culture and sensitivity tests before starting therapy; repeat p.r.n.<br>Instruct patient to report visual disturbances; these usually disappear with reduced dose. Tell him to avoid undue exposure to sunlight. Photosensitivity may persist up to 3 months after discontinuing drug. |
| **nitrofurantoin**<br>50 to 100 mg P.O. q.i.d. | *Magnesium-containing antacids:* decreased nitrofurantoin absorption. Administer 1 hour apart.<br>*Probenecid, sulfinpyrazone:* increased blood levels and decreased urine levels of nitrofurantoin | Nausea, vomiting, diarrhea, pulmonary sensitivity reactions (cough, chest pains, fever, chills, dyspnea) | Obtain clean-catch urine specimen for culture and sensitivity tests before starting therapy, and repeat p.r.n. Give drug with food or milk to minimize GI distress. Monitor pulmonary status. Tell patient that nitrofurantoin may cause brown urine. |
| **sulfisoxazole**<br>1 to 2 g P.O. q.i.d. | *Oral anticoagulants:* increased risk of bleeding. Monitor prothrombin time.<br>*Oral antidiabetics:* increased pharmacologic effect. Monitor for hypoglycemia.<br>*PABA-containing drugs:* inhibited antibacterial action. Don't use together.<br>*Phenytoin:* increased blood levels. Monitor for phenytoin toxicity. | Nausea, vomiting, diarrhea, erythema multiforme (Stevens-Johnson syndrome), generalized skin eruptions, epidermal necrolysis, exfoliative dermatitis, blood dyscrasias | Tell patient to drink a full glass of water with each dose and plenty of water during the day to prevent crystalluria. Monitor fluid intake and urinary output. In adults, daily output should be 3,000 to 4,000 ml.<br>Tell patient to report early signs of blood dyscrasias (sore throat, fever, pallor) immediately and to stop taking the drug. Initial loading dose, although often given, is not pharmacologically necessary. |

## Anti-infectives (continued)

| Drug, dose, and route | Interactions | Side effects | Special considerations |
|---|---|---|---|
| **tobramycin**<br>1.5 mg/kg I.M. or I.V. q 8 hours | *Bumetanide, ethacrynic acid, furosemide:* increased ototoxicity. Use cautiously together.<br>*I.V. penicillins:* separate tobramycin dose by at least 1 hour. Also, don't mix together in same I.V. container.<br>*Nondepolarizing muscle relaxants:* increased neuromuscular blocking effects. Use together cautiously. | Nephrotoxicity (directly related to high blood levels), ototoxicity, skin rash | Before therapy begins, weigh patient and obtain baseline renal function studies (urine output, specific gravity urinalysis, BUN, creatinine levels, and creatinine clearance). Monitor renal function during therapy. Notify the doctor of signs of renal impairment. Evaluate patient's hearing before and during therapy. Notify doctor if the patient complains of tinnitus, vertigo, or hearing loss.<br>After I.V. infusion, flush line with normal saline solution. |

## Antipruritics

| Drug, dose, and route | Interactions | Side effects | Special considerations |
|---|---|---|---|
| **cyproheptadine**<br>4 mg P.O. t.i.d. or q.i.d. | *Metyrapone:* invalidates pituitary-adrenal function diagnostic test. Avoid concomitant use. | Drowsiness, mouth dryness, weight gain | Warn patient against drinking alcohol during therapy and about driving or other activities that require alertness until CNS response to drug is determined. Tell him coffee or tea may reduce drowsiness; sugarless gum, hard candy, or ice chips may relieve dry mouth. |
| **trimeprazine**<br>2.5 mg P.O. q.i.d. | *Phenothiazines:* increased effects. Don't use together. | Drowsiness, nausea, dry mouth and throat | Warn patient against drinking alcohol and about driving or other activities that require alertness until CNS response to drug is determined. Reduce GI distress by giving with food or milk. Tell patient that coffee or tea may reduce drowsiness, and sugarless gum, sour hard candy, or ice chips may relieve dry mouth. |

## Cholinergics

| Drug, dose, and route | Interactions | Side effects | Special considerations |
|---|---|---|---|
| **bethanechol**<br>10 to 30 mg P.O. t.i.d. or q.i.d. or 2.5 to 5 mg S.C. t.i.d. or q.i.d., if necessary | *Procainamide, quinidine:* may reverse therapeutic effect. Observe for lack of response. | Abdominal cramps, diarrhea, sweating, lacrimation | Never give bethanechol I.M. or I.V.; it can cause circulatory collapse, hypotension, severe abdominal cramping, bloody diarrhea, shock, or cardiac arrest. Watch closely for side effects, especially with subcutaneous administration. Frequently monitor vital signs, especially respirations. Keep atropine available. Be prepared to give atropine 0.5 mg subcutaneously or by slow I.V. push as ordered, and provide respiratory support if needed.<br>Before treatment for urinary retention, ensure that a bedpan is close by. Monitor intake and output. |
| **neostigmine**<br>0.25 to 1 mg I.M. or S.C. q 4 to 6 hours | *Procainamide, quinidine:* may reverse cholinergic effect on muscle. Observe for lack of drug effect. | Nausea, vomiting, diarrhea, abdominal cramps, muscle cramps, excessive salivation, sweating | Lack of response within 1 hour of first dose requires patient catheterization. Frequently monitor vital signs, especially respirations. Keep atropine injection available. Be prepared to give atropine 0.5 mg subcutaneously or by slow I.V. push as ordered, and provide respiratory support as needed.<br>Before giving drug for postoperative distention or urinary retention, rule out mechanical obstruction. |

## Hematinics

| Drug, dose, and route | Interactions | Side effects | Special considerations |
|---|---|---|---|
| **ferrous sulfate**<br>325 mg P.O. t.i.d. | *Antacids, aluminum salts, cholestyramine resin, pancreatic extracts, vitamin E:* decreased iron absorption. Give separate doses if possible.<br>*Chloramphenicol:* delayed response to iron therapy<br>*Doxycycline:* decreased absorption. Give doxycycline 2 hours before or 3 hours after iron administration.<br>*Vitamin C:* may increase iron absorption; beneficial drug interaction | Nausea, vomiting, constipation | Between-meal dosing of drug is preferable. However, drug can be given with some foods even though absorption may be decreased. Enteric-coated products reduce GI upset but also reduce amount of iron absorbed. Dilute liquid preparations in juice (preferably orange juice) or water but not in milk or antacids. Give tablets with orange juice to promote iron absorption. Give liquid iron preparations with glass straw to avoid staining teeth.<br>Check for constipation; record color and amount of stool. Teach dietary measures to prevent constipation. Tell patient that oral iron may turn stools black. |
| **iron dextran**<br>250 mg (50 ml) I.M. by Z-track injection or direct, slow I.V. push not exceeding 50 mg/minute | None significant | Soreness and inflammation at I.M. injection site, brown skin discoloration at I.M. injection site, local phlebitis with I.V. injection, peripheral vascular flushing with rapid I.V. administration, hypotension, anaphylaxis | Give test dose of 25 mg. Monitor vital signs. Varied and severe reactions range from pain, inflammation, and myalgia to hypotension, shock, and death. Inject deeply into upper outer quadrant of buttock—never into arm or other exposed area—with a 2" to 3", 19G or 20G needle. Use Z-track technique to avoid leakage into subcutaneous tissue and tattooing of skin.<br>Give I.V. in patients with insufficient muscle mass for deep I.M. injection; with impaired absorption from muscle due to stasis or edema; with uncontrolled I.M. bleeding from trauma (possible in hemophilia); and with massive, prolonged parenteral therapy. |

## Immunosuppressants

| Drug, dose, and route | Interactions | Side effects | Special considerations |
|---|---|---|---|
| **azathioprine**<br>Initially, 3 to 5 mg/kg P.O. daily. Maintenance dose: 1 to 2 mg/kg daily, depending on patient response | *Allopurinol:* impaired inactivation of azathioprine. Decrease azathioprine dose to one-quarter or one-third normal dose. | Bone marrow depression (leukopenia, macrocytic anemia, pancytopenia, thrombocytopenia), risk of infection due to immuno-suppression, nausea, vomiting | Obtain hemoglobin, WBC, and platelet count at least weekly and more often at beginning of treatment. Azathioprine is a potent immunosuppressive; warn patient to report even mild infections (coryza, fever, sore throat, malaise). Give with meals to improve GI tolerance. Warn patient about possible thinning of hair.<br>Avoid all I.M. injections when platelets are low. |
| **cyclophosphamide**<br>1 to 5 mg/kg P.O. daily. Dose varies with patient response. | *Corticosteroids, chloramphenicol:* reduced activity of cyclophosphamide. Use cautiously.<br>*Succinylcholine:* may cause apnea. Don't use together. | Leukopenia, thrombocytopenia, nausea, vomiting, hemorrhagic cystitis, alopecia | Monitor CBC regularly. Advise male and female patients to practice contraception during and for 4 months after therapy; this drug is potentially teratogenic. Warn patient that alopecia is likely but reversible.<br>Avoid all I.M. injections when platelets are low. |
| **cyclosporine**<br>Before transplantation: 15 mg/kg P.O. After transplantation, continue dose daily for 1 to 2 weeks. Then reduce gradually to maintenance dose: 5 to 10 mg/kg daily. Or administer I.V. until patient can tolerate oral solution. | *Ketoconazole, amphotericin B:* possible increased blood levels of cyclosporine. Monitor for increased toxicity. | Tremor, hypertension, nephrotoxicity, gum hyperplasia, hirsutism | Cyclosporine may cause nephrotoxicity up to 3 months after transplantation. Monitor BUN and serum creatinine levels, and report findings to doctor. He may reduce dose. Cyclosporine and adrenal corticosteroids are given concomitantly. Measure oral doses carefully in an oral syringe. Mix with whole or chocolate milk or fruit juice to increase palatability. Use a glass container to minimize adherence to container walls. Give drug once daily in the morning. Instruct patient to take drug at the same time each day. Tell patient to use hair remover cream if hirsutism occurs. |

## Miscellaneous

| Drug, dose, and route | Interactions | Side effects | Special considerations |
|---|---|---|---|
| **aluminum hydroxide**<br>*For hyperphosphatemia:* 500 mg to 2 g P.O. b.i.d. to q.i.d. | *Iron salts:* decreased hematinic response. Separate administration times.<br>*Phenothiazines, penicillamine:* decreased absorption. Separate administration times.<br>*Sodium polystyrene sulfonate:* systemic alkalosis, reduced potassium exchange capability. Don't use together. | Constipation, hypophosphatemia | Monitor serum phosphate levels. Watch for symptoms of hypophosphatemia with prolonged use (anorexia, malaise, muscle weakness). Aluminum hydroxide can cause calcium resorption and bone demineralization. |
| **calcitriol**<br>*For hypocalcemia:* 0.25 to 1.25 mcg P.O. daily or alternate days<br><br>**dihydrotachysterol**<br>*For hypocalcemia:* 0.2 to 2 mg P.O. daily | None significant | Vitamin D intoxication (weakness, headache, somnolence, nausea, vomiting, metallic taste, muscle and bone pain) | Monitor serum and urine calcium levels. Watch for signs of hypercalcemia. Tell patient to immediately report weakness, nausea, vomiting, mouth dryness, constipation, muscle or bone pain, or metallic taste—early symptoms of Vitamin D intoxication. Instruct patient to adhere to diet and calcium supplementation. |
| **nandrolone decanoate**<br>*For refractory anemias:* 100 to 200 mg I.M. weekly | *Oral anticoagulants:* increased risk of bleeding. Monitor prothrombin time. | Reversible hepatotoxicity, virilization (acne, hirsutism, hoarseness, menstrual irregularities), edema | Control edema with salt restrictions and/or diuretics. Watch for symptoms of jaundice. Dose adjustment may reverse condition. Abnormal liver function tests require discontinuation of therapy. Observe patient receiving concomitant anticoagulant therapy for ecchymotic areas, petechiae, or abnormal bleeding. Monitor prothrombin time. |
| **phenazopyridine**<br>*For urinary analgesia:* 100 to 200 mg P.O. t.i.d. | None significant | Nausea, headache | Use only as an analgesic. Use with an antibiotic to treat urinary tract infection. Stop drug if skin or sclera becomes yellow-tinged. This may stem from impaired renal excretion. Tell patient that phenazopyridine causes red or orange urine and may stain fabrics. |
| **sodium polystyrene sulfonate**<br>*For hyperkalemia:* 15 g in water or sorbitol P.O. or 30 to 50 g/100 ml of sorbitol by rectal administration one to four times daily | *Antacids and laxatives (nonabsorbable, cation-donating type, including magnesium hydroxide):* systemic alkalosis, reduced potassium exchange capability. Don't use together. | Constipation, fecal impaction in the elderly, diarrhea (with sorbitol emulsions), hypokalemia | Monitor serum potassium at least once daily. Watch for signs of hypokalemia: irritability, confusion, cardiac dysrhythmias, EKG changes, severe muscle weakness and possible paralysis, and digitalis toxicity in digitalized patients. Potassium level below 4 mEq/liter usually requires stopping drug. Watch for signs of hypernatremia. About one third of resin's sodium is retained.<br>Use only fresh suspensions, stir just before use, and discard unused portion after 24 hours. Do not heat resin. This impairs drug's effectiveness. Mix resin only with water or sorbitol for P.O. administration. *Never* mix with orange juice (high K+ content) to disguise taste. Chill oral suspension for palatability. |

# Recommended drug dosage in renal failure

This table lists recommended dosage adjustments in mild, moderate, and severe renal failure. These adjustments are necessary because impaired renal function may modify a drug's bioavailability, distribution, pharmacologic action, or elimination, thereby predisposing the patient to drug toxicity. For example, digoxin toxicity can follow impaired renal function because digoxin is eliminated from the body almost exclusively by the kidneys (via glomerular filtration).

| Drug | Mild renal impairment (GFR > 50 ml/min) | | Moderate renal impairment (GFR 10 to 50 ml/min) | | Severe renal impairment (GFR < 10 ml/min) | |
|---|---|---|---|---|---|---|
| | % of normal dose | Interval | % of normal dose | Interval | % of normal dose | Interval |
| acetaminophen | 100% | q 4 hr | 100% | q 6 hr | 100% | q 8 hr |
| acetazolamide | 100% | q 6 hr | 100% | q 12 hr | Avoid | Avoid |
| acetohexamide | 100% | q 12 hr | Avoid | Avoid | Avoid | Avoid |
| acyclovir | 100% | q 8 hr | 100% | q 24 hr | 100% | q 48 hr |
| allopurinol | 100% | q 8 hr | 75% | q 8 hr | 50% | q 8 hr |
| amantadine | 100% | q 12 to 24 hr | 100% | q 48 to 72 hr | 100% | q 7 days |
| amikacin | 60% to 90% | q 8 to 12 hr | 30% to 70% | q 12 hr | 20% to 30% | q 24 hr |
| amoxicillin | 100% | q 6 hr | 100% | q 6 to 12 hr | 100% | q 12 to 16 hr |
| amphotericin B | 100% | q 24 hr | 100% | q 24 hr | 100% | q 24 to 36 hr |
| ampicillin | 100% | q 6 hr | 100% | q 6 to 12 hr | 100% | q 12 to 16 hr |
| aspirin | 100% | q 4 hr | 100% | q 4 to 6 hr | Avoid | Avoid |
| atenolol | 100% | q 24 hr | 100% | q 48 hr | 100% | q 96 hr |
| azathioprine | 100% | q 24 hr | 100% | q 24 hr | 100% | q 36 hr |
| azlocillin | 100% | q 4 to 6 hr | 100% | q 6 to 8 hr | 100% | q 8 hr |
| bleomycin | 100% | Varies | 100% | Varies | 50% | Varies |
| bretylium | 100% | Continuous infusion | 25% to 50% | Continuous infusion | Avoid | Avoid |
| captopril | 100% | t.i.d. | 100% | t.i.d. | 50% | t.i.d. |
| carbamazepine | 100% | q 6 to 8 hr | 100% | q 6 to 8 hr | 75% | q 6 to 8 hr |
| carbenicillin | 100% | q 8 to 12 hr | 100% | q 12 to 24 hr | 100% | q 24 to 48 hr |
| cefaclor | 100% | q 6 hr | 50% to 100% | q 6 hr | 33% | q 6 hr |
| cefadroxil | 100% | q 8 hr | 100% | q 12 to 24 hr | 100% | q 24 to 48 hr |
| cefamandole | 100% | q 6 hr | 100% | q 6 to 8 hr | 100% | q 8 hr |
| cefazolin | 100% | q 8 hr | 100% | q 12 hr | 100% | q 24 to 48 hr |
| cefotaxime | 100% | q 6 to 8 hr | 100% | q 8 to 12 hr | 100% | q 12 to 24 hr |
| cefoxitin | 100% | q 8 hr | 100% | q 8 to 12 hr | 100% | q 24 to 48 hr |
| cephalexin | 100% | q 6 hr | 100% | q 6 to 8 hr | 100% | q 12 hr |
| cephalothin | 100% | q 6 hr | 100% | q 6 hr | 100% | q 8 to 12 hr |
| cephapirin | 100% | q 6 hr | 100% | q 6 to 8 hr | 100% | q 12 hr |
| cephradine | 100% | q 6 hr | 50% | q 6 hr | 25% | q 6 hr |
| chloral hydrate | 100% | At bedtime | Avoid | Avoid | Avoid | Avoid |
| chlorpropamide | 100% | q 24 hr | Avoid | Avoid | Avoid | Avoid |
| chlorthalidone | 100% | q 24 hr | 100% | q 24 hr | 100% | q 48 hr |

## Recommended drug dosage in renal failure (continued)

| Drug | Mild renal impairment (GFR > 50 ml/min) | | Moderate renal impairment (GFR 10 to 50 ml/min) | | Severe renal impairment (GFR < 10 ml/min) | |
|---|---|---|---|---|---|---|
| | % of normal dose | Interval | % of normal dose | Interval | % of normal dose | Interval |
| cimetidine | 100% | q 6 hr | 100% | q 8 hr | 100% | q 12 hr |
| cisplatin | 100% | Varies | 75% | Varies | 50% | Varies |
| clofibrate | 100% | q 6 to 12 hr | 100% | q 12 to 18 hr | 100% | q 24 to 48 hr |
| clonidine | 100% | b.i.d. | 100% | b.i.d. | 50% to 75% | b.i.d. |
| colchicine | 100% | Varies | 100% | Varies | 50% | Varies |
| cyclacillin | 100% | q 6 hr | 100% | q 6 to 12 hr | 100% | q 12 to 24 hr |
| cyclophosphamide | 100% | q 12 hr | 100% | q 12 hr | 100% | q 18 to 24 hr |
| diflunisal | 100% | q 12 hr | 100% | q 12 hr | 50% | q 12 hr |
| digitoxin | 100% | q 24 hr | 100% | q 24 hr | 50% to 75% | q 24 hr |
| digoxin | 100% | q 24 hr | 100% | q 36 hr | 100% | q 48 hr |
| diphenhydramine | 100% | q 6 hr | 100% | q 6 to 9 hr | 100% | q 9 to 12 hr |
| disopyramide | 100% | q 6 hr | 100% | q 12 to 24 hr | 100% | q 24 to 40 hr |
| doxycycline | 100% | q 12 hr | 100% | q 12 to 18 hr | 100% | q 18 to 24 hr |
| ethacrynic acid | 100% | q 6 hr | 100% | q 6 hr | Avoid | Avoid |
| ethambutol | 100% | q 24 hr | 100% | q 24 to 36 hr | 100% | q 48 hr |
| ethosuximide | 100% | q 12 hr | 100% | q 12 hr | 75% | q 12 hr |
| flucytosine | 100% | q 6 hr | 100% | q 12 to 24 hr | 100% | q 24 to 48 hr |
| gemfibrozil | 100% | b.i.d. | 50% | b.i.d. | 25% | b.i.d. |
| gentamicin | 60% to 90% | q 8 to 12 hr | 30% to 70% | q 12 hr | 20% to 30% | q 24 hr |
| guanethidine | 100% | q 24 hr | 100% | q 24 hr | 100% | q 24 to 36 hr |
| hydralazine | 100% | q 8 hr | 100% | q 8 hr | 100% | q 8 to 16 hr (fast acetylators) q 12 to 24 hr (slow acetylators) |
| hydroxyurea | 100% | Varies | 100% | Varies | 50% | Varies |
| isoniazid | 100% | q 24 hr | 100% | q 24 hr | 66% to 75% | q 24 hr |
| kanamycin | 60% to 90% | q 8 to 12 hr | 30% to 70% | q 12 hr | 20% to 30% | q 24 hr |
| lincomycin | 100% | q 6 hr | 100% | q 12 hr | 100% | q 24 hr |
| lithium carbonate | 100% | t.i.d. to q.i.d. | 50% to 75% | t.i.d. to q.i.d. | 25% to 50% | t.i.d. to q.i.d. |
| lorazepam | 100% | t.i.d. to q.i.d. | 100% | t.i.d. to q.i.d. | 50% | t.i.d. to q.i.d. |
| meprobamate | 100% | q 6 hr | 100% | q 9 to 12 hr | 100% | q 12 to 18 hr |
| methadone | 100% | q 6 to 8 hr | 100% | q 6 to 8 hr | 50% to 75% | q 6 to 8 hr |
| methenamine mandelate | 100% | q.i.d. | Avoid | Avoid | Avoid | Avoid |
| methicillin | 100% | q 4 hr | 100% | q 4 to 8 hr | 100% | q 8 to 12 hr |
| methotrexate | 100% | Varies | 50% | Varies | Avoid | Avoid |
| methyldopa | 100% | q 6 hr | 100% | q 9 to 18 hr | 100% | q 12 to 24 hr |
| metoclopramide | 100% | Varies | 75% | Varies | 50% | Varies |

## Recommended drug dosage in renal failure (continued)

| Drug | Mild renal impairment (GFR > 50 ml/min) | | Moderate renal impairment (GFR 10 to 50 ml/min) | | Severe renal impairment (GFR < 10 ml/min) | |
|---|---|---|---|---|---|---|
| | % of normal dose | Interval | % of normal dose | Interval | % of normal dose | Interval |
| metronidazole | 100% | q 8 hr | 100% | q 8 to 12 hr | 100% | q 12 to 24 hr |
| mezlocillin | 100% | q 4 to 6 hr | 100% | q 6 to 8 hr | 100% | q 8 hr |
| mithramycin | 100% | Varies | 75% | Varies | 50% | Varies |
| mitomycin C | 100% | Varies | 100% | Varies | 75% | Varies |
| moxalactam | 100% | q 8 hr | 100% | q 12 hr | 100% | q 12 to 24 hr |
| nadolol | 100% | q 24 hr | 50% | q 24 hr | 25% | q 24 hr |
| nalidixic acid | 100% | q.i.d. | Avoid | Avoid | Avoid | Avoid |
| neostigmine | 100% | q 6 hr | 100% | q 6 hr | 100% | q 12 to 18 hr |
| netilmicin | 60% to 90% | q 8 to 12 hr | 30% to 70% | q 12 hr | 20% to 30% | q 24 hr |
| nicotinic acid | 100% | t.i.d. | 50% | t.i.d. | 25% | t.i.d. |
| nitrofurantoin | 100% | q.i.d. | Avoid | Avoid | Avoid | Avoid |
| oxazepam | 100% | q.i.d. | 100% | q.i.d. | 75% | q.i.d. |
| penicillin G | 100% | q 6 to 8 hr | 100% | q 8 to 12 hr | Avoid over 10 million units/day | q 12 to 16 hr |
| phenobarbital | 100% | t.i.d. | 100% | t.i.d. | 100% | q 12 to 16 hr |
| phenylbutazone | 100% | t.i.d. to q.i.d. | 100% | t.i.d. to q.i.d. | Avoid | Avoid |
| piperacillin | 100% | q 4 to 6 hr | 100% | q 6 to 8 hr | 100% | q 8 hr |
| primidone | 100% | q 8 hr | 100% | q 8 to 12 hr | 100% | q 12 to 24 hr |
| probenecid | 100% | q.i.d. | Avoid | Avoid | Avoid | Avoid |
| procainamide | 100% | q 4 hr | 100% | q 6 to 12 hr | 100% | q 8 to 24 hr |
| propoxyphene | 100% | q 4 hr | 100% | q 4 hr | 25% | q 4 hr |
| reserpine | 100% | q 24 hr | 100% | q 24 hr | Avoid | Avoid |
| spironolactone | 100% | q 6 to 12 hr | 100% | q 12 to 24 hr | Avoid | Avoid |
| streptomycin | 100% | q 24 hr | 100% | q 24 to 72 hr | 100% | q 72 to 96 hr |
| sulfamethoxazole | 100% | q 12 hr | 100% | q 18 hr | 100% | q 24 hr |
| sulfisoxazole | 100% | q 6 hr | 100% | q 8 to 12 hr | 100% | q 12 to 24 hr |
| sulindac | 100% | b.i.d. | 100% | b.i.d. | 50% | b.i.d. |
| terbutaline | 100% | t.i.d. | 50% | t.i.d. | Avoid | Avoid |
| thiazides | 100% | Daily to b.i.d. | 100% | Daily to b.i.d. | Avoid | Avoid |
| ticarcillin | 100% | q 8 to 12 hr | 100% | q 12 to 24 hr | 100% | q 24 to 48 hr |
| tobramycin | 60% to 90% | q 8 to 12 hr | 30% to 70% | q 12 hr | 20% to 30% | q 24 hr |
| triamterene | 100% | q 12 hr | 100% | q 12 hr | Avoid | Avoid |
| trimethoprim | 100% | q 12 hr | 100% | q 18 hr | 100% | q 24 hr |
| vancomycin | 100% | q 1 to 3 days | 100% | q 3 to 10 days | 100% | q 10 days |
| vidarabine | 100% | Continuous infusion | 100% | Continuous infusion | 75% | Continuous infusion |

# Nephrotoxic drugs

| Drug | Reaction | Pathophysiologic effects | Special considerations |
|---|---|---|---|
| **allopurinol** | Hypersensitivity | Drug injures tubular epithelial cells, resulting in necrosis of the proximal convoluted tubular cells with fibrinoid deposits. Drug also causes interstitial nephritis. | Use cautiously in patients with renal disease. Discontinue drug at first sign of a rash, which may precede nephrotoxicity.<br><br>Check renal function before therapy and periodically thereafter. Monitor intake and output, and encourage fluids unless contraindicated. Maintain daily urine output of at least 2 liters and a neutral or slightly alkaline urine pH. |
| **aminoglycosides** (amikacin, gentamicin, kanamycin, neomycin, netilmicin, streptomycin, tobramycin) | Dose-related | These drugs produce proximal tubular necrosis resulting from cellular vacuolation. Drug accumulation in the renal cortex leads to pathologic changes. | Aminoglycosides vary widely in relative toxicity. Neomycin is thought to be the most nephrotoxic, followed by amikacin, gentamicin, kanamycin, tobramycin, netilmicin, and streptomycin. The nephrotoxic effects of aminoglycosides are reversible with early detection and immediate dosage reduction.<br><br>To prevent nephrotoxicity, frequently monitor renal status. Before therapy, weigh the patient and ensure baseline renal function studies are performed. During therapy, weigh the patient daily and regularly monitor blood urea nitrogen (BUN) and serum creatinine levels and urinary output. Encourage fluids. Immediately report cells or casts in the urine, proteinuria, decreased creatinine clearance, or elevated serum creatinine or BUN levels. |
| **amphotericin B** | Dose-related | Drug causes renal vasoconstriction and glomerular and tubular damage. Distal tubular damage may lead to reduced urine concentrating ability; renal tubular acidosis; and electrolyte disturbances, especially hypokalemia. | Nephrotoxicity occurs in most patients treated with this drug but is reversible with drug discontinuation or dosage reduction. Concomitant use of other nephrotoxic antibiotics, such as aminoglycosides, may increase risk of toxicity.<br><br>During therapy, monitor intake and output, and report any change in urine appearance or volume. Obtain renal function studies weekly. If BUN level exceeds 40 mg/dl or serum creatinine level exceeds 3 mg/dl, inform the doctor; he may reduce dosage or stop drug until renal function improves. Frequently monitor serum potassium level, and watch for any signs of hypokalemia, such as muscle weakness, flaccid paralysis, and hypotension. Periodically monitor serum calcium and magnesium levels. |
| **analgesics** (acetaminophen, aspirin, choline magnesium trisalicylate, choline salicylate, magnesium salicylate, salicylamide, salsalate, sodium salicylate, sodium thiosalicylate) | Dose-related | These drugs produce analgesic nephropathy (a syndrome of papillary necrosis and progressive renal medullary impairment). This commonly leads to proteinuria, reduced urine concentrating ability, and the presence of white blood cells (WBCs) in the urine. | Mild analgesic nephropathy is reversible, but severe nephropathy may persist even after stopping drug and may cause chronic renal failure. Although analgesic syndrome has been associated with phenacetin, elimination of this drug from combination products hasn't significantly reduced the incidence of analgesic nephropathy. |
| **captopril** | Idiosyncratic | Drug produces membranous glomerulonephritis with thickening of the glomerular basement membrane and deposition of immune complex. | Use cautiously in renal impairment, autoimmune disease (especially systemic lupus erythematosus), or drug therapy that suppresses the immune response.<br><br>Proteinuria accompanies membranous glomerulonephritis in 1% to 3% of patients treated with this drug, but it usually subsides despite continuation of therapy. However, persistent proteinuria or proteinuria that exceeds 1 g/day requires reevaluation of captopril therapy. |
| **cephalosporins** (cefaclor, cefadroxil, cefamandole, cefazolin, cefoperazone, cefotaxime, cefoxitin, cephalexin, cephalothin, cephapirin, cephradine, moxalactam) | Hypersensitivity | These drugs damage renal tissue, leading to interstitial nephritis. They cause thickening of the renal cortex, focal or diffuse interstitial infiltration with leukocytes, and tubular degeneration. | Use cautiously in renal impairment. Concomitant use of aminoglycosides or diuretics may increase risk of nephrotoxicity. |
| **cisplatin** | Dose-related | Drug causes widespread necrosis of the proximal convoluted tubular cells. Affected tubules contain interluminal casts of necrotic cells and debris. | Use cautiously in renal impairment. Concomitant use of aminoglycosides increases risk of nephrotoxicity.<br><br>Because prehydration and diuresis may reduce risk of renal toxicity, infuse normal saline solution to maintain urine output of 100 ml/hour for 4 hours before, and for 24 hours after, therapy. Also give 12.5 g mannitol I.V. bolus before starting cisplatin infusion. Follow with mannitol infusion at rate of up to 10 g/hour p.r.n. during cisplatin infusion and up to 24 hours thereafter.<br><br>Do not repeat dose unless platelet count exceeds 100,000/mm³, WBC count is over 4,000/mm³, serum creatinine level is under 1.5 mg/dl, or BUN level is under 25 mg/dl. Monitor complete blood count, platelets, and renal function studies before initial and subsequent doses. Risk of nephrotoxicity increases with repeated doses. Renal function must return to normal before next dose. |

## Nephrotoxic drugs (continued)

| Drug | Reaction | Pathophysiologic effects | Special considerations |
|---|---|---|---|
| dextrans | Dose-related | Drug produces tubular vacuolation (osmotic nephrosis). | Don't give drug in extreme dehydration or in renal disease with severe oliguria or anuria. Monitor urine flow rate during administration. If oliguria or anuria occurs and is not relieved by fluid infusion, stop dextrans and give osmotic diuretic. |
| D-penicillamine | Hypersensitivity | Drug causes membranous glomerulo-nephritis resulting from deposition of antigen-antibody complexes on the basement membrane. This may lead to nephrotic syndrome. | Monitor renal function every 2 weeks for first 6 months of therapy, then monthly thereafter. Check for hematuria and proteinuria, which may indicate glomerulonephritis. These signs may persist for 1 year or longer after discontinuing therapy. |
| gold salts | Hypersensitivity and dose-related | Gold salts can cause membranous glomerulonephritis resulting from deposition of immune complexes on the basement membrane. | Don't give gold salts in renal disease. Tell patient that close medical follow-up and frequent urine tests are necessary during therapy. Before each injection, check for proteinuria and urine sediment changes. Persistent proteinuria or microscopic hematuria requires discontinuation of drug until sediment clears. |
| lithium | Dose-related | Drug can induce nephrogenic diabetes insipidus (resulting from renal tubular resistance to vasopressin), interstitial nephritis, renal fibrosis, and glomerular atrophy. | Nephrogenic diabetes insipidus is usually reversible with discontinuation of lithium. Typically, renal tissue damage occurs only after 1 year of therapy. Schedule renal function tests every 6 to 12 months.<br>Polyuria (over 5 liters daily) or urine specific gravity below 1.015 may indicate diabetes insipidus. |
| methotrexate | Dose-related | Drug causes widespread necrosis of the proximal convoluted tubular cells. This can lead to renal failure and uremic syndrome. | Monitor intake and output daily, and promote fluids (2 to 3 liters daily). Maintain urine pH above 6.5 with $NaHCO_3$ tablets to prevent precipitation of drug. Reduce dose if BUN exceeds 20 mg/dl or serum creatinine exceeds 1.2 mg/dl. Stop drug if BUN exceeds 30 mg/dl or serum creatinine exceeds 2 mg/dl. |
| methoxyflurane | Dose-related | Drug causes nephrogenic diabetes insipidus, proximal tubular damage, interstitial nephritis, and oxalate crystals. Nephrotoxicity may result from increased fluoride ion concentrations. | Drug may enhance nephrotoxic effects of tetracyclines and aminoglycosides. Don't use this drug in obese diabetic patients because of increased risk of nephrotoxicity. |
| nitrosoureas (carmustine, lomustine, semustine) | Dose-related | These drugs cause interstitial nephritis with thickening of the renal cortex, focal or diffuse interstitial infiltration with leukocytes, and tubular degeneration. | Almost all patients on long-term therapy develop interstitial nephritis. Use cautiously with other nephrotoxic drugs. Monitor renal function tests. |
| nonsteroidal anti-inflammatory agents (fenoprofen, ibuprofen, indomethacin, mefenamic acid, naproxen, phenylbutazone, piroxicam, tolmetin) | Dose-related | These drugs alter renal circulation—probably by inhibiting prostaglandin synthesis. This leads to reduced creatinine clearance rate and nonoliguric renal failure. Interstitial nephritis and nephrotic syndrome can also occur. | Nephrotoxicity is reversible with discontinuation of the drug. Nephrotoxic effects occur most commonly in volume depletion, shock, septicemia, congestive heart failure, and cirrhosis.<br>Use these drugs cautiously in renal disease. Check renal function periodically in long-term therapy. Stop drug if abnormalities occur. |
| penicillins (amoxicillin, ampicillin, azlocillin, bacampicillin, carbenicillin, cloxacillin, cyclacillin, dicloxacillin, hetacillin, methicillin, mezlocillin, nafcillin, oxacillin, penicillin G, penicillin V, piperacillin, ticarcillin) | Hypersensitivity | Penicillins, especially methicillin, can cause interstitial nephritis with thickening of the renal cortex, interstitial infiltration with leukocytes, and tubular degeneration. | Penicillin-induced interstitial nephritis most commonly occurs in long-term therapy, even though it isn't usually considered dose-dependent. Typically, it's accompanied by fever, rash, eosinophilia, and hematuria.<br>Use penicillins cautiously in impaired renal function. In prolonged therapy, frequently check renal function tests. Renal impairment ranges from mild elevations in BUN and serum creatinine levels to oliguria or anuria, requiring hemodialysis. |
| phenazopyridine | Dose-related | Drug may accumulate in renal tubules and interstitial tissues, causing phenazopyridine stones. | Signs of nephrotoxicity include yellow-tinged skin or sclera, oliguria, casts, elevated BUN level, and decreased creatinine clearance. Nephrotoxicity usually occurs with high dosage or prolonged therapy. |
| polymyxin B | Dose-related | Drug produces tubular necrosis and interstitial nephritis, which can result in renal failure and uremic syndrome. | Nephrotoxicity occurs in about 20% of patients receiving drug. Renal damage is usually reversible, but deterioration can continue even after stopping the drug. Monitor renal function tests before and during therapy. Maintain urine output of 3,000 to 4,000 ml/day for adults. Discontinue drug if BUN level rises and urine output falls. |
| tetracyclines (demeclocycline, methacycline, oxytetracycline, tetracycline) | Idiosyncratic or dose-related | Tetracyclines increase azotemia in preexisting renal impairment. Demeclocycline can cause nephrogenic diabetes insipidus. | Use with extreme caution in impaired renal function. Concomitant use of methoxyflurane may increase risk of nephrotoxicity. Monitor carefully. |
| trimethadione | Idiosyncratic | Drug can cause nephrotic syndrome with proteinuria. | Nephrotic syndrome can occur after months or years of therapy. It's usually reversible with early discontinuation of the drug. Check urinalysis before starting therapy and monthly thereafter. |

# Selected References and Acknowledgments

## Selected References

Arbeit, L.A., and Weinstein, S.W. "Acute Tubular Necrosis: Pathophysiology and Management," *Medical Clinics of North America* 65:147-63, 1981.

◆

Bennett, William M., et al. "Drug Prescribing in Renal Failure: Dosing Guidelines for Adults," *American Journal of Kidney Diseases*, pp. 155-193, November 1983.

◆

Brundage, Dorothy J. *Nursing Management of Renal Problems,* 2nd ed. St. Louis: C.V. Mosby Co., 1980.

◆

Del Greco, F., and Krumlovsky, F.A. "Role of the Laboratory in Management of Acute and Chronic Renal Failure," *Annals of Clinical and Laboratory Science* 11:283-91, 1981.

◆

Earley, Lawrence E., and Gottschalk, Carl W. *Strauss and Welt's Diseases of the Kidney,* 2 vols., 3rd ed. Boston: Little, Brown, & Co., 1979.

◆

First, M. Roy. *Chronic Renal Failure.* (Contemporary Patient Management Series.) New Hyde Park, N.Y.: Medical Examination Publishing Co., 1982.

◆

Folk-Lighty, M. "Solving the Puzzles of Patients' Fluid Imbalances," *Nursing84* 14(2):34-41, February 1984.

◆

Guzzetta, C.E., and Dossey, B.M. "Nursing Diagnosis: Framework, Process, and Problems," *Heart & Lung* 12 (3):281-91, May 1983.

◆

Hickey, Joanne V.X. *The Clinical Practice of Neurological and Neurosurgical Nursing.* Philadelphia: J.B. Lippincott Co., 1981.

◆

Hoeprich, Paul. *Infectious Diseases: A Modern Treatise of Infectious Processes,* 3rd ed. Philadelphia: J.B. Lippincott Co., 1983.

◆

Kunin, Calvin M. *Detection, Prevention and Management of Urinary Tract Infections,* 3rd ed. Philadelphia: Lea & Febiger, 1979.

◆

Lancaster, Larry E. *The Patient with End-Stage Renal Disease,* 2nd ed. New York: John Wiley & Sons, 1984.

Lerner, Judith, and Khan, Zafar. *Mosby's Manual of Urologic Nursing.* St. Louis: C.V. Mosby Co., 1982.

◆

Lewis, S.M. "Symposium on Chronic Renal Failure. Pathophysiology of Chronic Renal Failure," *Nursing Clinics of North America* 16:501-13, September 1981.

◆

McConnell, Edwina A., and Zimmerman, Mary F. *Care of Patients with Urologic Problems.* Philadelphia: J.B. Lippincott Co., 1982.

◆

Malasanos, Lois. *Health Assessment,* 2nd ed. St. Louis: C.V. Mosby Co., 1981.

◆

Marchant, D.J. "Urinary Incontinence in the Female," *Hospital Medicine* 19(6):49-64, June 1983.

◆

Netter, Frank. *Kidneys, Ureters and Urinary Bladder,* Vol. 6 in *The CIBA Collection of Medical Illustrations,* West Caldwell, N.J.: CIBA Medical Education Division, 1974.

◆

Petersdorf, Robert G., and Adams, Raymond D. *Harrison's Principles of Internal Medicine,* 10th ed. New York: McGraw-Hill Book Co., 1983.

◆

Saxton, Dolores F., et al. *The Addison-Wesley Manual of Nursing Practice: Prescriptions for Patient Care.* Reading, Mass.: Addison-Wesley Publishing Co., 1983.

◆

Schrier, R.W., et al. "Acute Renal Failure: Pathogenesis, Diagnosis and Treatment," *Advances in Nephrology* 10:213-40, 1981.

◆

Smith, Donald R. *General Urology,* 10th ed. Los Altos, Calif.: Lange Medical Pubns., 1981.

◆

Stein, Jay H. *Nephrology.* (The Science and Practice of Clinical Medicine Series.) New York: Grune & Stratton, 1980.

◆

Stone, William J., and Rabin, Pauline L., eds. *Chronic End-Stage Renal Diseases.* Orlando, Fla.: Academic Press, 1983.

◆

Tilkian, Sarko M., et al. *Clinical Implications of Laboratory Tests,* 3rd ed. St. Louis: C.V. Mosby Co., 1983.

◆

Tresler, Kathleen M. *Clinical Laboratory Tests: Significance and Nursing Implications.* Englewood Cliffs, N.J.: Prentice-Hall, 1982.

## Acknowledgments

◆ p. 53 Graph adapted from Lancaster, Larry E., "Home Study Program—Renal Failure: Pathophysiology, Assessment and Intervention," *Critical Care Nurse* 2(1):38-40, January/February 1982.

◆ p. 56 (top) Photo courtesy of North Penn Hospital, Department of Radiology, Lansdale, Pa.

◆ p. 56 (bottom left and right) Photos courtesy of Marc S. Lapayowker MD, Chairman, Department of Radiology, Abington (Pa.) Memorial Hospital

◆ p. 57 Photos courtesy of Armed Forces Institute of Pathology, Neg. No. 61-8528, 80-1115, 65-2074-4.

◆ p. 59 Photos courtesy of Marc S. Lapayowker, MD, Chairman, Department of Radiology, Abington (Pa.) Memorial Hospital

◆ p. 131 (bottom) Photo by Hank Morgan.

◆ p.136 (top row) Photo by W. Grayson Henry with permission of Ames Division, Miles Laboratory, Elkhart, Ind.

◆ p. 136 (middle and bottom rows) Adapted with permission from photos in *Urine under the Microscope.* Nutley, N.J.: ROCOM Press, Division of Hoffman-LaRoche Inc., 1979

◆ p. 144 Adapted with permission from Noel R. Rose, "Autoimmune Disease," Copyright © February 1981 by *Scientific American, Inc.* All rights reserved.

◆ p. 170 Adapted with permission of American Medical Systems, Inc., Minnetonka, Minn.

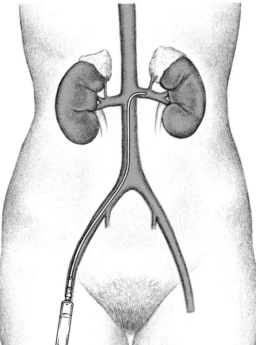

i = illustration; t = table

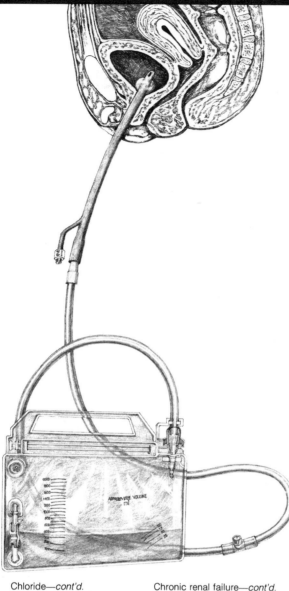

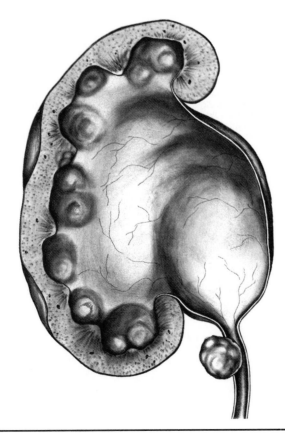

i = illustration; t = table

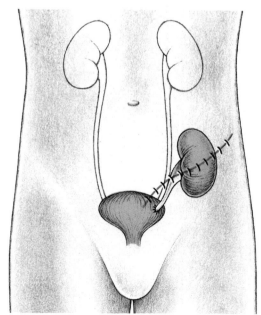

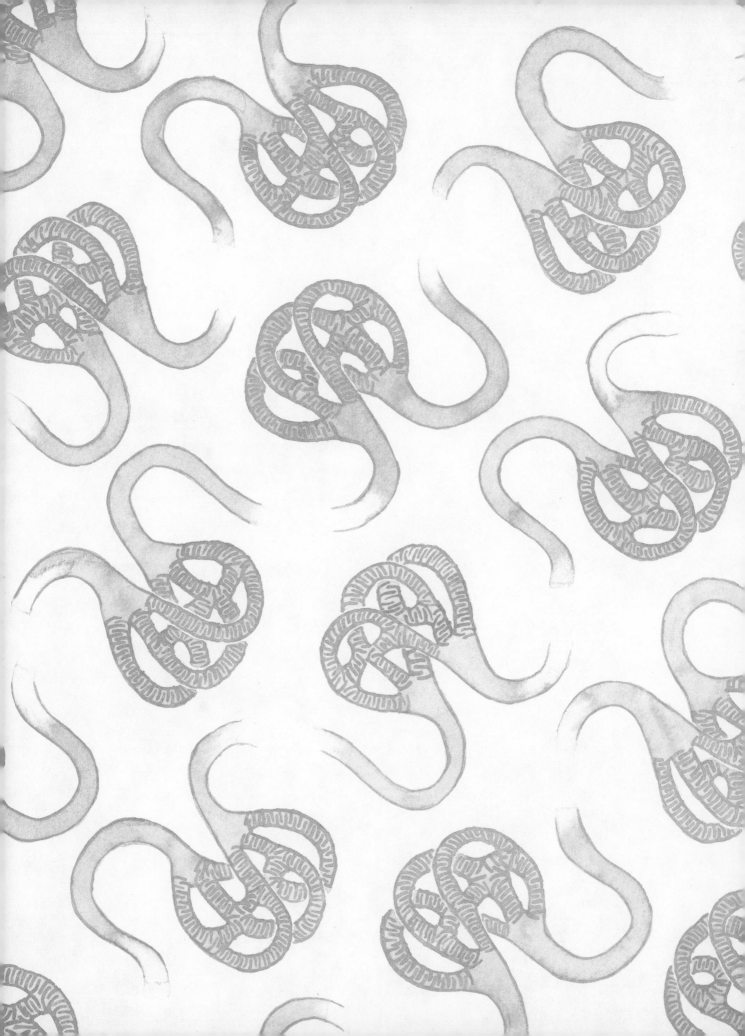